Treatment for
POSTTRAUMATIC STRESS DISORDER
in Military and Veteran Populations

Initial Assessment

Committee on the Assessment of Ongoing Efforts in the Treatment of Posttraumatic Stress Disorder

Board on the Health of Select Populations

INSTITUTE OF MEDICINE
OF THE NATIONAL ACADEMIES

THE NATIONAL ACADEMIES PRESS
Washington, D.C.
www.nap.edu

THE NATIONAL ACADEMIES PRESS 500 Fifth Street, N.W. Washington, DC 20001

NOTICE: The project that is the subject of this report was approved by the Governing Board of the National Research Council, whose members are drawn from the councils of the National Academy of Sciences, the National Academy of Engineering, and the Institute of Medicine. The members of the committee responsible for the report were chosen for their special competences and with regard for appropriate balance.

This study was supported by Contract No. W81XWH-10-C-0290 between the National Academy of Sciences and the Department of Defense. Any opinions, findings, conclusions, or recommendations expressed in this publication are those of the author(s) and do not necessarily reflect the view of the organizations or agencies that provided support for this project.

International Standard Book Number-13: 978-0-309-25421-2
International Standard Book Number-10: 0-309-25421-3

Additional copies of this report are available from the National Academies Press, 500 Fifth Street, NW, Keck 360, Washington, DC 20001; (800) 624-6242 or (202) 334-3313; http://www.nap.edu.

For more information about the Institute of Medicine, visit the IOM home page at: **www.iom.edu.**

Printed in the United States of America

The serpent has been a symbol of long life, healing, and knowledge among almost all cultures and religions since the beginning of recorded history. The serpent adopted as a logotype by the Institute of Medicine is a relief carving from ancient Greece, now held by the Staatliche Museen in Berlin.

Suggested citation: IOM (Institute of Medicine). 2012. *Treatment for posttraumatic stress disorder in military and veteran populations: Initial assessment.* Washington, DC: The National Academies Press.

"Knowing is not enough; we must apply.
Willing is not enough; we must do."
—Goethe

INSTITUTE OF MEDICINE
OF THE NATIONAL ACADEMIES

Advising the Nation. Improving Health.

THE NATIONAL ACADEMIES

Advisers to the Nation on Science, Engineering, and Medicine

The **National Academy of Sciences** is a private, nonprofit, self-perpetuating society of distinguished scholars engaged in scientific and engineering research, dedicated to the furtherance of science and technology and to their use for the general welfare. Upon the authority of the charter granted to it by the Congress in 1863, the Academy has a mandate that requires it to advise the federal government on scientific and technical matters. Dr. Ralph J. Cicerone is president of the National Academy of Sciences.

The **National Academy of Engineering** was established in 1964, under the charter of the National Academy of Sciences, as a parallel organization of outstanding engineers. It is autonomous in its administration and in the selection of its members, sharing with the National Academy of Sciences the responsibility for advising the federal government. The National Academy of Engineering also sponsors engineering programs aimed at meeting national needs, encourages education and research, and recognizes the superior achievements of engineers. Dr. Charles M. Vest is president of the National Academy of Engineering.

The **Institute of Medicine** was established in 1970 by the National Academy of Sciences to secure the services of eminent members of appropriate professions in the examination of policy matters pertaining to the health of the public. The Institute acts under the responsibility given to the National Academy of Sciences by its congressional charter to be an adviser to the federal government and, upon its own initiative, to identify issues of medical care, research, and education. Dr. Harvey V. Fineberg is president of the Institute of Medicine.

The **National Research Council** was organized by the National Academy of Sciences in 1916 to associate the broad community of science and technology with the Academy's purposes of furthering knowledge and advising the federal government. Functioning in accordance with general policies determined by the Academy, the Council has become the principal operating agency of both the National Academy of Sciences and the National Academy of Engineering in providing services to the government, the public, and the scientific and engineering communities. The Council is administered jointly by both Academies and the Institute of Medicine. Dr. Ralph J. Cicerone and Dr. Charles M. Vest are chair and vice chair, respectively, of the National Research Council.

www.nationalacademies.org

COMMITTEE ON THE ASSESSMENT OF ONGOING EFFORTS IN THE TREATMENT OF POSTTRAUMATIC STRESS DISORDER

Sandro Galea (*Chair*), Professor and Chair of the Department of Epidemiology, Mailman School of Public Health, Columbia University, New York, NY

Kathryn Basham, Professor and Editor, Co-Director of the PhD Program, College of Social Work, Smith College, Northampton, MA

Larry Culpepper, Professor and Chairman of the Department of Family Medicine, Boston University School of Medicine; Chief of Family Medicine, Boston Medical Center, MA

Jonathan Davidson, Emeritus Professor, Department of Psychiatry, Duke University Medical Center, Durham, NC

Edna Foa, Professor, Department of Psychiatry; Director, Center for the Treatment and Study of Anxiety, University of Pennsylvania School of Medicine, Philadelphia

Kenneth Kizer, Director, Institute for Population Health Improvement; Professor, School of Medicine and Nursing, University of California, Davis

Karestan Koenen, Associate Professor, Department of Epidemiology, Mailman School of Public Health, Columbia University, New York, NY

Douglas Leslie, Professor, Department of Public Health Sciences and Department of Psychiatry, Pennsylvania State University, State College

Richard McCormick, Senior Scholar, Center for Health Care Research and Policy, Case Western Reserve University, MetroHealth Medical Center, Cleveland, OH

Mohammed Milad, Associate Professor, Department of Psychiatry, Harvard Medical School; Director of Behavioral Neuroscience Laboratory, Associate in Research Psychiatry, Massachussets General Hospital, Boston

Elspeth Cameron Ritchie, Professor, Department of Psychiatry, Uniformed Services University of the Health Sciences; Chief Clinical Officer, Washington, DC, Department of Mental Health

Albert "Skip" Rizzo, Associate Director, Institute for Creative Technologies; Research Professor, Department of Psychiatry and School of Gerontology, University of Southern California, Los Angeles

Barbara O. Rothbaum, Associate Vice Chair of Clinical Research, Department of Psychiatry; Director, Trauma and Anxiety Recovery Program, Emory University School of Medicine, Atlanta, GA

Douglas Zatzick, Professor, University of Washington School of Medicine; Associate Vice Chair for Health Services Research, Medical Director of the Inpatient Consultation Liaison Service, University of Washington Harborview Level I Trauma Center, Seattle

Consultant

Carol Tamminga, Professor, Chairman, University of Texas Southwestern Medical Center, Dallas

Study Staff

Roberta Wedge, Study Director
Margot Iverson, Program Officer (through January 2012)
Anne Styka, Associate Program Officer
Rebecca Hebner, Senior Program Assistant (through March 2012)
Joi Washington, Senior Program Assistant (since April 2012)
Heidi Murray-Smith, Program Officer, Board on Environmental Studies and Toxicology
Norman Grossblatt, Senior Editor
Frederick Erdtmann, Director, Board on the Health of Select Populations

Reviewers

This report has been reviewed in draft form by individuals chosen for their diverse perspectives and technical expertise, in accordance with procedures approved by the National Research Council's Report Review Committee. The purpose of this independent review is to provide candid and critical comments that will assist the institution in making its published report as sound as possible and to ensure that the report meets institutional standards for objectivity, evidence, and responsiveness to the study charge. The review comments and draft manuscript remain confidential to protect the integrity of the deliberative process. We wish to thank the following individuals for their review of this report:

Christopher K. Cain, Nathan Kline Institute for Psychiatric Research
Joseph T. Coyle, Harvard Medical School
Johanna T. Dwyer, Tufts Medical Center
Mardi J. Horowitz, University of California, San Francisco
Israel Liberzon, University of Michigan
John Parrish, Massachusetts General Hospital
Alan Peterson, University of Texas Health Science Center at San Antonio
Gale S. Pollock, Pollock Associates, LLC
William E. Schlenger, Abt Associates Inc.
Murray Stein, University of California, San Diego

Although the reviewers listed above have provided many constructive comments and suggestions, they were not asked to endorse the conclusions or recommendations, nor did they see the final draft of the report before its release. The review of this report was overseen by **Floyd E. Bloom,** The Scripps Research Institute, and **Jacquelyn C. Campbell,** The Johns Hopkins University School of Nursing. Appointed by the National Research Council and Institute of Medicine, they were responsible for making certain that an independent examination of this report was carried out in accordance with institutional procedures and that all review comments were carefully considered. Responsibility for the final content of this report rests entirely with the authoring committee and the institution.

Contents

Appendixes

Preface

Posttraumatic stress disorder (PTSD) is one of the signature injuries of the U.S. engagements in Iraq and Afghanistan. Of the more than 2.6 million active-duty, National Guard, and reserve service members who have been deployed to Operation Enduring Freedom (OEF) in Afghanistan since 2001 and Operation Iraqi Freedom (OIF) since 2003, an estimated 13–20% of them have or may develop PTSD. Managing PTSD in those populations is a huge task for the Department of Defense (DoD) and the Department of Veterans Affairs (VA). The DoD and the VA have responded with substantial funding to foster research, develop programs, and initiate services to combat PTSD. Both departments are making strides in identifying and treating people who have PTSD, but there are many obstacles to the achievement of effective and timely treatments, from identifying those at risk for PTSD to using the best evidence-based treatments—psychotherapy, pharmacotherapy, or some combination. Diagnostic procedures and treatment options are not standardized with respect to who uses which approach and when. There is a need to ensure that service members and veterans who seek treatment receive it in a timely and thorough manner, and to make treatments available to those who are in remote locations or for whom access to treatment is difficult. Research is being conducted to identify the physiologic bases of reactions to trauma and to identify biomarkers for preventing and diagnosing PTSD, and for treating it.

The present two-phase Institute of Medicine (IOM) study is particularly timely, given the recent conclusion of OIF and the expectation that OEF will be winding down in the next few years. The charge given to this committee represents a serious commitment of the DoD and the VA to address health care issues surrounding service members and veterans who have PTSD. This phase 1 report summarizes much of the literature on the burden of PTSD in service members and veterans, including National Guard and reservists, and explores the options available in the DoD and the VA for the prevention of, diagnosis of, and treatment for PTSD. In the second phase of its work, the committee will focus on the evaluation of data provided by the DoD and the VA and will investigate cost considerations, new neurobiologic findings, and the use of complementary and alternative treatments. Although the committee did visit one congressionally mandated site for this report (Fort Hood, Texas), in phase 2 it will undertake visits to at least two other Army sites—Fort Bliss, Texas, and Fort Campbell, Tennessee—and it hopes to visit other military bases and VA medical facilities to gain an appreciation of real-world successes and problems related to the diagnosis of and treatment for PTSD in these settings. The committee recognizes the burden that PTSD poses for many service members, veterans, and their families, and the pressing need to prevent it, diagnosis it, and treat for it in those who have given so much for this country.

The committee gratefully acknowledges the many individuals and groups who generously gave their time and expertise to share their insights on particular aspects of PTSD, who provided reports and data, and who answered queries about their work and experience in dealing, personally and professionally, with PTSD. Among the many people who helped the committee are staff of the DoD and the VA, researchers, staff of veteran and service member organizations, and members of the public who attended the committee's open meetings. The committee also visited U.S. Army Garrison Fort Hood in Killeen, Texas, and expresses its appreciation for the time, insights, and personal stories offered by a variety of base staff, mental health providers, and service members who have PTSD and their families. The committee is also grateful to Roberta Wedge, who served as study director for this project, and to the IOM staff members who contributed to this project: Rebecca Hebner, Margot Iverson, Heidi Murray-Smith, Anne Styka, and Joi Washington. A thank you is also extended to William McLeod, who conducted database and literature searches.

Sandro Galea, *Chair*
Committee on the Assessment of Ongoing Efforts in the Treatment of Posttraumatic Stress Disorder

Acronyms

ACT	acceptance and commitment therapy
AFQT	Armed Forces Qualification Test
APA	American Psychiatric Association
ASD	acute stress disorder
BDNF	brain-derived neurotrophic factor
BHOP	Behavioral Health Optimization Program
BICEPS	brevity, immediacy, centrality or contract, expectancy, proximity, and simplicity
CAM	complementary and alternative medicine
CAPS	Clinician-Administered PTSD Scale
CBCT	cognitive-behavioral conjoint therapy
CBT	cognitive behavioral therapy
CBT-MVA	cognitive behavioral therapy–motor vehicle accident
CI	confidence interval
CIDI	Composite International Diagnostic Interview
CISD	critical incident stress debriefing
COSC	combat and operational stress control
COSR	combat and operational stress reaction
CPT	cognitive processing therapy
CRT	cognitive rehabilitation therapy
CSC	combat stress control
CSF	Comprehensive Soldier Fitness
CT	cognitive therapy

CWT	compensated work therapy
DART	deployment anxiety reduction training
DCoE	Defense Centers of Excellence for Psychological Health and Traumatic Brain Injury
DCS	D-cycloserine
DIS-IV	Diagnostic Interview Schedule
DNA	deoxyribonucleic acid
DoD	Department of Defense
DSM-IV	*Diagnostic and Statistical Manual of Mental Disorders–Fourth Edition*
EFT	emotional freedom technique
EMDR	eye movement and desensitization reprocessing
FOCUS	Families OverComing Under Stress
FORT	functional and occupational rehabilitation treatment
FY	fiscal year
GABA	gamma-aminobutyric acid
GAF	global assessment of function
GAO	Government Accountability Office
GAT	global assessment tool
HBOT	hyperbaric oxygen therapy
HOPE	Helping to Overcome PTSD with Empowerment
HPA	hypothalamic-pituitary-adrenal
HT	hydroxytryptamine
IED	improvised explosive device
IOM	Institute of Medicine
IPAP	International Psychopharmacology Algorithm Project
IPT	interpersonal therapy
IPV	intimate partner violence
IQ	intelligence quotient
IRT	imagery rehearsal therapy
ISTSS	International Society for Traumatic Stress Studies
MANSA	Manchester Short Assessment of Quality of Life
MAO	monoamine oxidase
MAOI	monoamine oxidase inhibitor
MHAT	Mental Health Advisory Team
MHS	military health system

MINI	Mini-International Neuropsychiatric Interview
MRI	magnetic resonance imaging
MST	military sexual trauma
mTBI	mild traumatic brain injury
MTF	military treatment facility
NCS	National Comorbidity Study
NCS-R	National Comorbidity Study-Replication
NHMRC	National Health and Medical Research Council
NICE	National Institute for Health and Clinical Excellence
NIH	National Institutes of Health
NIMH	National Institute of Mental Health
NMDA	*n*-methyl-d-aspartate
NVVRS	National Vietnam Veterans Readjustment Study
OEF	Operation Enduring Freedom
OIF	Operation Iraqi Freedom
OMHO	Office of Mental Health Operations (VA)
OND	Operation New Dawn
OR	odds ratio
OSCAR	operational stress control and readiness
PCL	PTSD Checklist
PC-PTSD	Primary Care PTSD screen
PDHA	Post-Deployment Health Assessment
PDHRA	Post-Deployment Health Reassessment
PE	prolonged exposure
PHA	Periodic Health Assessment
PSS-I	PTSD Symptom Scale—Interview Version
PTSD	posttraummatic stress disorder
RAS	reticular activating system
RCT	randomized controlled trial
REACH	Reaching Out to Educate and Assist Caring, Healthy Families
REM	rapid eye movement
RESPECT-Mil	Re-Engineering Systems for Primary Care Treatment of Depression and PTSD in the Military
RNA	ribonucleic acid
rTMS	repetitive transcranial magnetic stimulation
SCCIP-ND	Surviving Cancer Completely Intervention Program–Newly Diagnosed
SIP	Structured Interview for PTSD

SIT	stress inoculation training
SKY	Sudarshan Kriya yoga
SNRI	serotonin norepinephrine reuptake inhibitor
SPRINT	Short Post-Traumatic Stress Disorder Rating Interview
SRI	serotonin reuptake inhibitor
SSRI	selective serotonin reuptake inhibitor
STAIR	Skills Training in Affect and Interpersonal Regulation
STRONG STAR	South Texas Research Organizational Network Guiding Studies on Trauma and Resilience
TBI	traumatic brain injury
TMH	telemental health
USUHS	Uniformed Services University of the Health Sciences
VA	Department of Veterans Affairs
VBA	Veterans Benefit Administration
VHA	Veterans Health Administration
VISN	Veterans Integrated Service Network
VR	virtual reality
VRE	virtual reality exposure therapy
WHOQOL-100	World Health Organization Quality of Life Assessment
WL	wait list

Summary

The hallmarks of the recent conflicts in Iraq (2003–2011) and Afghanistan (2001–present) are blast injuries and the psychiatric consequences of combat, particularly posttraumatic stress disorder (PTSD), the subject of this report. According to the American Psychiatric Association's *Diagnostic and Statistical Manual of Mental Disorders, Fourth Edition, Text Revision* (*DSM-IV-TR*), PTSD symptoms must be manifested in three clusters:

1. Persistent re-experiencing, such as recurrent thoughts, nightmares, and flashbacks;
2. Persistent avoidance of trauma-associated stimuli (for example, avoiding related thoughts, feelings, conversations, or places) and emotional numbing that was not present before the trauma; and
3. Persistent hyperarousal that may be manifested as hypervigilance, an exaggerated startle response, or difficulty in concentrating.

Those symptoms must persist for at least a month and cause clinically significant distress or functional impairment. PTSD is unique among psychiatric disorders in that it is linked to a specific trigger—a traumatic event—such as combat, natural and accidental disasters, and victimization and abuse.

Recent estimates of the prevalence of PTSD in 2.6 million U.S. service members who have served in Iraq or Afghanistan since 2001 (including those who are currently there and 900,000 of whom have been deployed more than once) range from 13% to 20%.

The risk of developing PTSD after exposure to a traumatic event depends on many factors, including sex, age, ethnicity, sexual orientation, education attainment, intelligence quotient, annual income, childhood behavioral problems, prior exposure to a traumatic event, and a family history of psychologic disorders. Known risk factors for PTSD in military populations include experiencing combat, being wounded or injured, witnessing death, serving on graves registration duty or handling remains, being taken captive or tortured, experiencing unpredictable and uncontrollable stressful exposure, and experiencing sexual harassment or assault. Severe combat stressors include an increased number of unpredictable insurgent attacks in the form of suicide and car bombs, improvised explosive devices, sniper fire, and rocket-propelled grenades, which all increase the risk of being wounded or killed and thereby exacerbate the psychologic stress. Higher rates of PTSD and depression are associated with longer deployments, multiple deployments, and greater time away from base camp. Conversely, protective factors for PTSD include good leadership, unit support, and training, all of which may help promote positive mental health and well-being during deployment and thus reduce the risk for PTSD.

The current military population is all volunteer and has more women and racial or ethnic minorities than the military population in the Vietnam War or the 1990–1991 Gulf War. More National Guard and reservists have been deployed than in prior conflicts.

COMMITTEE'S STATEMENT OF TASK AND APPROACH

The National Defense Authorization Act for Fiscal Year 2010, reflecting congressional concern about the number of service members and veterans who were at risk for or had received a diagnosis of PTSD, required the Secretary of Defense, in consultation with the Secretary of Veterans Affairs, to sponsor this study of PTSD programs in the Department of Defense (DoD) and the Department of Veterans Affairs (VA). This report is the first of the two mandated in the legislation; the committee's statement of task is shown in Box S-1.

This phase 1 report is based on an extensive literature search, including government documents and data; two public information-gathering sessions with presentations from representatives of the DoD, the VA, veterans' organizations, and individual service members and veterans who had PTSD; meetings with a variety of mental health providers and with PTSD patients and their families at U.S. Army base Fort Hood in Killeen, Texas; and information from the Veterans Health Administration provided in response to the committee's request. The committee was unable to obtain comparable information from the DoD in time to include it in this phase 1 report. The

BOX S-1
Statement of Task

Phase 1 (initial report):

The IOM will convene a committee to conduct a study of ongoing efforts in the treatment of posttraumatic stress disorder (PTSD). The study will be conducted in two phases: the focus in phase 1 will be on data gathering and will result in the initial study as noted in the congressional legislation; the focus in phase 2 will be on the analysis of data and result in the updated study. The work of the committee is dependent upon the timely delivery of data, in a usable format, from the DoD and the VA on their current PTSD programs.

In phase 1 of the study, the committee will collect data from the DoD and the VA on programs and methods available for the prevention, screening, diagnosis, treatment, and rehabilitation of PTSD. The committee will highlight collaborative efforts between the DoD and the VA in those areas. Additionally, the committee will consider the status of studies and clinical trials involving innovative treatments of PTSD that are conducted by the DoD, the VA, or the private sector, with regard to

- efforts to identify physiological markers of PTSD;
- efforts to determine causation of PTSD, using brain imaging studies and studies looking at the correlation between brain region physiology and PTSD diagnoses and the results (including any interim results) of such efforts;
- the effectiveness of alternative therapies in the treatment of PTSD, including the therapeutic use of animals;
- the effectiveness of administering pharmaceutical agents before, during, or after a traumatic event in the prevention and treatment of PTSD; and
- identification of areas in which the DOD and the VA may be duplicating studies, programs, or research with respect to PTSD.

Phase 2 (updated report):

In phase 2 of the study, the committee will analyze the data received in phase 1 specifically to determine the rates of success for each program or method; and an estimate of the number of members of the Armed Forces and veterans diagnosed by the DoD or the VA as having PTSD and the number of such veterans who have been successfully treated.

In addition, the committee will focus on targeted interventions at Fort Hood, Texas; Fort Bliss, Texas; Fort Campbell, Tennessee; and any other locations the committee deems necessary, including VA facilities. The committee will also examine gender-specific and racial and ethnic group-specific mental health treatment services available for members of the Armed Forces, including the availability of such treatment and services; the access to such treatment and services; the need for such treatment and services; and the efficacy and adequacy of such treatment and services.

Finally, the committee will examine the current and projected future annual expenditures by the DoD and the VA for the treatment and rehabilitation of PTSD; and provide recommendations for areas for future research with respect to PTSD.

committee expects to receive information from the DoD in time to complete phase 2 of the study.

The committee did not develop an exhaustive list of all the available PTSD programs and services in the DoD; such a list may be found in the 2011 RAND report *Programs Addressing Psychological Health and Traumatic Brain Injury Among U.S. Military Servicemembers and Their Families*. The committee did obtain a list of many PTSD programs in the VA. Although PTSD in military and veteran populations has a huge impact on spouses, children, parents, caregivers, and others, this report covers children and families only in the context of treatment of service members or veterans.

NEUROBIOLOGIC RESEARCH ON PTSD

Understanding of the neurobiology of PTSD is in a period of growth, but there is much to be learned before this knowledge can become the basis of effective treatments. The advent of neuroimaging tools and preclinical research has provided a platform upon which to begin to examine the neurobiology of PTSD. Research has generally concentrated on the sympathetic nervous system and the hypothalamic-pituitary-adrenal axis, but other neurobiologic systems—such as the serotonin system, the opiate system, and sex steroidal systems—have been implicated in pathologic and protective responses to stress. More research is needed to link any neurobiologic mechanism to PTSD risk or resilience, to identify environmental and biologic factors that contribute to the onset and severity of PTSD symptoms, to apply biomarkers and neuroimaging models to the diagnosis of PTSD (which would help to reduce the dependence on self-reported symptoms), and to locate potential targets for future pharmacologic treatment of PTSD or pharmacologic agents that could enhance current treatment therapies.

Both the DoD and the VA fund research on the neurobiology of PTSD. For example, the DoD is funding a study on multimodal neurodiagnostic imaging of traumatic brain injury (TBI) and PTSD and a study on the neurobiology of tinnitus with PTSD as a secondary outcome, but these studies are ongoing and results are not available. The VA is funding studies that include examinations of memory and the hippocampus in twins, brain imaging of psychotherapy for PTSD, and neural correlates of cognitive rehabilitation in PTSD.

DOD AND VA PROGRAMS FOR PTSD

The DoD and the VA provide an array of prevention, screening, diagnosis, treatment, and rehabilitation options to maintain force readiness for the DoD and to enable veterans to function well in daily life.

The DoD Military Health System (MHS) provides many health programs and services for active-duty service members, retired personnel, and their families, including National Guard members and reservists when on active duty. TRICARE, a major component of the MHS, is a wide-reaching health care provider that delivers *direct care* through military treatment facilities and *purchased care* through network and non-network civilian health professionals, hospitals, and pharmacies. In 2011, about 9.7 million beneficiaries were eligible for DoD medical care, and 5.5 million were enrolled in TRICARE. TRICARE provides a spectrum of mental health practitioners, including psychiatrists, clinical psychologists, certified psychiatric nurse specialists, clinical social workers, certified marriage and family therapists, pastoral counselors, and mental health counselors. Those practitioners deliver inpatient or outpatient care (including mental health care, such as psychotherapy, psychoanalysis, testing, and medication management), acute care, psychiatric partial hospitalization, and residential treatment center care. All the services have some type of PTSD treatment program, but no single source within DoD or any of the service branches maintains a complete listing of such programs, tracks the development of new or emerging programs, or has appropriate resources in place to direct service members to programs that may best meet their individual needs.

PTSD treatment is an important part of the VA's mission. During 2010, 438,091 veterans were treated for PTSD in the VA medical system. Although the VA has a system of specialized treatment programs that focus exclusively on PTSD, most PTSD-related services are offered in general mental health and medical settings, including primary care. The VA also supports Vet Centers that are staffed with social workers, clinical psychologists, mental health counselors, and professionally trained counselors and therapists.

Collaborative activities between the DoD and the VA with respect to the prevention, screening, diagnosis, and treatment of PTSD are reflected in the joint *VA/DoD Clinical Practice Guideline for Management of Post-Traumatic Stress*, originally developed in 2004 and updated in 2010. The VA and the DoD have also issued joint guidelines for other medical conditions that are frequently comorbid with PTSD, such as postdeployment health, concussion and mild TBI, substance use disorder, major depressive disorder, and several types of pain. Other collaborative efforts between the DoD and the VA include multiple joint executive councils, coordinating offices, working groups, and direct sharing agreements between VA medical centers and DoD medical facilities as well as a number of conferences on military health issues. In 2011, the VA and the DoD released the *VA/DoD Collaboration Guidebook to Healthcare Research* as part of the VA/DoD Joint Strategic Plan for 2009–2011.

Prevention

The two primary approaches to prevention of PTSD are to prepare service members for combat and other deployment-related stressors and to intervene quickly after exposure. All of the services have instituted prevention programs that promote resilience and training for the rigors of deployment, including the Army's Comprehensive Soldier Fitness program, the Navy's Combat and Operational Stress Continuum program, the Marine Corps's Operational Stress Control and Readiness (OSCAR) program, and the Air Force's Total Force Resiliency Program. Each of those programs has several layers of training for enlisted service members and officers and includes concepts of positive psychology and individual hardiness, and factors such as a positive command climate, unit cohesion, social support, and confidence in the military mission and training. At present, however, there is no empirical evidence regarding the effectiveness of these approaches.

Several of the DoD predeployment PTSD programs also have components to help service members and their families prevent the development of PTSD after deployment, including the Army Comprehensive Soldier Fitness program and the Navy and Marine Corps Families OverComing Under Stress (FOCUS) program. FOCUS is a family-centered and evidence-based resilience training program adapted for use by Marine Corps and Navy families. It helps families cope with the stresses and uncertainties of deployment and reintegration after deployment. Since 2009, FOCUS Family Resiliency Services have been made available to Army and Air Force families at some installations. The preventive interventions include psychoeducation, emotional regulation skills, problem-solving skills, communication skills, and management of traumatic stress reactions.

The VA has several programs to prevent PTSD after exposure to trauma, including Life Guard and Moving Forward. The VA also refers veterans and their families to prevention programs such as FOCUS. Vet Centers also provide prevention services to veterans.

Some clinical prevention efforts seek to detect and treat PTSD in its early stages (for example, treat those who meet the criteria for acute stress disorder) often before it presents clinically as chronic PTSD. Several studies have demonstrated that early interventions for acute stress disorder result in significant reductions of symptoms and the prevention of the onset of PTSD in the majority of individuals treated. Cognitive behavioral therapy and other interventions may be used when people show severe PTSD symptoms within the first month after trauma. Prevention may also involve mitigating the consequences of existing symptoms by improving functioning and reducing complications.

Screening

The 2010 *VA/DoD Clinical Practice Guideline for Management of Post-Traumatic Stress* found that screening improves health outcomes and that the benefits outweigh the potential harm or costs. Although screening may lead to anxiety and further testing, there are adverse implications of *not* screening: allowing problems to go undetected may compound them and lead to increased disability. Screening for PTSD is ineffective unless there is adequate follow-up to confirm or refute a positive screen and adequate capability to provide appropriate treatment.

Many PTSD screening instruments are available, but the evidence is insufficient to support recommending one tool over another. The VA/DoD guideline recommends the use of one of the following instruments: the Primary Care PTSD screen (PC-PTSD), the PTSD Brief Screen, the Short Screening Scale for *DSM-IV* PTSD, and the PTSD Checklist (PCL). The four-item PC-PTSD is the most widely used screen in the VA. In the DoD, PC-PTSD screening questions are incorporated into the post-deployment health assessment (PDHA), which is administered immediately after deployment, and the post-deployment health reassessment (PDHRA), which is administered 3–6 months after deployment. The PDHA and the PDHRA require a credentialed health care provider to review and discuss a service member's responses during a face-to-face assessment. In DoD clinic settings, the PCL is commonly used to screen for PTSD, and the screening results are usually integrated into a more comprehensive assessment and require interpretation by qualified professionals.

Service members who received care in an integrated mental health and primary care setting had significantly reduced psychologic distress and improved clinical outcomes. The Army-specific RESPECT-Mil (Re-Engineering Systems for Primary Care Treatment of Depression and PTSD in the Military) program, in which primary care providers are trained to screen and treat soldiers for PTSD and depression at every visit, is one example of a successful screening program. The Air Force and Navy have also implemented programs that integrate mental health and primary care.

The VA has increased the number of mental health professionals who work in integrated primary care teams. Every veteran seen in a VA primary care setting is screened for PTSD, depression, suicidality, sexual trauma that occurred during military service, and problem drinking, usually during the first appointment. PTSD screening occurs annually for the first 5 years and every 5 years thereafter.

Diagnosis

The diagnosis of PTSD ultimately rests on a careful and comprehensive clinical evaluation performed by a qualified professional (a psychologist, social worker, psychiatrist, or psychiatric nurse practitioner) under conditions of privacy and confidentiality. It may take some time to elicit the information necessary to determine the diagnosis. Such information should include chief complaints; lifetime history of exposures to trauma and physical injury to self or others; frequency and severity of symptoms of PTSD and other morbidity; level of function; quality of life and ongoing life stressors; medical history and present health; prior psychiatric diagnosis and treatment; details regarding family, recreation, and supports; personal strengths and vulnerabilities; coping styles; and details concerning experiences in the military. Several structured interviews have been validated for the diagnosis of PTSD, including the Clinician-Administered PTSD Scale, which is recommended by the VA/DoD guideline and widely, although not exclusively, used by the VA and the DoD; the Structured Clinical Interview for DSM-IV; and the Composite International Diagnostic Interview.

Treatment

There are numerous psychosocial and pharmacologic interventions for chronic PTSD, and the evidence supporting them varies considerably. The committee considered a wide variety of treatments that are used for PTSD from those with strong evidence bases such as exposure therapies, to pharmacologic agents such as serotonin reuptake inhibitors, and emerging therapies such as complementary and alternative medicines.

Psychosocial Therapies

The vast majority of treatments that have been examined via randomized controlled trials (RCTs) are in the general group of psychosocial therapies called cognitive behavioral therapy (CBT). They include exposure therapies such as prolonged exposure (PE), stress inoculation training or anxiety-management programs, cognitive therapies such as cognitive processing therapy, and eye movement desensitization and reprocessing (EMDR). Many treatment programs combine components of each of those general treatment groups.

Exposure therapies are first-line treatments designed to reduce PTSD symptoms and related problems such as depression, anger, and guilt, by helping patients confront their trauma-related memories, feelings, and stimuli. Exposure interventions may include imaginal exposure, in vivo exposure, or both types of exposure; programs such as PE that include both kinds of exposure tend to have better outcomes than those with only a single component. PE is effective for chronic PTSD as well as acute stress disorder and improvements are generally maintained at a year or more. Variations of exposure therapy, such as narrative exposure therapy and imagery rescripting, have also been shown to be efficacious in RCTs.

In cognitive therapy, the therapist helps the patient who has PTSD identify and modify negative thoughts and beliefs related to the traumatic event (for example, survival guilt, self-blame for causing the trauma, or feelings of personal inadequacy) that are believed to underlie pathological emotions and behaviors. RCTs have shown that cognitive therapy alone results in significant PTSD symptom reduction and improved mood and functioning. Cognitive processing therapy is a treatment that combines aspects of both cognitive therapy and PE.

Other effective treatments include EMDR and imagery rehearsal therapy. EMDR assists patients in accessing and processing traumatic memories while bringing them to an adaptive resolution. Imagery rehearsal therapy specifically targets nightmares, a common symptom of PTSD, by changing the content of the patient's nightmares to promote mastery over the content threat and thereby alter the importance of the nightmare. Imagery rehearsal therapy is an effective treatment for nightmares, but its efficacy as a treatment for PTSD is questionable.

The committee considered the evidence base for numerous other psychosocial therapies, including psychodynamic psychotherapy, brief eclectic psychotherapy, hypnosis, relaxation, stress inoculation training, interpersonal therapy, skills training in affect and interpersonal regulation, and group therapy. In particular, CBT-based group therapy has been studied in a number of RCTs that indicate that it is effective in reducing symptoms of PTSD. The efficacy of the other psychosocial therapies is supported by only a few RCTs or in some cases only one small RCT. Small RCTs and open trials of acceptance and commitment therapy have also been conducted because it is often used to address chronic PTSD experienced by veterans in many VA medical centers and warrants further review. Virtual reality exposure programs integrate computer graphics and head-mounted visual displays as a tool to deliver PE. For example, the Virtual Iraq/Afghanistan program is specific for combat-related PTSD and consists of a series of virtual scenarios designed to simulate service members' experiences during deployment to Iraq or Afghanistan and serve as digital contexts for delivering PE.

Pharmacologic Therapies

PTSD treatment guidelines, including the 2010 VA/DoD guideline, all recommend the use of antidepressants, specifically, a selective serotonin reuptake inhibitor (SSRI) or a serotonin norepinephrine reuptake inhibitor (SNRI), as a first-line treatment. However, although two studies of Bosnian and Iranian veterans demonstrated the efficacy of SSRI treatment for PTSD, no positive trials have been conducted in U.S. veterans. A 2008 IOM report on PTSD treatments concluded that neither SSRIs nor any other drugs could be considered effective for the treatment of PTSD, although one committee member dissented. A 2006 Cochrane review found that there was good evidence for SSRIs and SNRIs in chronic PTSD as both short-term and maintenance treatment. The evidence base for other antidepressants, tricyclic and monoamine oxidase inhibitors, and other drugs as effective pharmacotherapy for PTSD is at best mixed and generally inconclusive.

The committee examined the use of multiple drugs and combinations of traditional psychiatric medications with CBT for treatment of PTSD and found mixed evidence as to the effectiveness of this intervention. The majority of PTSD patients in the VA receive more than one psychotropic drug—about 80% of them receive an SSRI. Further research is needed on acute administration of novel medications, such as D-cycloserine, with psychotherapy as a combination treatment for PTSD.

Emerging Therapies

Some treatments that are being used for PTSD do not have a substantial evidence base with which to judge their efficacy. These treatments include couple and family therapy (such as cognitive behavioral conjoint therapy for couples) and numerous complementary and alternative medicine (CAM) treatments, including yoga, contemplative treatments, and acupuncture. Evidence of the effectiveness of these therapies for PTSD is based on small RCTs, case studies, or anecdotal reports. Nevertheless, the committee heard from numerous service members that they are using CAM treatments and that the treatments help to alleviate their PTSD symptoms. The VA offers a wide variety of CAM treatments at its facilities, and some military bases also offer CAM therapies, including animal-assisted therapy for service members who have mental health disorders.

CO-OCCURRING CONDITIONS AND PSYCHOSOCIAL COMPLEXITIES

Three categories of conditions frequently co-occur with PTSD: psychiatric (depression and substance use disorders), medical (chronic pain, TBI, and spinal-cord injury), and psychosocial (relationship problems, difficulties in social settings, intimate partner violence [IPV], child maltreatment, unemployment or lack of employment, homelessness, and incarceration). Because those conditions can interfere with effective PTSD treatment, their presence necessitates integrating treatment for them into a comprehensive PTSD management program.

Stepped-care approaches begin with low-intensity treatments, such as care management and support groups, and phase in more intensive procedures, such as CBT or pharmacotherapy for patients who have persistent or recurrent symptoms of PTSD and related comorbidities. Collaborative stepped-care interventions for PTSD, that is treatment by a team of health care providers, can help initiate early treatment, diminish such high-risk behaviors as binge drinking, and encourage the use of appropriate psychotherapy and pharmacotherapy. Established treatments, such as PE, can also address some psychologic comorbidities, such as depression, anger, guilt, and general anxiety.

Several medical conditions can occur with PTSD and result from the same traumatic event, such as explosions; these comorbidities include TBI and chronic pain. The overlapping symptoms of TBI and chronic pain (such as headache, irritability, sleep disturbance, and memory impairment) with PTSD often complicate diagnosis and treatment. Recent studies suggest that the co-occurrence of PTSD with mild TBI may prolong the duration of TBI symptoms and exacerbate them. No studies have examined treatment protocols that specifically target co-occurring TBI and PTSD symptoms. The effectiveness of CBT to treat both chronic pain and PTSD is supported by empirical evidence.

Veterans who have PTSD have higher incidences of IPV, divorce, and aggression and violence than veterans who do not. Psychosocial rehabilitation typically involves family psychoeducation and supported employment, education, and housing. Data support an integrated, collaborative treatment plan for PTSD that combines trauma-focused therapies with psychosocial rehabilitation. Preliminary findings suggest that programs such as the Navy and Marine Corps FOCUS project reduce the risk of IPV in military couples.

Veterans who have PTSD have higher rates of underemployment and unemployment than veterans who do not. Veterans who are disabled with combat-related PTSD may use the VA Vocational Rehabilitation and Employment Program, which includes funds for schooling or training, comprehensive vocational evaluation, work-readiness services, and case management and vocational placement services.

PTSD is commonly associated with drug abuse, alcohol abuse, anger, and aggressive behavior, all of which may lead to legal problems. Studies suggest that veterans who have PTSD and are incarcerated or were recently released from jail can benefit from comprehensive treatment and rehabilitation programs that address PTSD symptoms, substance abuse, and aggression. In general, the evidence base for treatment for PTSD and co-occurring problems—particularly such psychosocial conditions as homelessness, high-risk behaviors, and many medical conditions such as cardiovascular disease—is sparse.

ACCESS TO CARE

Of the U.S. service members and veterans who served in Iraq and Afghanistan and have screened positive for PTSD, only slightly more than half of those have received treatment. Barriers to care exist at the patient, provider, and institutional levels. Patients might not seek care because of concerns about the effects of seeking PTSD treatment on employment or military career, a perception that mental health care is ineffective, a lack of information on resources for care, financial concerns, and logistical problems, such as travel distance. For providers, barriers to treating patients with PTSD might include lack of training, lack of time, and treatment location issues, such as transportation in the theater of war. At the organizational level, barriers can include the treatment setting (for example, limited treatment opportunities in combat zones), restrictions on when and where pharmacotherapy for PTSD can be used, and logistical difficulty in getting to appointments (for example, getting to a mental health provider in a combat zone for service members or getting to a specialized VA PTSD clinic for a veteran living in a rural area).

The DoD and the VA have made progress in early identification of service members and veterans who have PTSD; this progress needs to be followed by timely access to the best evidence-based care. The DoD has increased the number of referrals to TRICARE mental health providers in an attempt to reduce waiting times for appointments. The VA has also increased the number of mental health providers and increased training in PTSD treatments for counselors in Vet Centers.

Treatment Delivery Technologies

New approaches are being used to improve the delivery of mental health services to military and veteran populations, including the use of computers to deliver person-to-person therapy. Telemental health approaches take advantage of recent advances in computing and information technology to support user interaction with clinicians via videoteleconferencing or interaction with websites via connectivity with the Internet. Telemental health methods may be used to deliver such services as screening assessments and general clinical information to users in remote locations. In some cases, guides allow users to self-manage mental health programs, often supported by interactions with a clinical provider. That approach decreases the burdens of travel time and costs and time away from work or family; it could improve access to services for traditionally underserved populations and for people in areas that may be difficult for therapists to access (such as combat zones). Several RCTs of Internet-based treatments for PTSD have found them to be effective in military populations.

FINDINGS AND RECOMMENDATIONS

The committee's findings led to recommendations that could, in the short and long terms, improve the management of PTSD for service members, veterans, and their families. To emphasize recommendations that were, in many cases, applicable to both the DoD and the VA and that addressed research topics, data collection, and gaps in DoD and VA programs, services, and facilities, the committee grouped its recommendations into five action items: analyze, implement, innovate, overcome, and integrate, which are delineated below.

A. Analyze

- **A1. To study the efficacy of treatment and to move toward measurement-based PTSD care in the DoD and the VA, assessment data should be collected before, during, and after treatment and should be entered into patients' medical records. This information should be made accessible to researchers with appropriate safeguards to ensure patient confidentiality.**
- **A2. The DoD and the VA should institute programs of research to evaluate the efficacy, effectiveness, and implementation of all their PTSD screening, treatment, and rehabilitation services, including research in different populations of active-duty personnel and veterans; the effectiveness of DoD prevention services should also be assessed. The DoD and the VA should coordinate, evaluate, and review these efforts continually and routinely and should disseminate the findings widely.**

B. Implement

- **B1. PTSD screening should be conducted at least once a year when primary care providers see service members at DoD military treatment facilities or at any TRICARE provider locations, as is currently done when veterans are seen in the VA.**

C. Innovate

- **C1. Specialized intensive PTSD programs and other approaches for the delivery of PTSD care, including combining different treatment approaches and such emerging treatments as complementary and alternative medicine and couple and family therapy, need to be rigorously evaluated throughout DoD facilities** (including TRICARE providers) and VA facilities for efficacy, effectiveness, and cost. More rigorous assessment of symptom improvements (for example, such outcome metrics as follow-up rates) and of functional improvements (for example, improvements in physical comorbidities, memory, and return to duty) is needed. The evaluations of these programs should be made publicly available.

- C2. The DoD and the VA should support neurobiology research that might help translate current knowledge of the neurobiology of PTSD to screening, diagnosis, and treatment approaches and might increase understanding of the biologic basis of evidence-based therapies.

D. Overcome

- D1. The DoD and the VA should support research that investigates emerging technologic approaches (mobile, telemedicine, Internet-based, and virtual reality) that may help to overcome barriers to awareness, accessibility, availability, acceptability, and adherence to evidence-based treatments and disseminate the outcomes to a wide audience.

E. Integrate

- E1. Research to create an evidence base to guide the integration of treatment for comorbidities with treatment for PTSD should be encouraged by the DoD and the VA. PTSD treatment trials should incorporate assessment of comorbid conditions and the value of concurrent and sequential care. Effective treatments should be included in updates of the *VA/DoD Clinical Practice Guideline for Management of Post-Traumatic Stress.*

PHASE 2

The committee understood its objectives as given in the Statement of Task to be a comprehensive review and synthesis of the available literature and data on the prevention, screening, diagnosis, treatment, and rehabilitation of PTSD in military and veteran populations. Based on this review and synthesis, the recommendations in this phase 1 report are intended to be actionable by the DoD and the VA, ahead of the phase 2 report. Although the committee found a variety of information in the published literature and from other sources, particularly DoD, VA, and other government reports, this information was insufficient to make judgments on the efficacy of many of the PTSD services and programs offered by these departments. A variety of information has been requested from the DoD and the VA, including numbers of service members and veterans, respectively, who have PTSD, the treatments that they are receiving, the outcomes of those treatments, the programs that are being evaluated (or not), and the costs for those programs. With the receipt of all these data in phase 2, the committee hopes to capitalize on the new DoD- and VA-specific information to refine the phase 1 findings and recommendations.

Phase 2 calls for visits to three Army bases: Fort Hood and Fort Bliss in Texas and Fort Campbell in Tennessee. The committee has already visited Fort Hood and will visit the other two Army bases in phase 2. Because a large number of marines have deployed to Iraq and Afghanistan, the committee also hopes to visit a Marine Corps base. To increase its understanding of veterans with PTSD, the committee expects to visit at least one VA medical center.

The committee also anticipates that new information will continue to be published on many of the programs, treatments, and research covered in this report—including neurobiology and the use of complementary and alternative treatments for PTSD. Thus additional literature searches and discussions with researchers and patients will be conducted in phase 2 so that the growing body of evidence on the need for, use of, and outcomes from the programs and promising research on PTSD can be assessed.

1

Introduction

In response to the terrorist attacks of September 11, 2001, the U.S. military engaged in conflicts in the Middle East. Operation Enduring Freedom (OEF) began in October 2001 with troops stationed in and around Afghanistan for military and humanitarian purposes. Operation Iraqi Freedom (OIF) began in March 2003 as American-led coalition forces invaded Iraq, and it officially ended on August 31, 2010. Operation New Dawn (OND) was initiated on September 1, 2010, to reflect the changing mission of and reduction in U.S. military personnel in Iraq and officially ended on December 15, 2011; the last U.S. military personnel left that country on December 18, 2011. The conflict continues in Afghanistan, where 90,000 service members were deployed as of January 20, 2012 (ISAF, 2012). Since the beginning of the OEF and the OIF/OND conflicts, approximately 2.6 million U.S. service members have been deployed, 900,000 of them more than once (GAO, 2011b). Table 1-1 shows the breakdown of deployed service members by component and branch through April 2009 (IOM, 2010). As of April 30, 2012, a total of 1,831 American service members had been killed and 15,713 wounded in OEF. Casualty totals for OIF and OND are 4,475 military deaths and 32,225 wounded (DoD, 2012). Hereafter in this report, the term *OIF* will encompass both OIF and OND, unless otherwise stated.

The engagements of the U.S. military in Iraq and Afghanistan have been markedly different from prior conflicts with regard to both the service populations and the signature injuries sustained. Unlike previous wars and conflicts, OEF and OIF are distinguished by the large number of National Guard and reservists that have been deployed to Iraq and Afghanistan in

TABLE 1-1 Service Members Deployed by Component as of April 30, 2009

	Army	Navy	Air Force	Marine Corps	Coast Guard	Total
Active component	582,733	320,140	269,220	209,175	3,539	1,384,807
National Guard*	239,336	N/A	65,295	N/A	N/A	304,631
Reserves	125,595	33,891	38,056	37,602	228	235,372
Total	947,664	354,031	372,571	246,777	3,767	1,924,810

* Unlike the Army and Air Force, the Navy, Marine Corps, and Coast Guard do not have National Guard components.
SOURCE: Adapted from IOM, 2010.

addition to active-duty service members from all the services. Whereas infectious diseases and catastrophic gunshot wounds were the signature injuries of prior conflicts and wars, the hallmarks of the recent conflicts are blast injuries and the psychiatric consequences of exposure to combat, particularly posttraumatic stress disorder (PTSD). Recent estimates of prevalence of PTSD in service members deployed to OEF and OIF are 13% to 20% (Hoge et al., 2004; Seal et al., 2007; Tanielian and Jaycox, 2008; Vasterling et al., 2010).

Of growing concern to both the Department of Defense (DoD) and the Department of Veterans Affairs (VA) is the high prevalence of PTSD in active-duty and veteran populations. As the conflicts in the Middle East scale down and service members return home, the VA and the DoD may expect a commensurate rise in the number of OEF and OIF veterans needing services. To address this concern, the DoD and the VA have allocated substantial funding to foster research, develop programs, and initiate services to combat PTSD. The focus of the DoD is to maintain force readiness; therefore, it has invested heavily in building psychologic resilience, education, health maintenance, screening, and PTSD treatment services and programs. The VA has more than doubled its funding for PTSD research since 2005 (GAO, 2011a), targeting treatment and rehabilitation of veterans. Since FY 2005, the VA has added more than 7,500 full-time mental health staff and has trained, through national training initiatives, more than 3,400 VA clinicians in two evidence-based therapies for the treatment of PTSD—cognitive processing therapy (CPT) and prolonged exposure (PE). In addition, the VA has trained more than 900 DoD mental health providers in CPT and more than 120 in PE. The VA requires that all mental health services should be recovery-oriented, which means that services are strengths-based, individualized, and person-centered and allow veterans to have input into their own treatment within the range of evidence-based approaches (Schoenhard, 2011).

COMMITTEE'S CHARGE

In response to the number of service members and veterans who are at risk for and have received a diagnosis of PTSD, in 2009 Congress passed the National Defense Authorization Act for FY 2010. Section 726 of the act required the Secretary of Defense, in consultation with the Secretary of Veterans Affairs, to enter into an agreement with the Institute of Medicine (IOM) of the National Academy of Sciences to assess PTSD treatment programs and services in the DoD and the VA. The statement of task is shown in Box 1-1, and the legislative language calling for the study is in Appendix B.

COMMITTEE'S APPROACH

The present report is the first of two mandated in the legislation. During phase 1 the committee held six meetings over about 12 months. In the first two meetings, the committee held information-gathering sessions that were open to the public, and these meetings included presentations from the sponsor (the DoD), several subject-matter experts in the DoD and the VA, veterans organizations, and service members who have PTSD. As required by the authoring legislation, the committee also visited the U.S. Army base at Fort Hood in Killeen, Texas. During its visit, the committee heard from a variety of mental health providers and from PTSD patients and their families. Additional site visits—including congressionally mandated visits to Fort Bliss in Texas and Fort Campbell in Tennessee—will be conducted during phase 2.

The committee began its deliberations by determining what information would be necessary in order for it to assess the effectiveness of the multitude of treatments that are available to and used by service members and veterans who have PTSD. Information that the committee deemed important to collect included how many service members and veterans have been screened for and diagnosed with PTSD, what treatments (psychosocial, pharmacologic, and other) are they currently receiving, where do service members and veterans receive treatment (for example, primary care clinic, outpatient mental health clinic, specialized PTSD program, inpatient residential program), the duration and frequency of the treatment, what outcomes are tracked and for how long, what is the ratio of mental health providers to patients, and what training is given to health care providers

BOX 1-1
Statement of Task*

The Institute of Medicine will convene a committee to conduct a study of ongoing efforts in the treatment of posttraumatic stress disorder (PTSD). The study will be conducted in 2 phases: the focus in phase 1 will be on data gathering and will result in the initial study as noted in the congressional legislation; the focus in phase 2 will be on the analysis of data and result in the updated study. The work of the committee is dependent upon the timely delivery of data, in a usable format, from the DOD and the VA on their current PTSD programs.

Phase 1 (initial report):

In phase 1 of the study, the committee will collect data from the DoD and the VA on programs and methods available for the prevention (Chapter 5), screening (Chapter 6), diagnosis (Chapter 6), treatment (Chapter 7), and rehabilitation (Chapter 8) of post-traumatic stress disorder. The committee will highlight collaborative efforts between DoD and the VA in those areas (Chapter 4). Additionally, the committee will consider the status of studies and clinical trials involving innovative treatments of post-traumatic stress disorder that are conducted by the DoD, the VA, or the private sector, with regard to

- efforts to identify physiological markers of PTSD (Chapter 3);
- efforts to determine causation of PTSD, using brain imaging studies and studies looking at the correlation between brain region physiology and PTSD diagnoses and the results (including any interim results) of such efforts (Chapter 3);
- the effectiveness of alternative therapies in the treatment of PTSD, including the therapeutic use of animals (Chapter 7);
- the effectiveness of administering pharmaceutical agents before, during, or after a traumatic event in the prevention and treatment of PTSD (Chapter 5); and
- identification of areas in which the DoD and the VA may be duplicating studies, programs, or research with respect to PTSD.

Phase 2 (updated report):

In phase 2 of the study, the committee will analyze the data received in phase 1 specifically to determine the rates of success for each program or method; and an estimate of the number of members of the Armed Forces and veterans diagnosed by the DoD or the VA as having PTSD and the number of such veterans who have been successfully treated.

In addition, the committee will focus on targeted interventions at Fort Hood, Texas; Fort Bliss, Texas; Fort Campbell, Tennessee; and any other locations the committee deems necessary, including VA facilities. The committee will also examine gender-specific and racial and ethnic group-specific mental health treatment services available for members of the Armed Forces, including the availability of such treatment and services; the access to such treatment and services; the need for such treatment and services; and the efficacy and adequacy of such treatment and services.

Finally, the committee will examine the current and projected future annual expenditures by the DoD and the VA for the treatment and rehabilitation of PTSD; and provide recommendations for areas for future research with respect to PTSD.

---

* Chapter references were not part of the original statement of task and are intended to guide the reader to the chapter where this topic is discussed.

for treating PTSD. The committee also asked both the DoD and the VA to provide information on PTSD-related programs and services, including who is eligible for the program, where it is offered (for example, primary care, mental health clinic), what treatments are used in the program, how much it costs per participant, and what the program outcomes are. Any PTSD services and programs whether for screening, diagnosis, prevention, treatment, or rehabilitation were to be included. The committee encountered several barriers in obtaining information. The VA was helpful, and the committee was able to obtain much of the requested information from the Veterans Health Administration in a timely manner. Information received from the VA has been included in the report where relevant, but much of it may be found in Chapter 4, "Programs and Services for PTSD in the Department of Defense and the Department of Veterans Affairs," where the health systems of the VA and the DoD, their organizations, the communities they serve, and their PTSD services and programs, are described. It was more difficult to obtain information from the DoD, in part because committee's data requests had to go to each of the service branches who then had to task the request to various data repositories, and once tasked, the data needed to be collected, analyzed, and approved. Identifying the correct personnel to task with the request, in spite of the assistance and preliminary information given to the committee by the staff at the DoD Defense Center of Excellence for Psychological Health and Brain Injury, was difficult with the result that although the information requests eventually were tasked to the Army, Air Force, Navy, and Marine Corps, the data had not been received by the committee in time to include them in this phase 1 report. The information will be updated and included in the phase 2 report. Collaborative efforts between the DoD and the VA with regard to the prevention and treatment of PTSD are described in Chapter 4. This information was obtained from expert knowledge of the committee members, Internet searches, and discussions with DoD and VA staff.

During its deliberations, the committee conducted numerous focused searches of peer-reviewed literature, government reports, and books, manuals, and documents relevant to PTSD. Although it is not a comprehensive literature review itself, this report constitutes a synthesis of evidence with the intent of highlighting PTSD prevention, screening, diagnosis, treatment, and rehabilitation options that are or could be used in the DoD and the VA mental health care systems. The committee did not take its task to be an evaluation of the current guidelines for the management of PTSD that are available from several organizations such as the American Psychiatric Association and the joint guideline from the VA and the DoD. Therefore, although the committee considered many studies in this report, it did not systematically review and rank each study. The committee felt that to do so would essentially be preparing another guideline, which was unnecessary and beyond its charge. Rather, the goal of presenting the studies, particularly randomized controlled trials (RCTs) for the many treatment options described in Chapter 7, was to identify those widely used by the DoD and the VA as well as to help the committee identify treatments and approaches that may need further evaluation for phase 2. The term *evidence based* as used by the committee refers to the use of RCTs or other well-conducted studies that provide the basis for judging the efficacy of a particular treatment, program, or approach.

The report does not discuss every aspect of PTSD: the committee considered related disorders (such as acute stress disorder, depression, and adjustment disorders) and comorbidities (such as traumatic brain injury) only as they may complicate treatment for PTSD; this is not to minimize the impact of those conditions and disorders on service members and veterans but rather to note that attention to ancillary illnesses is outside the committee's charge. Furthermore, the committee did not develop an exhaustive list of all of the available PTSD programs and services available through the DoD or the VA, although both the DoD and the VA were asked to provide information on their programs in the data requests discussed earlier. However, such a list for the DoD may be found in the recent RAND report *Programs Addressing Psychological Health and Traumatic Brain Injury Among U.S. Military Servicemembers and Their Families* (Weinick et al., 2011). The VA provided examples of prevention and specialized treatment programs, and these are described in Chapter 4. Because of the lack of information from the DoD, the committee was unable to compare all DoD services, programs, and research with those of the VA as required in the statement of task. The committee will consider the feasibility of doing this in phase 2.

This report is centered on PTSD in service members and veterans that has resulted from their time in service and acknowledges that some service members may have entered the military with symptoms of PTSD and that PTSD may result from exposure to traumatic events not related to military service. PTSD in military and veteran populations has a huge impact on spouses, children, parents, and others; however, these populations do not fall within the purview of this report. The impact of PTSD on service members' and veterans' caregivers is presented when relevant information is available.

Finally, the committee concluded that it was important to include some recommendations for the DoD and the VA in this phase 1 report rather than waiting until the completion of the phase 2 report. There are several reasons for this. First, the committee concluded that many of its recommendations could be implemented relatively quickly and that the DoD and the VA (and thus service members and veterans) should not have to wait 4 years to learn of them. Some of the recommendations might initiate or reinforce data-gathering and -tracking efforts in the DoD and the VA. Lastly, the recommendations provide action items for the DoD and the VA.

ORGANIZATION OF THE REPORT

This report addresses the committee's tasks. In Chapter 2, the committee summarizes the criteria necessary for a diagnosis of PTSD, discusses the epidemiology of the disorder, and introduces some of the challenges faced by mental health care providers in the diagnosis of and treatment for PTSD in military and veteran populations. Chapter 3 explains adaptive and maladaptive responses to stress and the neurobiology of PTSD and addresses some of the research being conducted to identify physiological markers of PTSD. The chapter also includes a discussion of innovative work to determine who is at risk for PTSD and techniques such as brain imaging that may be used to more effectively diagnose and treat it. The intent of these chapters is to provide an overview of the science as the basis of prevention and treatment for PTSD. Chapter 4 offers a summary of the DoD and the VA health care systems and examples of PTSD programs and services offered in both departments. It also describes some examples of collaborative efforts between the DoD and the VA with regard to PTSD services, programs, and research. The chapter provides a summary of some the research currently or recently being funded by the DoD, the VA, and the National Institutes of Health. Approaches to the prevention of PTSD both before and after exposure to a traumatic event, including the use of pharmacologic agents, and particularly in the military, are described in Chapter 5. Chapter 6 discusses the goals of and considerations in screening for PTSD, including the most common tools and instruments used by the DoD and the VA. The second part of the chapter differentiates screening from diagnosis and reviews the types of clinician-administered interviews used to assess PTSD symptoms and severity. Chapter 7 evaluates the evidence supporting the many options for PTSD treatment. The chapter covers not only widely used evidence-based psychosocial and pharmacologic therapies but also the evidence supporting complementary and alternative therapies such as animal-assisted therapy, and emerging treatments, such as couple therapy and virtual reality exposure. Chapter 8 is a continuation of the treatment discussion but with a focus on the treatment and rehabilitation needs of service members and veterans who have both PTSD and comorbid medical and psychiatric conditions and psychosocial treatment needs. Novel and emerging interventions are addressed where pertinent in Chapters 7 and 8, although the innovative and emerging approaches will be tackled more fully in the phase 2 report. The barriers to PTSD diagnosis and effective care encountered by service members, veterans, and their families are discussed in detail in Chapter 9. This chapter also includes a description of some facilitators for the treatment of PTSD such as the use of the Internet to deliver therapy. The report ends with a summary of the committee's key findings and recommendations and a brief discussion of plans for phase 2.

REFERENCES

DoD (Department of Defense). 2012. *DoD casualty reports.* http://www.defense.gov/news/casualty.pdf (accessed January 20, 2012).

GAO (U.S. Government Accountability Office). 2011a. *VA health care—VA spends millions on post-traumatic stress disorder research and incorporates research outcomes into guidelines and policy for post-traumatic stress disorder services.* Washington, DC: GAO.

GAO. 2011b. *VA mental health: Number of veterans receiving care, barriers faced, and efforts to increase access.* GAO 12-12. Washington, DC: GAO.

Hoge, C. W., C. A. Castro, S. C. Messer, D. McGurk, D. I. Cotting, and R. L. Koffman. 2004. Combat duty in Iraq and Afghanistan, mental health problems, and barriers to care. *New England Journal of Medicine* 351(1):13-22.

IOM (Institute of Medicine). 2010. *Returning home from Iraq and Afghanistan: Preliminary assessment of readjustment needs of veterans, service members, and their families.* Washington, DC: The National Academies Press.

ISAF (International Security Assistance Force). 2012. *Troop numbers & contributions: United States.* http://www.isaf.nato.int/troop-numbers-and-contributions/united-states/index.php (accessed January 20, 2012).

Schoenhard, W. 2011. *Statement to the Senate Committee on Veterans' Affairs.* July 14, 2011. http://veterans.senate.gov/hearings.cfm?action=release.display&release_id=796c41ee-3006-4647-b461-920653c6425e (accessed April 27, 2012).

Seal, K. H., D. Bertenthal, C. R. Miner, S. Sen, and C. Marmar. 2007. Bringing the war back home: Mental health disorders among 103,788 US veterans returning from Iraq and Afghanistan seen at Department of Veterans Affairs facilities. *Archives of Internal Medicine* 167(5):476-482.

Tanielian, T. L., and L. Jaycox. 2008. *Invisible wounds of war: Psychological and cognitive injuries, their consequences, and services to assist recovery.* Arlington, VA: RAND Corporation.

Vasterling, J. J., S. P. Proctor, M. J. Friedman, C. W. Hoge, T. Heeren, L. A. King, and D. W. King. 2010. PTSD symptom increases in Iraq-deployed soldiers: Comparison with nondeployed soldiers and associations with baseline symptoms, deployment experiences, and postdeployment stress. *Journal of Traumatic Stress* 23(1):41-51.

Weinick, R. M., E. B. Beckjord, C. M. Farmer, L. T. Martin, E. M. Gillen, J. D. Acosta, M. P. Fisher, J. Garnett, G. C. Gonzalez, T. C. Helmus, L. Jaycox, K. A. Reynolds, N. Salcedo, and D. M. Scharf. 2011. *Programs addressing psychological health and traumatic brain injury among U.S. military servicemembers and their families.* Santa Monica, CA: RAND Corporation.

2

History, Diagnostic Criteria, and Epidemiology

This chapter provides an overview of the epidemiology of posttraumatic stress disorder (PTSD). It begins with a brief history of the disorder in the American military, which is followed by a discussion of its diagnostic criteria. The remainder of the chapter presents factors associated with trauma and PTSD, first in the general population and then in military and veteran populations, with an emphasis on combat as the traumatic event that triggered the development of PTSD. Although other traumatic events—such as the terrorist attacks of September 11, 2001, and Hurricane Katrina—have increased knowledge about PTSD, this chapter does not focus on civilian populations or nonmilitary related trauma. The chapter concludes with special epidemiologic considerations regarding PTSD in military populations and their implications for screening, diagnosis, and treatment.

HISTORY OF PTSD

Prior to the codifying of PTSD by the American Psychiatric Association (APA) as a distinct mental health disorder in 1980 (APA, 1980), characteristic symptoms of PTSD had been recognized and documented in the 19th century in civilians involved in catastrophic events, such as railway collisions, and in American soldiers fighting in the Civil War (Birmes et al., 2003; Jones, 2006; Welke, 2001). Many Civil War soldiers had diagnoses of nostalgia or melancholia, characterized by lethargy, withdrawal, and "excessive emotionality" (Birmes et al., 2003). Others had diagnoses of exhaustion, effort syndrome, or heart conditions variously called "irritable heart," "soldier's heart," and "cardiac muscular exhaustion." Many medical professionals and surgeons at the time believed that those conditions arose from the heavy packs that soldiers carried, insufficient time for new recruits to acclimatize to the military lifestyle, homesickness, and, as one army surgeon stated, poorly motivated soldiers who had unrealistic expectations of war (Jones, 2006). For much of the 20th century, psychologic conditions and impairments in military personnel were not accorded high medical priority because of the high fatality rates from disease, infection, and accidental injuries during war.

During World War I, shell shock and disordered action of the heart were commonly diagnosed in combat veterans (Jones, 2006). Symptoms of shell shock included tremors, tics, fatigue, memory loss, difficulty in sleeping, nightmares, and poor concentration—similar to many of the symptoms associated with PTSD. What is now known as delayed-onset PTSD was termed *old-sergeant syndrome* during the era of the world wars, when after prolonged combat, experienced soldiers were no longer able to cope with the constant threats of death or serious injury (Shephard, 2000). Stemming from the World War I definition of shell shock, other common diagnoses of soldiers during World War II included exhaustion, battle exhaustion, flying syndrome, war neurosis, cardiac neurosis, and psychoneurosis (Jones, 2006).

It was not until after the Vietnam War that research and methodical documentation of what was then termed *combat fatigue* began to accelerate in response to the many veterans suffering from chronic psychologic problems that resulted in social and occupational dysfunction (IOM, 2008a). The National Vietnam Veterans Readjustment Survey (NVVRS) was one of the first large-scale studies to examine PTSD and other combat-related psychologic issues in a veteran population (Kulka, 1990). The NVVRS helped to illuminate PTSD as a signature wound of the Vietnam War and resulted in greater recognition of PTSD as a mental health disorder. The findings contributed to the formal recognition of PTSD as a distinct disorder by the APA and later refining of the characteristic symptoms and diagnostic criteria.

DIAGNOSTIC CRITERIA FOR PTSD

Since 1980, PTSD has been the focus of much epidemiologic and clinical research, which in turn has led to modifications in the defining diagnostic criteria for PTSD. The current diagnostic criteria, taken from the *Diagnostic and Statistical Manual of Mental Disorders, Fourth Edition, Text Revision* (*DSM-IV-TR*), can be found in Box 2-1 (APA, 2000). The Department of Defense (DoD) and the Department of Veterans Affairs

BOX 2-1
***DSM-IV-TR* Diagnostic Criteria for Posttraumatic Stress Disorder**

A1. The person experienced, witnessed, or was confronted with an event or events that involved actual or threatened death or serious injury, or a threat to the physical integrity of self or others
A2. The person's response involved intense fear, helplessness, or horror

B. Re-experiencing Symptoms (requires one or more of):
B1. Intrusive recollections
B2. Distressing nightmares
B3. Acting/feeling as though event were recurring (flashbacks)
B4. Psychological distress when exposed to traumatic reminders
B5. Physiological reactivity when exposed to traumatic reminders

C. Avoidant/Numbing Symptoms (requires three or more of):
C1. Avoidance of thoughts, feelings, or conversations associated with the stressor
C2. Avoidance of activities, places, or people associated with the stressor
C3. Inability to recall important aspects of traumatic event
C4. Diminished interest in significant activities
C5. Detachment from others
C6. Restricted range of affect
C7. Sense of foreshortened future

D. Hyperarousal Symptoms (requires two or more of):
D1. Sleep problems
D2. Irritability
D3. Concentration problems
D4. Hypervigilance
D5. Exaggerated startle response

E. Duration of the disturbance is at least 1 month
Acute—when the duration of symptoms is less than 3 months
Chronic—when symptoms last 3 months or longer
With Delayed Onset—at least 6 months have elapsed between the traumatic event and onset of symptoms

F. Requires significant distress or functional impairment

SOURCE: American Psychiatric Association (2000) with permission.

(VA) both use these criteria in diagnosing the condition in service members and veterans.

PTSD is unique among psychiatric disorders in that it is linked to a specific trigger: a traumatic event (Criterion A1). Traumatic events known to trigger PTSD include combat, natural and accidental disasters (for example, tsunamis, earthquakes, and vehicle and airplane crashes), and victimization or abuse (for example, sexual assault, armed robbery, and torture) (Basile et al., 2004; Harrison and Kinner, 1998; Hoge et al., 2004; Neria et al., 2007; Punamaki et al., 2010). PTSD may be of acute, chronic, or delayed onset. In acute PTSD, symptoms develop immediately or soon after experiencing a traumatic event and persist longer than a month but less than 3 months. If symptom duration is longer than 3 months, a person has chronic PTSD.

In delayed-onset PTSD, a person does not express symptoms for months or even years after the traumatic event (APA, 2000). The condition is considered partial or subthreshold PTSD if a person does not meet the full diagnostic criteria—exposure to a traumatic event and at least six symptoms: at least one B criterion of re-experiencing, at least three C criteria of numbing or avoidance, and at least two D criteria of hyperarousal—or if symptoms are not in the correct distribution. Changes to the diagnostic criteria for PTSD proposed for the next version of the DSM are shown in Box 2-2.

BOX 2-2
Proposed Changes in Diagnostic Criteria for PTSD in *DSM-5*

Research on PTSD and acute stress reactions has progressed, and diagnostic criteria are expected to change to reflect the updated version of *DSM-5*. One of the changes affects Criterion A1: it is proposed to expand it from experiencing or witnessing threatened or actual death or serious injury to oneself or others to include *learning about* such an event that happened to a relative or close friend and to include first responders or others who are continuously exposed to or experience details of traumatic events (Friedman et al., 2010). Because of the characteristics of the statistical association and predictive value of experiencing intense fear, helplessness, or horror during the event and onset of PTSD (Brewin et al., 2000a) and because some persons—for example, military personnel, who are trained to not have an emotional response during such an event—it has been proposed that Criterion A2 be eliminated (Friedman et al., 2010).

Other proposed changes for PTSD in *DSM-5* include replacing the current three-pronged model with a four-pronged model. In the proposed model, Criterion B would become "Intrusion Symptoms," Criterion C "Persistent Avoidance," Criterion D "Alterations in Cognition and Mood," and Criterion E "Hyperarousal and Reactivity Symptoms." Although all 17 symptoms of *DSM-IV* would be kept in the proposed *DSM-5*, some of them would be revised or regrouped (such as including anger and aggressive behavior with irritability), and three symptoms would be added: erroneous self-blame or other blame regarding the cause or consequences of trauma, pervasive negative emotional states, and reckless and self-destructive behavior. The final proposed change in *DSM-5* is to omit the distinction between acute and chronic PTSD. There is no proposal to include cases of subthreshold, or subsyndromal, PTSD as a distinct disorder in *DSM-5* (Friedman et al., 2010).

EPIDEMIOLOGY OF PTSD IN THE GENERAL POPULATION

This section begins with a brief discussion of factors associated with the experience of trauma in the general population, inasmuch as this is a main criterion in the diagnosis of PTSD, before considering the epidemiology of PTSD in the general population. The next major section deals with trauma and epidemiology specific to military and veteran populations.

Men are more likely than women to experience potential traumatic events overall, although the types of traumatic events differ by sex (Tolin and Foa, 2006). Studies assessing the role of race and ethnicity have had mixed results but have found that whites have higher risks of exposure to any traumatic event than Hispanics and blacks (Noris, 1992; Roberts et al., 2011). Other factors found to be associated with increased risk of experiencing traumatic events include lower education attainment (less than a 4-year college degree), lower annual income (less than $25,000), and nonheterosexual orientation (Breslau et al., 1998; Roberts et al., 2010). Three prospective studies have documented that externalizing behavioral problems (for example, difficult temperament and antisocial behavior) in early childhood increase the risk of traumatic-event exposure—particularly assaultive violence—over a lifetime (Breslau et al., 2006; Koenen et al., 2007; Storr et al., 2007).

Trauma type and severity are central determinants of the risk of development of PTSD. Experiencing physical injuries (penetrating and assault), viewing the event as a true threat to one's life, and suffering major losses are all associated with a higher risk of PTSD (Holbrook et al., 2001; Ozer et al., 2003). The occurrence of dissociation itself during a traumatic event does not appear to predict development of PTSD as much as dissociation that persists after the event (Panasetis and Bryant, 2003) or the experience of perievent emotional reactions (Galea et al., 2003). As recognized by the *VA/DoD Clinical Practice Guideline for Management of Post-Traumatic Stress* (2010), lack of social support, trauma severity, and ongoing life stress increase the risk of PTSD. Lack or loss of social support (for example, spouse, friends, or family) after a traumatic event and ongoing life stress—including loss of employment, financial strain, and disability—have been associated with increased risk of PTSD (Brewin et al., 2000a; Ozer et al., 2003).

Several large, nationally representative surveys have provided estimates of the prevalence of PTSD in the general population. The National Comorbidity Survey (NCS), conducted from 1990 to 1992, was one of the first large-scale surveys to examine the distribution of and factors associated with psychiatric disorders in the United States. Using a structured diagnostic interview, the NCS found that the lifetime prevalence of PTSD was 7.8% overall (Kessler et al., 1995). In the National Comorbidity Survey–Replication (NCS–R) conducted 10 years after the original, the prevalence of lifetime PTSD was estimated to be 6.8% overall and that of current (12-month) PTSD 3.6% overall (Kessler et al., 2005). The 2004–2005 National Epidemiologic Survey on Alcohol and Related Conditions estimated lifetime prevalence of PTSD to be 7.3% overall (Roberts et al., 2011).

Sex and trauma type are two risk factors associated with PTSD (protective factors are discussed in Chapter 5). PTSD prevalence has consistently been shown to differ by sex in the civilian population (Kessler et al., 1995, 2005; Tolin and Foa, 2006). The original NCS found PTSD prevalence to be twice as great in women as in men, and the NCS–R estimated it to be 2.7 times greater in women than in men (Harvard Medical School, 2007b; Kessler et al., 1995). The type of trauma experienced may lead to the discrepancy between the sexes. For example, Tolin and Foa (2006) found no sex differences associated with PTSD in persons who experienced assaultive violence or nonsexual child abuse or neglect, but there were marked differences between men and women who experienced combat, accidents, and disasters. Men were more likely to report having experienced a traumatic event over their lifetimes, but women were more likely to meet criteria for PTSD (Tolin and Foa, 2006), have PTSD symptoms four times as long as men (48 months vs. 12 months) (Breslau et al., 1998), have a poorer quality of life if they have PTSD (Holbrook et al., 2001; Seedat et al., 2005), and develop more comorbid psychiatric disorders (Seedat et al., 2005).

There is some evidence on the effect of race and ethnicity on the development of PTSD although findings are inconsistent among studies. Results from the 2004–2005 wave of the National Epidemiologic Survey on Alcohol and Related Conditions showed that whites were more likely to have experienced any trauma, and lifetime prevalence of PTSD was highest in blacks and lowest in Asians. Even after adjustment for characteristics related to trauma, the risk of PTSD was significantly higher in blacks and lower in Asians than in whites in the sample (Roberts et al., 2011). Marshall et al. (2009) found that in a sample of survivors of physical trauma, Hispanic whites reported greater symptoms related to cognitive and sensory perception (for example, hypervigilance and emotional reactivity) and overall symptom severity than non-Hispanic whites. Other work has shown that Hispanic whites are more likely to report PTSD after a traumatic event than are non-Hispanic whites (Galea et al., 2004). In a study of adults 18–45 years old in the Detroit area, Breslau et al. (1998) found that nonwhites were not at higher risk for PTSD than whites.

PTSD can affect people of any age. In the NCS–R, people were divided into four cohorts: 18–29, 30–44, 45–59, and older than 59 years old. The highest lifetime and 12-month prevalences of PTSD were in the group 45–59 years old (9.2% and 5.3%, respectively), and the lowest prevalences (2.8% and 1.0%, respectively) were in the group over 59 years old (Harvard Medical School, 2007a,b). Results from the earlier NCS showed a different distribution of lifetime prevalence of PTSD by age group. The lowest prevalence was in men 15–24 years old (2.8%) and women 45–54 years old (8.7%) (Kessler et al., 1995). However, most of those studies examined the association between current age of the participants and PTSD symptoms or diagnostic threshold, and the strength of association between age and development of PTSD is unknown. Prevalence estimates of PTSD by age groups may also be confounded by historical events, such as the Vietnam War.

Sexual orientation has been associated with risk of PTSD. The National Epidemiologic Survey of Alcohol and Related Conditions found that the risk of PTSD was significantly higher in lesbians and gays, bisexuals, and heterosexuals with any same-sex partners than it was in the heterosexual reference group. After adjusting for demographic factors, the higher risk of PTSD was largely explained by nonheterosexuals' greater exposure to violence, exposure to more potentially traumatic events, and earlier age at trauma exposure (Roberts et al., 2010).

Cognitive reserve—individual differences in brain structure and function that are thought to provide resilience against damage from neuropathology—is thought to be one important etiologic factor in the development and severity of PTSD and other neuropsychiatric disorders (Barnett et al., 2006). Intelligence quotient (IQ), a marker of cognitive reserve, has been shown to be inversely related to risk of PTSD and other psychiatric disorders (Batty et al., 2005; Walker et al., 2002). In a 17-year prospective study of randomly selected newborns in southeastern Michigan, Breslau et al. (2006) found that children who at the age of 6 years had an IQ of greater than 115 had a decreased conditional risk of PTSD after trauma exposure; however, the risk increased for children that experienced anxiety disorders and whom teachers rated as high for externalizing problems. Overall, the authors found that high IQ (115 or higher) protected exposed persons from developing PTSD in this cohort (Breslau et al., 2006).

Similarly, Koenen et al. (2007) examined the association between early childhood neurocognitive factors and risk of PTSD in a New Zealand birth cohort that was followed through the age of 32 years. The authors found that IQ assessed at the age of 5 years was inversely associated with risk for developing PTSD by the age of 32 years. No associations were found between PTSD and other neurodevelopmental factors assessed in the cohort, suggesting that the IQ–PTSD association was not a marker of broader neurodevelopmental deficits.

The findings on the strength of association between family psychiatric history and PTSD are mixed. In one analysis of NCS data, after controlling for previous traumatic events, parental mental health disorders were associated with increased risk of PTSD in both men and women (Bromet et al., 1998). Although Breslau et al. (1991) found statistically significant associations between PTSD after a traumatic event and family psychiatric history of depression, anxiety, and psychosis, a meta-analysis of risk factors for PTSD did not find this association in either civilian or military population studies (Brewin et al., 2000b). A family history of psychiatric disorders may be indicative of adverse family environment, which may increase the risk of experiencing a traumatic event, such as abuse, during childhood (Breslau et al., 1995; Brewin et al., 2000b). A positive association was found between reported family history of psychopathologic conditions and higher rates of PTSD symptoms or diagnosis, but the strength of this relationship differed by the type of traumatic experience of the target event (stronger after noncombat interpersonal violence than after combat exposure) and method of PTSD assessment (stronger when symptoms were determined in interviews than in self-reports) (Ozer et al., 2003). In a study that followed a New Zealand birth cohort and assessed for PTSD at the age of 26 years and again at the age of 32 years, maternal depression before the age of 11 years was associated with increased risk of PTSD through the age of 32 years (Koenen et al., 2007).

Family and twin studies of PTSD have produced two major findings. First, PTSD has a genetic component. Modern genetic studies of PTSD began with the observation that relatives of probands (persons serving as index cases in genetic investigations of families) who had PTSD had a higher risk of the disorder than relatives of similarly trauma-exposed controls who did not develop PTSD. Twin studies established that genetic influences explain much of the vulnerability to PTSD, from about 30% in male Vietnam veterans (True et al., 1993) to 72% in young women (Sartor et al., 2011), even after genetic influences on trauma exposure are accounted for. Second, both family and twin studies suggest that there is strong overlap for genetic influences on PTSD and those of other mental disorders including major depression, generalized anxiety disorder, and alcohol and drug dependence. For example, in a sample of Vietnam veterans, common genetic influences explained 63% of the major depression–PTSD comorbidity and 58% genetic variance in PTSD (Koenen et al., 2008a). Other studies using the Vietnam Era Twin Registry found genetic influences of generalized anxiety disorder and panic disorder symptoms (Chantarujikapong et al., 2001), alcohol dependence and drug dependence (Xian et al., 2000), and nicotine dependence (Koenen et al., 2005b) account for a substantial proportion of the genetic variance for PTSD. Those results suggest that most of the genes that affect the risk of PTSD also influence the risk of these psychiatric disorders and vice versa. A more complete discussion of genetic influences on PTSD is found in Chapter 3.

Several prospective studies have implicated pretrauma psychopathology in increasing the risk of PTSD. In a cohort of randomly selected newborns in southeastern Michigan followed for 17 years, children who at the age of

6 years were rated as having externalizing problems above the normal range were more likely to develop PTSD than children who were rated as normal externalizers; young adults who had received a diagnosis of any anxiety disorder at the age of 6 years were significantly more likely to develop PTSD than those who had not (Breslau et al., 2006). Another prospective study in a cohort of children of similar age entering first grade over a 2-year period and followed for 15 years, those who in first grade were categorized as highly anxious or having depressive mood were at higher risk for PTSD among those exposed to traumatic events than their peers who did not have these psychologic problems; exhibiting aggressive or disruptive behaviors, concentration problems, and low social interaction were not found to be associated with increased risk of PTSD in this cohort (Storr et al., 2007). A third prospective study, which followed a New Zealand birth cohort and assessed for trauma exposure and PTSD at the ages of 26 and 32 years, found several childhood risk factors to be associated with PTSD. Childhood temperament ratings were made at the ages of 3 and 5 years, and behavior ratings were made by teachers biannually from the ages of 5 through 11 years. Children who had difficult temperaments or antisocial behavior and who were unpopular were statistically more likely to develop PTSD than their peers who did not have these characteristics. Antisocial behavior assessed before the age of 11 years predicted development of PTSD at the age of 26 years and at the age of 32 years. Childhood poverty and high levels of internalizing symptoms in mothers were also associated with development of PTSD (Koenen et al., 2007).

Childhood abuse may have an effect on the development of PTSD. A meta-analysis that considered nine studies suggests that abuse during childhood is a risk factor for PTSD (Brewin et al., 2000b). Desai et al. (2002) found that physical or sexual childhood victimization or both increased the risk of adult victimization by an intimate partner. This aligns with NCS findings that women who experienced physical abuse during childhood had the highest risk of lifetime PTSD (Kessler et al., 1995).

In addition to pretrauma psychopathology or childhood abuse, prior trauma has been shown to increase the risk of PTSD. Ozer et al. (2003) found a significant association between a history of prior trauma and PTSD symptoms or diagnosis. Persons who experienced a traumatic event before the target stressor reported higher levels of PTSD symptoms on the average than persons who did not. Prior trauma was more strongly associated with PTSD in connection with traumatic experiences of noncombat interpersonal violence than with combat exposures (Ozer et al., 2003). However, more recent data from prospective studies offer evidence against the hypothesis that prior trauma alone increases the risk of PTSD. Using a random sample from a large health maintenance organization in southeastern Michigan, Breslau et al. (2008) found that prior experience of trauma does not necessarily increase the risk of PTSD in response to a subsequent trauma. Only those persons who developed PTSD in response to a prior trauma had an increased risk of PTSD after a later trauma. A follow-up study on assaultive violence found that it was the development of prior PTSD after a trauma that was predictive of the development of current PTSD after a later trauma (Breslau and Peterson, 2010).

Trajectory of PTSD

The course of PTSD may remit with time, with steepest remission in the first 12 months after diagnosis. In a nonrandomized, observational, retrospective analysis based on the NCS, the median time until diagnostic criteria were no longer met in those who received treatment was 36 months compared with 64 months in those who did not receive treatment (Kessler et al., 1995). However, approximately one-third of PTSD cases do not remit even after many years of treatment. A prospective study of PTSD in rape victims found that half recovered spontaneously, with the steepest declines from the first to the fourth assessment (mean, 35 days after the assault), whereas victims who had a diagnosis of PTSD 2 months or more after the trauma (rape) were unlikely to recover without treatment (Rothbaum et al., 1992). Other studies have shown remission of PTSD after particular traumatic events, such as disasters, in the first 6 months after exposure to the event (Galea and Resnick, 2005). Although PTSD is triggered by the initial exposure to a traumatic event, several studies have shown that exposure to ongoing stressors and other traumatic events throughout life contributes to the persistence of PTSD in the general population (Galea et al., 2008).

Few studies have investigated the chronicity of PTSD, most conducted before some current therapies were available; therefore, they are relatively dated. Two similarly designed prospective observational studies of people who had diagnosed PTSD and who were seeking care in tertiary care psychiatric practices (Zlotnick et al., 1999) or primary care practices (Zlotnick et al., 2004) had similar findings. Over the 5-year follow-up of the 54 persons in the tertiary care study, the probability of experiencing full remission was 18%. Chronicity of PTSD was associated with a history of alcohol abuse or dependence and childhood trauma (Zlotnick et al., 1999). In the primary care study, the authors considered full and partial remission separately. The findings were similar to those of the tertiary care study: over the 2-year follow-up of the 84 primary care subjects, the probability of full remission was 18% and the probability of partial remission 69%. Both full remission and partial remission were associated with fewer comorbid anxiety disorders and a smaller degree of psychosocial impairment. The authors also evaluated the type, dose, and duration of treatment. The treatment was not randomized, but there was no association between the use of selective serotonin reuptake inhibitors or serotonin norepinephrine reuptake inhibitors and PTSD status at any point during the follow-up period (Zlotnick et al., 2004).

Men who reported combat as their worst trauma in the NCS were more likely to have lifetime PTSD, delayed onset of PTSD symptoms, and unresolved PTSD symptoms than men who named other types of trauma as their worst (Prigerson et al., 2001). Veterans enrolled in the NVVRS who had ever had full or partial PTSD reported they had experienced symptoms 63% of the time during the preceding 5 years (data collected between 1994–1996); 55% reported having symptoms every month, and 17% reported having no symptoms. In the 3 months before assessment, 78% had been symptomatic (Schnurr et al., 2003).

PTSD is associated with several adverse outcomes, including lower quality of life, work-related impairment, and medical illness throughout its course (Marshall et al., 2001; Resnick and Rosenheck, 2008; Zatzick et al., 1997). Several studies have shown an adverse effect of PTSD on physical health (Weiss et al., 2011), and others have found that exposure to a traumatic event increases the risk of adverse physical health, including many of the leading causes of premature death, such as cardiovascular disease and stroke (Boscarino, 2008; Cohen et al., 2009, 2010; Dirkzwager et al., 2007; Dong et al., 2004; Kubzansky et al., 2007, 2009). The associations are thought to be mediated in part by health behaviors, such as smoking, alcohol use, and physical inactivity (Breslau et al., 2003; Dobie et al., 2004). Because it would be unethical to expose humans to major trauma experimentally, randomized studies of the trajectory of PTSD are not feasible. The only available studies of trajectory of PTSD are natural history and observational studies, so the inference of findings to the general populaton is limited, and this makes it difficult to project future care and treatment needs.

Comorbidities of PTSD

People who have PTSD often have co-occurring psychologic disorders, such as depressive disorders, substance dependence, panic disorder, agoraphobia, generalized anxiety disorder, social phobia, bipolar disorder, and somatization (APA, 2000). People who have diagnoses of more than one mental health disorder have greater impairment than those who have a single diagnosis (IOM, 2008b). Those additional disorders can precede or present simultaneously with PTSD, and they may also resolve before, after, or simultaneously with PTSD. A prospective study that used data from a New Zealand birth cohort found that 96.3% of all adults who at the age of 32 years had a diagnosis of PTSD in the preceding year and 93.5% of those meeting criteria for lifetime diagnosis of PTSD at the age of 26 years had met criteria for diagnosis of another mental health disorder (major depression, an anxiety disorder, conduct disorder, marijuana dependence, or alcohol dependence) between the ages of 11 and 21 years (Koenen et al., 2008b).

An analysis of 23 studies found small but significant effect sizes of a relationship between PTSD and prior adjustment problems, including mental health treatment; pretrauma emotional problems, anxiety, or affective disorders; and, in particular, depression (Ozer et al., 2003). The strength of the relationship between prior adjustment problems and PTSD symptoms or diagnosis changed as a function of type of traumatic experience (stronger for noncombat interpersonal violence and accidents than for combat exposure), amount of time elapsed (stronger for less time between the event and PTSD assessment), and method of assessment for PTSD symptoms or diagnosis (stronger for interview studies than for self-reported measures) (Ozer et al., 2003). In an Australian study of people involved in motor vehicle incidents and later hospitalized, a personal history of psychiatric treatment was significantly associated with all trauma measures, including PTSD symptoms, 6 months after the event (Jeavons et al., 2000). In a meta-analysis of 22 studies, psychiatric history was found to be a significant predictor of PTSD (Brewin et al., 2000b).

Many studies have documented the association between PTSD and suicide ideation, attempts, and completions. In a study of civilians who had chronic PTSD and were attending a clinic, Tarrier and Gregg (2004) found that 38.3% reported suicide ideation and 9.6% reported having made a suicide attempt since experiencing the traumatic event. A comparison of those results with the NCS suggested higher suicidal tendencies among persons who had PTSD. Further support for the finding comes from a study by Marshall et al. (2001), who showed a linear increase in current suicide ideation with increased number of PTSD symptoms.

PTSD and drug or alcohol use is often associated. The lifetime prevalence of substance use disorders in NCS participants who had PTSD was more than twice that in people who did not have PTSD—a significant finding overall and also in comparing men with women. Comparing men who had PTSD to those who did not have PTSD, the odds ratio (OR) for having comorbid alcohol abuse or dependence was 2.06 (95% confidence interval [CI] 1.14–3.70), and the OR was 2.97 (95% CI 1.52–5.79) for comorbid drug abuse or dependence; for women, the ORs were 2.48 (95% CI 1.78–3.45) and 4.46 (95% CI 3.11–6.39), respectively (Kessler et al., 1995). In an in-depth investigation of three possible causal pathways linking PTSD and drug use disorders, which included a longitudinal design of a randomly selected sample in a health maintenance organization in Michigan, Chilcoat and Breslau (1998) suggested that the most plausible pathway was self-medication. In this pathway, PTSD-affected persons are thought to initiate use of drugs and other psychoactive substances use after symptom development to cope with and manage their memories and symptoms of PTSD (Brown and Wolfe, 1994; Khantzian, 1985; Stewart, 1996). That hypothesis was supported by the finding that people who had a history of PTSD were four times more likely to have drug use or dependence than those who did not have a PTSD diagnosis (Chilcoat and Breslau, 1998).

In civilian studies of smoking and psychiatric disorders, on the basis of data from the Tobacco Supplement of the NCS, current psychiatric disorders were found to increase the risk of onset of daily smoking in nonsmokers. In current smokers, the disorders were found to increase the risk of progression to nicotine dependence (Breslau et al., 2004). Another analysis of NCS smoking data found that the rates of current and lifetime smoking in people who had current and lifetime mental illness were significantly higher than in those who never reported having a mental illness. The study also concluded that people who have mental illness are twice as likely to smoke as those who do not (Lasser et al., 2000). Similarly, studies of the Vietnam-era twins cohort have concluded that active PTSD increased the risk of smoking independently of genetic makeup (Koenen et al., 2006) and that pre-existing nicotine dependence increased the risk of PTSD in male veterans (Koenen et al., 2005b).

EPIDEMIOLOGY OF PTSD IN MILITARY AND VETERAN POPULATIONS

This section first describes the change in demographic profile and different stressors and trauma faced by members of the military since the Vietnam War. The epidemiology of PTSD in active duty, National Guard, and reserve military populations and in veteran populations is then presented. Finally, some special considerations of PTSD in the military and veteran populations and their implications for screening, diagnosis, and treatment are highlighted.

Military-Related Stressors and Trauma

The current military population and veterans of Operation Enduring Freedom (OEF) and Operation Iraqi Freedom (OIF) differ from military personnel and veterans of other eras, such as those of the Vietnam War and the 1990–1991 Gulf War. One of the largest differences between the military in the Vietnam War and in OEF and OIF is selection into military service. Roughly one-third of Vietnam service members were drafted, whereas the military in OEF and OIF is all volunteer. Demographics of the military (and therefore veteran) population have also changed since the Vietnam War. The female-to-male ratio has increased; only 0.2% of service members in Vietnam were women compared with 12.7% of the deployed force in OEF and OIF (Maguen et al., 2010). Currently, 15.5% of all military personnel and nearly one-fourth of Army reserves are women (DoD, 2010). The racial and ethnic composition of the military has also evolved since the 1960s: 87% of military personnel in Vietnam were non-Hispanic white compared with 75% of current personnel (DoD, 2008).

Stressors and traumatic events have likewise shifted over time. As chronicled in detail in the Institute of Medicine *Gulf War and Health* series, stressors experienced by 1990–1991 Gulf War combat troops included uncertainty about possible exposures to chemical and biologic weapons, environmental exposures (such as to oil-well fire smoke and petroleum-based combustion products), incomplete knowledge of enemy troops, the harsh desert climate, separation from family, and crowded and difficult living conditions (for example, lack of privacy, infrequent access to hot water and laundry facilities, and constant vigilance for scorpions and snakes) (IOM, 2008a, 2010). OEF and OIF are occurring in a similar geographic location, and service members are subject to many of the same stressors. However, one of the largest differences between the current conflicts and prior engagement in the Middle East is the increasing number of insurgent attacks in the form of suicide bombs and car bombs, improvised explosive devices, sniper fire, and rocket-propelled grenades. Attacks are difficult to predict, often occurring in civilian areas where identification of enemy combatants is extremely challenging. As such, service members face increased risks of being wounded and killed and consequent exacerbation of the psychologic stressors that they experience. In contrast with the 1990–1991 Gulf War, where most military personnel were deployed for 9 months or less, troops deployed in OEF and OIF are subject to longer and repeated deployments with shorter rest and recovery times between deployments (MacGregor et al., 2012; Wieland et al., 2010). A recent study that examined the association between dwell time—the time between the end of one deployment and the start of the next—and diagnosed mental health disorders in more than 65,000 marines deployed to OIF found that those with two deployments had significantly higher rates of PTSD only, PTSD with another mental health disorder, and other mental health disorders than marines deployed only once. Further, longer dwell time—at least two times longer than the period of deployment—was associated with significantly reduced odds of PTSD (MacGregor et al., 2012). With the conflict in Iraq having ended and the conflict in Afghanistan expected to wind down, more service members will be returning home; as a result, the number seeking treatment for psychologic issues is expected to increase.

In addition to the many stressors encountered by service members while serving in the military, there are protective factors specific to military service that should not be overlooked. Unit cohesion, the close bond and culture of interdependence developed among groups of service members (Tanielian and Jaycox, 2008), has been cited as one of the most important factors for preventing mental problems (Helmus and Glenn, 2004). See Chapter 5 for more discussion on risk and protective factors.

Epidemiologic Studies of Military and Veteran Populations

Estimates of lifetime PTSD prevalence in service members deployed to OEF and OIF are two to three times those in the general population. Estimates of current prevalence of PTSD in OEF and OIF service members range from 13% to 20% (Hoge et al., 2004; Seal et al., 2007; Tanielian and Jaycox, 2008; Vasterling et al., 2010). In a survey of 18,305 Army veterans who had returned from Iraq or Afghanistan, Thomas et al. (2010) found the PTSD prevalence at 3 months after deployment to be 7.7% in the active component and 6.7% in National Guard members and at 12 months to be 8.9% and 12.4%, respectively, on the basis of a strict definition of PTSD with serious functional impairment. Results of the NVVRS, conducted in 1988 with a representative sample of 1,200 veterans, found that 30.9% of men who served in Vietnam had developed PTSD at some point and 15.2% were currently living with it (Kulka, 1990). A reanalysis of the NVVRS by Dohrenwend et al. (2006) found reduced rates: an estimated lifetime PTSD prevalence of 18.7% and a current prevalence (when the survey was originally conducted) of 9.1%. Despite the difference, the prevalence of PTSD in the veteran population is still several times higher than that observed in the general population.

A study of 103,788 returning OEF and OIF veterans seen in VA health care facilities during September 2001–December 2005 showed that nearly one-third of them received at least one mental health or psychosocial diagnosis, and 13% of them had a diagnosis of PTSD (Seal et al., 2007). It is estimated that 23% to 40% of service members and veterans in need of mental health services receive care (Hoge et al., 2004); therefore, estimates of mental health burden based on service records probably underestimate the burden in these populations.

Combat Stress Severity

Known risk factors for PTSD specific to military populations include experiencing combat, high combat severity, being wounded or injured, witnessing death (especially grotesque death), serving on graves registration duty or handling remains, being taken captive or tortured, experiencing unpredictable and uncontrollable stressful exposure, experiencing sexual harassment or assault, combat preparedness, and deployment to a war zone without combat (IOM, 2007). In the NCS, 38% of men who had experienced combat-related trauma had PTSD (Kessler et al., 1995). A positive dose–response relationship between severity of combat stressor exposure and clinically diagnosed PTSD was found in the NVVRS (see Figure 2-1). In addition to experiencing combat-related traumas, having experienced sexual assault while in the military is also of concern, especially in women. In the nationally representative VA Women's Health Project, 55% of the female veterans in ambulatory care reported being sexually harassed, and 23% reported being sexually assaulted while they were in the military (Skinner et al., 2000).

Many studies assessing PTSD onset and duration in service members have used the 1990–1991 Gulf War veteran population because that war was the first large U.S. military engagement undertaken after PTSD was officially recognized as a psychologic disorder in 1980. During the 9-month conflict, about 697,000 U.S. military personnel were deployed to the Persian Gulf. In a large survey of Gulf War deployed veterans compared with era veterans from all services, 12.1% of those deployed had a diagnosis of PTSD compared with 4.3% of era veterans, and the risk of PTSD increased as a function of stress severity. Of those who had experienced minimal stress (were activated but not deployed or not activated reservists), 3.3%

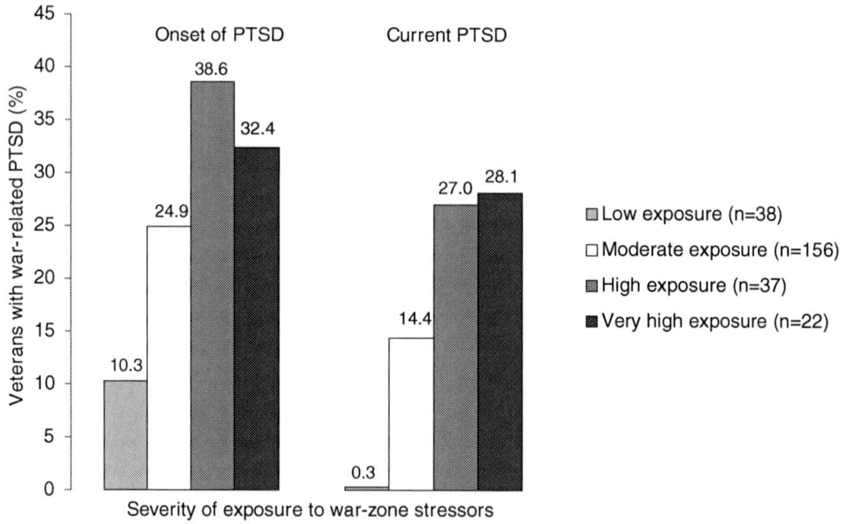

FIGURE 2-1 Dose–response relationship of combat severity and clinically diagnosed PTSD.
SOURCE: Dohrenwend et al., 2006; reprinted with permission from AAAS.

had a diagnosis of PTSD, whereas 22.6% of those who were classified as having experienced high stress (having worn chemical protective gear, been involved in combat, or witnessed death) received the diagnosis (Kang et al., 2003). In the same sample population 10 years after the war, 6.2% of deployed veterans and 1.1% of nondeployed veterans had received a diagnosis of service-related PTSD (Toomey et al., 2007).

Sex

Although women are prohibited from serving in direct ground combat, they are subject to combat exposure while deployed. Of 329,049 OEF and OIF veterans who received care at a VA health care facility, females were significantly less likely than their male counterparts to receive a diagnosis of PTSD (17% vs. 22%, respectively) but significantly more likely to receive a diagnosis of depression (23% vs. 17%, respectively) (Maguen et al., 2010). Although Vogt et al. (2011) found that men were significantly more likely to report combat-related stressors (such as combat exposure, aftermath of battle, and difficult living environment), no sex differences were found in combat-associated stressors for predicting posttraumatic stress symptoms. In a sample of National Guard service members 1 month before deployment, no differences between males and females were found in posttraumatic stress symptoms (mean scores on the PTSD Checklist—Civilian version were 26.0 and 27.4, respectively) although females were significantly more likely to screen positive for depression symptoms (mean scores on the Beck Depression Inventory-II were 5.6 for men and 9.5 for women) (Carter-Visscher et al., 2010). Similarly, in a study of OEF and OIF veterans seen in VA health care facilities from 2001 through 2005, women and men were equally likely to receive at least one mental health diagnosis (26% and 25%, respectively), but men were significantly more likely to receive a diagnosis of PTSD (risk ratio 1.14, 95% CI 1.08–1.10) (Seal et al., 2007). However, in a prospective study that used a deployed and nondeployed Millennium Cohort sample, new onset of self-reported PTSD symptoms was proportionally higher in women than in men overall (3.8% and 2.4%, respectively) and significantly higher after stratification by service branch, except for the marines (Smith et al., 2008).

Age

Unlike the civilian population, in which 16.7% of people are 18–29 years old (Howden and Meyer, 2011), more than 60% of active-duty service members are 30 years old or younger (DoD, 2008). In a study of mental health diagnoses in OEF and OIF veterans seen in VA health care facilities in 2001–2005, veterans 18–24 years old had the highest risk of receiving a diagnosis of PTSD, followed by the 30–39-year age group and the 25–29-year age group, compared with veterans 40 years and older (Seal et al., 2007).

Sexual Assault

Sexual assault is a leading risk factor for PTSD (Kessler et al., 1995). Prevalence estimates vary by method of assessment, sample type (clinical, research, or benefit-seeking), and definition used (Suris and Lind, 2008). Military sexual trauma (MST) is a term used specifically in the VA and is defined as "sexual harassment that is threatening in character or physical assault of a sexual nature that occurred while the victim was in the military, regardless of geographic location of the trauma, gender of the victim, or the relationship to the perpetrator" (VA, 2012). MST surveillance data collected by the VA on nearly 1.7 million veterans showed that about 22% of women and 1% of men experienced MST. However, it has been estimated that about 54% of all VA users that screen positive for MST are men (Suris and Lind, 2008). Other convenience and small-sample studies of experiencing rape and sexual assault during military service have estimated the prevalence in women to range from 23% to 41% (Coyle et al., 1996; Frayne et al., 1999; Sadler et al., 2000). In a small study of female veterans that compared MST with other types of trauma, 60% of those who reported MST had received a diagnosis of PTSD compared with 43% of those who experienced other traumas (with or without MST) (Yaeger et al., 2006). In a follow-up analysis, MST was compared with nonmilitary sexual trauma for predicting PTSD. Although sexual trauma is significantly associated with PTSD, MST was more likely to result in PTSD than sexual assault occurring outside of military service (Himmelfarb et al., 2006). In a small convenience sample of female veterans, Suris et al. (2004) found that women who had a history of sexual assault were nine times more likely to have PTSD than women who did not experience sexual assault. In a large sample of deployed OEF and OIF veterans who separated from the military by October 2006 and later used VA health care services, 15.1% of females and 0.7% of males screened positive for MST. Women who screened positive for MST were 3.8 times more likely than women who did not report MST to receive a diagnosis of PTSD. Men who screened positive for MST were 2.5 times more likely than men who did not to receive a diagnosis of PTSD (Kimerling et al., 2010).

Race

In a large sample of OEF and OIF veterans seen at VA health care facilities over a 4-year period, Seal et al. (2007) found that blacks were more likely to receive a diagnosis of PTSD than other racial or ethnic groups. In a subsample of the NVVRS, Dohrenwend et al. (2008) examined racial differences in current (chronic) PTSD attributed to service in the military. Black veterans' high prevalence of PTSD was explained by their greater exposure to war-zone stressors, and Hispanic veterans' higher prevalence of current PTSD was explained by several factors, including younger age at deployment to Vietnam, lower education, and lower Armed Forces Qualification Test (AFQT) scores. A subsample of the NVVRS found that the higher prevalence of chronic PTSD in Hispanic veterans persists after adjustment for exposure to war-zone stressors. Levels of impairment due to current PTSD in those Hispanic veterans were not statistically different from those in other racial groups; this suggests that cultural factors of "greater expressiveness" cannot explain the higher prevalence of PTSD in this population (Lewis-Fernandez et al., 2008).

IQ

As lower IQ scores have been associated with increased risk of developing PTSD in the civilian population, so are lower scores on the AFQT associated with increased risk of PTSD. Some researchers have argued that low IQ and other cognitive deficits may be sequelae of PTSD (De Bellis, 2001), but prospective studies of military samples that have used measures of cognitive ability from military records (for example, the AFQT) show that premilitary IQ is inversely associated with risk of combat-related PTSD (Kremen et al., 2007; Macklin et al., 1998; Pitman et al., 1991). In a study of veterans exposed to potentially traumatic events recruited from the Vietnam Era Twin Registry after controlling for confounders, persons who had the highest AFQT scores (76–99 and 56–75) had significantly less risk of PTSD than persons who had the lowest category of AFQT scores (0–33) (Kremen et al., 2007). In a large-scale prospective study of a military sample, Gale et al. (2008) replicated the link between low IQ and PTSD but found a stronger link between low IQ and PTSD with comorbidities, including generalized anxiety disorder and substance abuse or dependence. Those results suggest that the severity of the psychiatric disorder may play a role in the IQ–PTSD link.

Psychopathology

Premilitary psychopathology is also a risk factor for PTSD in military populations. Data from the NVVRS (Kulka, 1990) and the Vietnam Era Twin Registry suggest that negative juvenile conduct increases the risk of both level of combat and PTSD (Fu et al., 2007; Koenen et al., 2002, 2005a). Those results are similar to those of prospective civilian studies that found that externalizing behavior problems in childhood increase the risk of PTSD in adulthood (Gregory et al., 2007; Koenen et al., 2007). The findings are further supported by a meta-analysis of seven military or veteran population studies that associated adverse childhood risk factors with PTSD (Brewin et al., 2000b).

Koenen et al. (2002) examined familial and individual risk factors and their associations with exposure to trauma and PTSD in a cohort of Vietnam era twins. Although a family history of mood disorders was associated with increased risk of exposure to traumatic events, people who had a pre-existing mood disorder were less likely to be exposed to traumatic events. Family history of paternal depression and pre-existing psychologic disorders (conduct disorder, panic or generalized anxiety disorder, and major depression) were all associated with an increased risk of PTSD. Those findings suggest that the association of family psychiatric history and PTSD may be mediated by individual-level risks of traumatic exposure and pre-existing psychologic disorders (Koenen et al., 2002).

Genetics

Several studies of Vietnam Era Twin Registry data have also shown associations between familial risk factors and PTSD. In one study that examined genetic and environment effects on conduct disorder, major depression, and PTSD, Fu et al. (2007) found that the three outcomes correlated strongly. Those who had a history of conduct disorder or major depression were more likely to have a lifetime diagnosis of PTSD than those who did not have such a history. Although there was no genetic covariance between conduct disorder and PTSD, common genetic influences alone could be attributed to the association between major depression and PTSD. Koenen et al. (2008a) examined the genetic and individual-specific environmental correlation between comorbid major depression and PTSD in Vietnam veterans. Environmental influences did not explain much of the comorbid correlation, but shared genetic factors explained 62.5% of comorbid major depression and PTSD. Furthermore, genetic influences common to major depression explained 58% of the genetic variation in PTSD; this suggests that genes associated with one of these disorders are good candidates for studies of the other disorder. In a related study of genetic and environmental associations of internalizing and externalizing dimensions of psychiatric comorbidity in Vietnam veteran twins, specifically PTSD, Wolf et al. (2010) found that shared genetic factors explained a significant proportion of variance for both internalizing and externalizing comorbidity. Although the authors found greater genetic association with the internalizing spectrum and only modest genetic association with the externalizing factors and PTSD, commonly shared or experienced factors (including immediate family environment and socioeconomic status) may influence the externalizing psychopathology, which may then influence the expression of psychiatric conditions, such as PTSD.

Comorbidities of PTSD

Comorbid conditions—including depressive symptoms, alcohol use, and other high-risk behaviors—are present in more than 50% of OEF and OIF veterans who have PTSD (Hoge et al., 2004; Santiago et al., 2010). Recent estimates of PTSD and substance use disorders in military populations have varied. In a study of 151 Iraq and Afghanistan veterans who were seeking primary care, 39.1% screened positive for PTSD only and 15.9% screened positive for alcohol problems and PTSD, and PTSD symptoms and severity of alcohol problems correlated significantly (McDevitt-Murphy et al., 2010). Using a VA medical database of OEF and OIF veterans enrolled in VA services from 2001 to 2006, Stecker et al. (2010) found that 12.0% had a PTSD-only diagnosis and 4.2% had a diagnosis of PTSD and alcohol misuse. The authors suggest that the rate probably underreported substance use disorders greatly.

Several studies of combat experience in the Vietnam War have also found higher proportions of suicide ideation, attempts, and completions among those who have PTSD (Farberow et al., 1990; Fontana and Rosenheck, 1995; Hendin and Haas, 1991; Kramer et al., 1994). Those findings are of particular importance in light of the large numbers of service members that have served in OEF and OIF and have had a diagnosis of PTSD; the number of suicides among active-duty and reserve service members has continued to rise since the beginning of the conflicts. A study that examined PTSD as a risk factor for suicidal ideation among 407 OEF and OIF veterans who were referred to the VA health care system for mental health services found that veterans who screened positive for PTSD were about 4.5 times more likely to report suicidal ideation than veterans who did not have PTSD (Jakupcak et al., 2009). Furthermore, among the 202 veterans that screened positive for PTSD, those who also screened positive for two or more comorbid disorders were 5.7 times more likely to report suicidal ideation that those who had fewer comorbidities (Jakupcak et al., 2009). Beginning in 2003, DoD Mental Health Advisory Teams have been conducting mental health surveillance for service members in Iraq and Afghanistan combat environments. Although the most recent report shows the percentage of positive responses to a question about suicide ideation among Army and Marine Corps personnel is unchanged from previous survey results, there have been significant increases in the adjusted percentage of those who report acute stress (MHAT VII, 2011).

Special Considerations

Many unique concerns surround the diagnosis of and treatment for PTSD in the military, particularly service members and veterans who have served in OEF and OIF. Some of the concerns pertain to time in the theater of war and the traumatic events that service members experience there, such as traumatic brain injury, physical wounds, experience of firefights, and the deaths of close companions. The effects of those will be discussed further in Chapter 8. Societal and cultural influences (Lewis-Fernandez et al., 2010) and premorbid factors peculiar to military populations also affect diagnosis and treatment course. Chapter 9 elaborates on the particular barriers to PTSD care in military populations, and Chapter 8 discusses the challenges to rehabilitation that result from the comorbidity of PTSD with other psychiatric illnesses in military populations. The present section addresses issues that are of concern to members of the military who have PTSD.

Underrecognized and Underreported

The true prevalence of PTSD in military populations is probably higher than the available estimates. Generally, prevalence estimates for PTSD in the populations have ranged from 13% to 20% (Hoge et al., 2004; Seal et al., 2007; Tanielian and Jaycox, 2008; Vasterling et al., 2010). However, those may be underestimates of the prevalence of PTSD in the military and veteran populations. The fear of negative consequences for a military career, including decreased potential for promotion and perceived stigma by peers and leaders (Hoge et al., 2004), may lead to underreporting of PTSD symptoms.

Despite rigorous screening efforts by the DoD, underreporting of symptoms may be common. In one study by Warner et al. (2011), a brigade of Army soldiers first completed the post-deployment health assessment (PDHA) on returning from Iraq, and a subsample completed an anonymous survey that consisted of the same mental health questions as were on the PDHA. The number of positive responses to the mental health questions overall and to the PTSD-specific questions more than doubled, and in some cases quadrupled, in the anonymous survey (7.7% screened positive) compared with the PDHA (3.3% screened positive); of those who screened positive for either PTSD or depression on the anonymous survey, 20.3% reported that they were not comfortable in reporting their answers honestly on the PDHA. Those results indicate a high level of underreporting of mental health symptoms, which may have negative implications for the health and readiness of the armed forces.

The positive-screen group from the Warner et al. (2011) study also indicated they were less likely to seek treatment for these issues (one-third believing that it would harm their careers) than the group that screened negative for PTSD or depression. Kim et al. (2010) found that active-duty service members who had been deployed were less likely to use mental health services for any reported mental health problems and were more conscious of a stigma associated with seeking care than National Guard members who had been deployed. This underutilization of treatment is another barrier to the effective treatment of PTSD (see Chapters 6 and 9 for additional discussion).

A diagnosis of PTSD may be more likely in a particular military population. For example, in a sample of combat-injured and non–combat-injured service members in OIF, those who had more serious injuries and those whose injuries were related to combat were more likely to have a diagnosis of PTSD than were service members who had less serious injuries and injuries that were not combat related (MacGregor et al., 2009). Thus, although the DoD and the VA mandate population screening for PTSD, its prevalence is probably underreported.

Nomenclature

One source of PTSD-associated stigma in the military may be the name itself (Nash et al., 2009). General Peter Chiarelli, the Army vice chief of staff and second-highest ranking Army officer, stated that the word *disorder* itself is problematic and carries a stigma that has discouraged many soldiers from seeking treatment (Sagalyn, 2011). General Chiarelli has proposed a change to "posttraumatic stress injury" to encourage afflicted soldiers and their commanders to support the importance of diagnosis and treatment. Veterans' service organizations have concurred in the name change. One reason that *disorder* was kept as part of the name of this condition when it was first included in the *DSM-III* was to legitimatize the pain and suffering of Vietnam War veterans (Sagalyn, 2011). However, there are several arguments against the name change, such as PTSD afflicts many persons, not only service members; removing *disorder* could confuse normal and abnormal (in need of treatment) responses to stress; and the belief that PTSD will be stigmatized no matter what it is called. Despite the controversy, there is no plan to change the name when the next version of the *DSM* is released.

Healthy Warrior Effect

The "healthy worker effect" suggests that employed persons generally have lower rates of serious illnesses, disabilities, and deaths than the general population because their better health status allows them to gain employment and remain employed. The "healthy warrior effect" is an extension of this concept (Arrighi and Hertzpicciotto, 1994). People who have poor physical health are unlikely to join the armed forces or to complete basic training, and the same should be true of people who have poor mental health. If such people are not medically discharged early in their military careers, they may be excluded from some deployments (Wilson et al., 2009).

Subthreshold PTSD

As discussed earlier in this chapter, *DSM-IV* lists 17 symptoms of PTSD, at least 6 of which are required—in the correct distribution (one re-experiencing, three numbing or avoidance, and two hyperarousal)—for a diagnosis of PTSD. However, several studies have indicated that even subthreshold PTSD is impairing and that people who have it may benefit from treatment (Grubaugh et al., 2005; Marshall et al., 2001; Stein et al., 1997; Zlotnick et al., 2002). If the purpose of diagnosing PTSD and treating it is to regain and maintain functioning, then it is clear that any symptoms that are potentially attributable to prior trauma and are accompanied by functional impairment warrant treatment. Subthreshold PTSD may also be a signal of other pathologic conditions, such as depression or an additional anxiety disorder, in that there is overlap in the defining symptoms of these conditions. Subthreshold symptoms have potential implications for screening, level of functioning, degree of distress, and treatment. A full discussion of the implications of subthreshold PTSD is beyond the scope of this report, but it merits mention as a subject of further inquiry.

Compensation Issues and Secondary Gain

PTSD in military and veteran populations is complicated by concerns about malingering and attempts to receive the diagnosis for secondary gain. This issue has become particularly important in military populations inasmuch as its presence is formally recognized as making someone eligible for DoD and VA benefits. Thus, a diagnosis of PTSD is problematic in both active-duty and veteran populations, and can lead to underreporting (for example, to remain in one's position) or to overreporting (for example, to gain benefits or to be excused from duty). A previous Institute of Medicine report on PTSD compensation and military service (IOM, 2007) noted that, apart from problems with the current procedures for assigning a disability rating to PTSD, other considerations include "barriers or disincentives to recovery, the effect of disability compensation on recovery, and the advisability of periodic re-examination of PTSD compensation beneficiaries." Although that committee found that compensation does not appear to serve as a disincentive to seeking treatment, periodic re-examinations for veterans who have a PTSD service-connected disability were regarded as inappropriate because research on misreporting and exaggeration of symptoms had not found evidence supporting a singling out of PTSD (IOM, 2007). This is an important and complicated issue, and the present committee will reconsider it if any new literature becomes available during phase 2.

SUMMARY

PTSD is prevalent in the general population in which it has a lifetime prevalence of about 8% in adults, but military and veteran populations are exposed to many more traumatic events than the general population, and service members who have served in OEF and OIF have a lifetime PTSD prevalence of 13% to 20%. Many factors increase a service member's risk of PTSD, some demographic—such as age; sex; prior exposure to trauma, particularly sexual assault and childhood maltreatment; lower education attainment; and lower IQ—and some combat-specific—such as killing someone, seeing someone killed, and being in an explosion or being badly injured. PTSD is often comorbid with other psychologic or medical conditions, such as depression, substance use (particularly alcohol use) disorder, and traumatic brain injury. Special considerations in the diagnosis of and treatment for PTSD in military and veteran populations include subthreshold PTSD, underreporting and overreporting of PTSD symptoms, the role of stigma in seeking care for PTSD, the healthy warrior effect, and compensation. The next chapter provides a discussion of the biologic basis of and factors that affect the development of PTSD.

REFERENCES

APA (American Psychiatric Association). 1980. *DSM-III: Diagnostic and statistical manual of mental disorders*. 3rd ed. Washington, DC: American Psychiatric Association.

APA. 2000. *Diagnostic and statistical manual of mental disorders, fourth edition, text revision (DSM-IV-TR)*. Washington, DC: American Psychiatric Association.

Arrighi, H. M., and I. Hertzpicciotto. 1994. The evolving concept of the healthy worker survivor effect. *Epidemiology* 5(2):189-196.

Barnett, J. H., C. H. Salmond, P. B. Jones, and B. J. Sahakian. 2006. Cognitive reserve in neuropsychiatry. *Psychological Medicine* 36(8):1053-1064.

Basile, K. C., I. Arias, S. Desai, and M. P. Thompson. 2004. The differential association of intimate partner physical, sexual, psychological, and stalking violence and posttraumatic stress symptoms in a nationally representative sample of women. *Journal of Traumatic Stress* 17(5):413-421.

Batty, G. D., E. L. Mortensen, and M. Osler. 2005. Childhood IQ in relation to later psychiatric disorder: Evidence from a Danish birth cohort study. *British Journal of Psychiatry* 187:180-181.

Birmes, P., L. Hatton, A. Brunet, and L. Schmitt. 2003. Early historical literature for posttraumatic symptomatology. *Stress and Health* 19(1):17-26.

Boscarino, J. A. 2008. A prospective study of PTSD and early-age heart disease mortality among Vietnam veterans: Implications for surveillance and prevention. *Psychosomatic Medicine* 70(6):668-676.

Breslau, N., and E. L. Peterson. 2010. Assaultive violence and the risk of posttraumatic stress disorder following a subsequent trauma. *Behaviour Research and Therapy* 48(10): 1063-1066.

Breslau, N., G. C. Davis, P. Andreski, and E. Peterson. 1991. Traumatic events and posttraumatic stress disorder in an urban population of young adults. *Archives of General Psychiatry* 48(3):216-222.

Breslau, N., G. C. Davis, and P. Andreski. 1995. Risk factors for PTSD-related traumatic events: A prospective analysis. *American Journal of Psychiatry* 152(4):529-535.

Breslau, N., R. C. Kessler, H. D. Chilcoat, L. R. Schultz, G. C. Davis, and P. Andreski. 1998. Trauma and posttraumatic stress disorder in the community—the 1996 Detroit area survey of trauma. *Archives of General Psychiatry* 55(7):626-632.

Breslau, N., G. C. Davis, and L. R. Schultz. 2003. Posttraumatic stress disorder and the incidence of nicotine, alcohol, and other drug disorders in persons who have experienced trauma. *Archives of General Psychiatry* 60(3):289-294.

Breslau, N., S. P. Novak, and R. C. Kessler. 2004. Daily smoking and the subsequent onset of psychiatric disorders. *Psychological Medicine* 34(2):323-333.

Breslau, N., V. C. Lucia, and G. F. Alvarado. 2006. Intelligence and other predisposing factors in exposure to trauma and posttraumatic stress disorder: A follow-up study at age 17 years. *Archives of General Psychiatry* 63(11):1238-1245.

Breslau, N., E. L. Peterson, and L. R. Schultz. 2008. A second look at prior trauma and the posttraumatic stress disorder effects of subsequent trauma. *Archives of General Psychiatry* 65(4):431-437.

Brewin, C. R., B. Andrews, and S. Rose. 2000a. Fear, helplessness, and horror in posttraumatic stress disorder: Investigating DSM-IV criterion A2 in victims of violent crime. *Journal of Traumatic Stress* 13(3):499-509.

Brewin, C. R., B. Andrews, and J. D. Valentine. 2000b. Meta-analysis of risk factors for posttraumatic stress disorder in trauma-exposed adults. *Journal of Consulting and Clinical Psychology* 68(5):748-766.

Bromet, E., A. Sonnega, and R. C. Kessler. 1998. Risk factors for DSM-III-R posttraumatic stress disorder: Findings from the national comorbidity survey. *American Journal of Epidemiology* 147(4):353-361.

Brown, P. J., and J. Wolfe. 1994. Substance abuse and post-traumatic stress disorder comorbidity. *Drug & Alcohol Dependence* 35(1):51-59.

Carter-Visscher, R., M. A. Polusny, M. Murdoch, P. Thuras, C. R. Erbes, and S. M. Kehle. 2010. Predeployment gender differences in stressors and mental health among U.S. National Guard troops poised for Operation Iraqi Freedom deployment. *Journal of Traumatic Stress* 23(1):78-85.

Chantarujikapong, S. I., J. F. Scherrer, H. Xian, S. A. Eisen, M. J. Lyons, J. Goldberg, M. Tsuang, and W. R. True. 2001. A twin study of generalized anxiety disorder symptoms, panic disorder symptoms and post-traumatic stress disorder in men. *Psychiatry Research* 103:133-145.

Chilcoat, H. D., and N. Breslau. 1998. Investigations of causal pathways between PTSD and drug use disorders. *Addictive Behaviors* 23(6):827-840.

Cohen, B. E., C. Marmar, L. Ren, D. Bertenthal, and K. H. Seal. 2009. Association of cardiovascular risk factors with mental health diagnoses in Iraq and Afghanistan war veterans using VA health care. *Journal of the American Medical Association* 302(5):489-492.

Cohen, B. E., P. Panguluri, B. Na, and M. A. Whooley. 2010. Psychological risk factors and the metabolic syndrome in patients with coronary heart disease: Findings from the heart and soul study. *Psychiatry Research* 175(1-2):133-137.

Coyle, B. S., D. L. Wolan, and A. S. Van Horn. 1996. The prevalence of physical and sexual abuse in women veterans seeking care at a Veterans Affairs medical center. *Military Medicine* 161(10):588-593.

De Bellis, M. D. 2001. Developmental traumatology: The psychobiological development of maltreated children and its implications for research, treatment, and policy. *Development and Psychopathology* 13:539-564.

Desai, S., I. Arias, M. P. Thompson, and K. C. Basile. 2002. Childhood victimization and subsequent adult revictimization assessed in a nationally representative sample of women and men. *Violence & Victims* 17(6):639-653.

Dirkzwager, A. J., P. G. van der Velden, L. Grievink, and C. J. Yzermans. 2007. Disaster-related posttraumatic stress disorder and physical health. *Psychosomatic Medicine* 69(5):435-440.

Dobie, D. J., D. R. Kivlahan, C. Maynard, K. R. Bush, T. M. Davis, and K. A. Bradley. 2004. Posttraumatic stress disorder in female veterans: Association with self-reported health problems and functional impairment. *Archives of Internal Medicine* 164(4):394-400.

DoD (Department of Defense). 2008. *Active duty demographic profile: Assigned strength, gender, race, marital, education and age profile of active duty force.* Defense Manpower Data Center.

DoD. 2010. *Demographics 2010: Profile of the military community.* Washington, DC: Office of the Deputy Under Secretary of Defense.

Dohrenwend, B. P., J. B. Turner, N. A. Turse, B. G. Adams, K. C. Koenen, and R. Marshall. 2006. The psychological risks of Vietnam for U.S. veterans: A revisit with new data and methods. *Science* 313(5789):979-982.

Dohrenwend, B. P., J. B. Turner, N. A. Turse, R. Lewis-Fernandez, and T. J. Yager. 2008. War-related posttraumatic stress disorder in black, Hispanic, and majority white Vietnam veterans: The roles of exposure and vulnerability. *Journal of Traumatic Stress* 21(2):133-141.

Dong, M., W. H. Giles, V. J. Felitti, S. R. Dube, J. E. Williams, D. P. Chapman, and R. F. Anda. 2004. Insights into causal pathways for ischemic heart disease: Adverse childhood experiences study. *Circulation* 110(13):1761-1766.

Farberow, N. L., H. K. Kang, and T. A. Bullman. 1990. Combat experience and postservice psychosocial status as predictors of suicide in Vietnam veterans. *Journal of Nervous & Mental Disease* 178(1):32-37.

Fontana, A., and R. Rosenheck. 1995. Attempted suicide among Vietnam veterans: A model of etiology in a community sample. *American Journal of Psychiatry* 152(1):102-109.

Frayne, S. M., K. M. Skinner, L. M. Sullivan, T. J. Tripp, C. S. Hankin, N. R. Kressin, and D. R. Miller. 1999. Medical profile of women Veterans Administration outpatients who report a history of sexual assault occurring while in the military. *Journal of Women's Health & Gender-Based Medicine* 8(6):835-845.

Friedman, M., P. A. Resick, R. A. Bryant, and C. R. Brewin. 2010. Considering PTSD for DSM-5. *Depression and Anxiety* 1(20).

Fu, Q., K. C. Koenen, M. W. Miller, A. C. Heath, K. K. Bucholz, M. J. Lyons, S. A. Eisen, W. R. True, J. Goldberg, and M. T. Tsuang. 2007. Differential etiology of posttraumatic stress disorder with conduct disorder and major depression in male veterans. *Biological Psychiatry* 62(10):1088-1094.

Gale, C. R., I. J. Deary, S. H. Boyle, J. Barefoot, L. H. Mortensen, and G. D. Batty. 2008. Cognitive ability in early adulthood and risk of 5 specific psychiatric disorders in middle age: The Vietnam experience study. *Archives of General Psychiatry* 65(12):1410-1418.

Galea, S., and H. Resnick. 2005. Posttraumatic stress disorder in the general population after mass terrorist incidents: Considerations about the nature of exposure. *CNS Spectrums* 10(2):107-115.

Galea, S., D. Vlahov, H. Resnick, J. Ahern, E. Susser, J. Gold, M. Bucuvalas, and D. Kilpatrick. 2003. Trends of probable post-traumatic stress disorder in New York City after the September 11 terrorist attacks. *American Journal of Epidemiology* 158(6):514-524.

Galea, S., D. Vlahov, M. Tracy, D. R. Hoover, H. Resnick, and D. Kilpatrick. 2004. Hispanic ethnicity and post-traumatic stress disorder after a disaster: Evidence from a general population survey after September 11, 2001. *Annals of Epidemiology* 14(8):520-531.

Galea, S., J. Ahern, M. Tracy, A. Hubbard, M. Cerda, E. Goldmann, and D. Vlahov. 2008. Longitudinal determinants of posttraumatic stress in a population-based cohort study. *Epidemiology* 19(1):47-54.

Gregory, A. M., A. Caspi, T. E. Moffitt, K. Koenen, T. C. Eley, and R. Poulton. 2007. Juvenile mental health histories of adults with anxiety disorders. *American Journal of Psychiatry* 164(2):301-308.

Grubaugh, A. L., K. M. Magruder, A. E. Waldrop, J. D. Elhai, R. G. Knapp, and B. C. Frueh. 2005. Subthreshold PTSD in primary care: Prevalence, psychiatric disorders, healthcare use, and functional status. *Journal of Nervous & Mental Disease* 193(10):658-664.

Harrison, C. A., and S. A. Kinner. 1998. Correlates of psychological distress following armed robbery. *Journal of Traumatic Stress* 11(4):787-798.

Harvard Medical School. 2007a. *12-month prevalence of DSM-IV/WMH-CIDI disorders by sex and cohort (n=9282).* http://www.hcp.med.harvard.edu/ncs/ftpdir/NCS-R_12-month_Prevalence_Estimates.pdf (accessed January 10, 2011).

Harvard Medical School. 2007b. *Lifetime prevalence DSM-IV/WMH-CIDI disorders by sex and cohort (n=9282).* http://www.hcp.med.harvard.edu/ncs/ftpdir/NCS-R_Lifetime_Prevalence_Estimates.pdf (accessed January 10, 2011).

Helmus, T. C., and R. W. Glenn. 2004. *Steeling the mind: Combat stress reactions and their implications for urban warfare.* Santa Monica, CA: RAND Corporation.

Hendin, H., and A. P. Haas. 1991. Suicide and guilt as manifestations of PTSD in Vietnam combat veterans. *American Journal of Psychiatry* 148(5):586-591.

Himmelfarb, N., D. Yaeger, and J. Mintz. 2006. Posttraumatic stress disorder in female veterans with military and civilian sexual trauma. *Journal of Traumatic Stress* 19(6):837-846.

Hoge, C. W., C. A. Castro, S. C. Messer, D. McGurk, D. I. Cotting, and R. L. Koffman. 2004. Combat duty in Iraq and Afghanistan, mental health problems, and barriers to care. *New England Journal of Medicine* 351(1):13-22.

Holbrook, T. L., D. B. Hoyt, M. B. Stein, and W. J. Sieber. 2001. Perceived threat to life predicts posttraumatic stress disorder after major trauma: Risk factors and functional outcome. *Journal of Trauma-Injury Infection & Critical Care* 51(2):287-292; discussion 292-283.

Howden, L. M., and J. A. Meyer. 2011. *Age and sex composition: 2010.* Washington, DC: U.S. Department of Commerce.

IOM (Institute of Medicine). 2007. *PTSD compensation and military service.* Washington, DC: The National Academies Press.

IOM. 2008a. *Gulf War and health: Physiologic, psychologic, and psychosocial effects of deployment-related stress.* Washington, DC: The National Academies Press.

IOM. 2008b. *Treatment of posttraumatic stress disorder: An assessment of the evidence.* Washington, DC: The National Academies Press.

IOM. 2010. *Gulf War and health: Update of health effects of serving in the Gulf War.* Washington, DC: The National Academies Press.

Jakupcak, M., J. Cook, Z. Imel, A. Fontana, R. Rosenheck, and M. McFall. 2009. Posttraumatic stress disorder as a risk factor for suicidal ideation in Iraq and Afghanistan war veterans. *Journal of Traumatic Stress* 22(4):303-306.

Jeavons, S., K. M. Greenwood, and D. J. Horne. 2000. Accident cognitions and subsequent psychological trauma. *Journal of Traumatic Stress* 13(2):359-365.

Jones, E. 2006. Historical approaches to post-combat disorders. *Philosophical Transactions of the Royal Society B: Biological Sciences* 361(1468):533-542.

Kang, H. K., B. H. Natelson, C. M. Mahan, K. Y. Lee, and F. M. Murphy. 2003. Posttraumatic stress disorder and chronic fatigue syndrome-like illness among Gulf War veterans: A population-based survey of 30,000 veterans. *American Journal of Epidemiology* 157(2):141-148.

Kessler, R. C., A. Sonnega, E. Bromet, M. Hughes, and C. B. Nelson. 1995. Posttraumatic stress disorder in the national comorbidity survey. *Archives of General Psychiatry* 52(12):1048-1060.

Kessler, R. C., P. Berglund, O. Demler, R. Jin, K. R. Merikangas, and E. E. Walters. 2005. Lifetime prevalence and age-of-onset distributions of *DSM-IV* disorders in the national comorbidity survey replication. *Archives of General Psychiatry* 62(6):593-602.

Khantzian, E. J. 1985. The self-medication hypothesis of addictive disorders: Focus on heroin and cocaine dependence. *American Journal of Psychiatry* 142(11):1259-1264.

Kim, P. Y., J. L. Thomas, J. E. Wilk, C. A. Castro, and C. W. Hoge. 2010. Stigma, barriers to care, and use of mental health services among active duty and National Guard soldiers after combat. *Psychiatric Services* 61:572-588.

Kimerling, R., A. E. Street, J. Pavao, M. W. Smith, R. C. Cronkite, T. H. Holmes, and S. M. Frayne. 2010. Military-related sexual trauma among Veterans Health Administration patients returning from Afghanistan and Iraq. *American Journal of Public Health* 100(8):1409-1412.

Koenen, K. C., R. Harley, M. J. Lyons, J. Wolfe, J. C. Simpson, J. Goldberg, S. A. Eisen, and M. Tsuang. 2002. A twin registry study of familial and individual risk factors for trauma exposure and posttraumatic stress disorder. *Journal of Nervous and Mental Disease* 190(4):209-218.

Koenen, K. C., Q. J. Fu, M. J. Lyons, R. Toomey, J. Goldberg, S. A. Eisen, W. True, and M. Tsuang. 2005a. Juvenile conduct disorder as a risk factor for trauma exposure and posttraumatic stress disorder. *Journal of Traumatic Stress* 18(1):23-32.

Koenen, K. C., B. Hitsman, M. J. Lyons, R. Niaura, J. McCaffery, J. Goldberg, S. A. Eisen, W. True, and M. Tsuang. 2005b. A twin registry study of the relationship between posttraumatic stress disorder and nicotine dependence in men. *Archives of General Psychiatry* 62(11):1258-1265.

Koenen, K. C., B. Hitsman, M. J. Lyons, L. Stroud, R. Niaura, J. McCaffery, J. Goldberg, S. A. Eisen, W. True, and M. Tsuang. 2006. Posttraumatic stress disorder and late-onset smoking in the Vietnam Era Twin Registry. *Journal of Consulting & Clinical Psychology* 74(1):186-190.

Koenen, K. C., T. E. Moffitt, R. Poulton, J. Martin, and A. Caspi. 2007. Early childhood factors associated with the development of post-traumatic stress disorder: Results from a longitudinal birth cohort. *Psychological Medicine* 37(2):181-192.

Koenen, K. C., Q. J. Fu, K. Ertel, M. J. Lyons, S. A. Eisen, W. R. True, J. Goldberg, and M. T. Tsuang. 2008a. Common genetic liability to major depression and posttraumatic stress disorder in men. *Journal of Affective Disorders* 105(1-3):109-115.

Koenen, K. C., T. E. Moffitt, A. Caspi, A. Gregory, H. Harrington, and R. Poulton. 2008b. The developmental mental-disorder histories of adults with posttraumatic stress disorder: A prospective longitudinal birth cohort study. *Journal of Abnormal Psychology* 117(2):460-466.

Kramer, T. L., J. D. Lindy, B. L. Green, M. C. Grace, and A. C. Leonard. 1994. The comorbidity of posttraumatic-stress-disorder and suicidality in Vietnam veterans. *Suicide and Life-Threatening Behavior* 24(1):58-67.

Kremen, W. S., K. C. Koenen, C. Boake, S. Purcell, S. A. Eisen, C. E. Franz, M. T. Tsuang, and M. J. Lyons. 2007. Pretrauma cognitive ability and risk for posttraumatic stress disorder: A twin study. *Archives of General Psychiatry* 64(3):361-368.

Kubzansky, L. D., K. C. Koenen, A. Spiro, 3rd, P. S. Vokonas, and D. Sparrow. 2007. Prospective study of posttraumatic stress disorder symptoms and coronary heart disease in the normative aging study. *Archives of General Psychiatry* 64(1):109-116.

Kubzansky, L. D., K. C. Koenen, C. Jones, and W. W. Eaton. 2009. A prospective study of posttraumatic stress disorder symptoms and coronary heart disease in women. *Health Psychology* 28(1):125-130.

Kulka, R. A. 1990. *Trauma and the Vietnam War generation: Report of findings from the National Vietnam Veterans Readjustment Study*. New York: Brunner/Mazel.

Lasser, K., J. W. Boyd, S. Woolhandler, D. U. Himmelstein, D. McCormick, and D. H. Bor. 2000. Smoking and mental illness: A population-based prevalence study. *Journal of the American Medical Association* 284(20):2606-2610.

Lewis-Fernandez, R., J. B. Turner, R. Marshall, N. Turse, Y. Neria, and B. P. Dohrenwend. 2008. Elevated rates of current PTSD among Hispanic veterans in the NVVRS: True prevalence or methodological artifact? *Journal of Traumatic Stress* 21(2):123-132.

Lewis-Fernandez, R., D. E. Hinton, A. J. Laria, E. H. Patterson, S. G. Hofmann, M. G. Craske, D. J. Stein, A. Asnaani, and B. Liao. 2010. Culture and the anxiety disorders: Recommendations for DSM-V. *Depression & Anxiety* 27(2):212-229.

MacGregor, A. J., R. A. Shaffer, A. L. Dougherty, M. R. Galarneau, R. Raman, D. G. Baker, S. P. Lindsay, B. A. Golomb, and K. S. Corson. 2009. Psychological correlates of battle and nonbattle injury among Operation Iraqi Freedom veterans. *Military Medicine* 174(3):224-231.

MacGregor, A. J., P. P. Han, A. L. Dougherty, and M. R. Galarneau. 2012. Effect of dwell time on the mental health of U.S. military personnel with multiple combat tours. *American Journal of Public Health* 102(Suppl 1):S55-S59.

Macklin, M. L., L. J. Metzger, B. T. Litz, R. J. McNally, N. B. Lasko, S. P. Orr, and R. K. Pitman. 1998. Lower precombat intelligence is a risk factor for posttraumatic stress disorder. *Journal of Consulting and Clinical Psychology* 66(2):323-326.

Maguen, S., L. Ren, J. O. Bosch, C. R. Marmar, and K. H. Seal. 2010. Gender differences in mental health diagnoses among Iraq and Afghanistan veterans enrolled in Veterans Affairs health care. *American Journal of Public Health* 100(12):2450-2456.

Marshall, G. N., T. L. Schell, and J. N. Miles. 2009. Ethnic differences in posttraumatic distress: Hispanics' symptoms differ in kind and degree. *Journal of Consulting and Clinical Psychology* 77(6):1169-1178.

Marshall, R. D., M. Olfson, F. Hellman, C. Blanco, M. Guardino, and E. L. Struening. 2001. Comorbidity, impairment, and suicidality in subthreshold PTSD. *American Journal of Psychiatry* 158(9):1467-1473.

McDevitt-Murphy, M. E., J. L. Williams, K. L. Bracken, J. A. Fields, C. J. Monahan, and J. G. Murphy. 2010. PTSD symptoms, hazardous drinking, and health functioning among U.S. OEF and OIF veterans presenting to primary care. *Journal of Traumatic Stress* 23(1):108-111.

MHAT VII (Mental Health Advisory Team VII). 2011. *Joint mental health advisory team 7 (J-MHAT 7) Operation Enduring Freedom 2010*. Washington, DC: Office of the Surgeon General, United States Army Medical Command, Office of the Command Surgeon HQ, USCENTCOM, Office of the Command Surgeon U.S. Forces Afghanistan.

Nash, W. P., C. Silva, and B. Litz. 2009. The historic origins of military and veteran mental health stigma and the stress injury model as a means to reduce it. *Psychiatric Annals* 39(8):789-794.

Neria, Y., R. Gross, B. Litz, S. Maguen, B. Insel, G. Seirmarco, H. Rosenfeld, E. J. Suh, R. Kishon, J. Cook, and R. D. Marshall. 2007. Prevalence and psychological correlates of complicated grief among bereaved adults 2.5-3.5 years after September 11th attacks. *Journal of Traumatic Stress* 20(3):251-262.

Norris, F. H. 1992. Epidemiology of trauma: Frequency and impact of different potentially traumatic events on different demographic groups. *Journal of Consulting & Clinical Psychology* 60(3):409-418.

Ozer, E. J., S. R. Best, T. L. Lipsey, and D. S. Weiss. 2003. Predictors of posttraumatic stress disorder and symptoms in adults: A meta-analysis. *Psychological Bulletin* 129(1):52-73.

Panasetis, P., and R. A. Bryant. 2003. Peritraumatic versus persistent dissociation in acute stress disorder. *Journal of Traumatic Stress* 16(6):563-566.

Pitman, R. K., S. P. Orr, M. J. Lowenhagen, M. L. Macklin, and B. Altman. 1991. Pre-Vietnam contents of posttraumatic stress disorder veterans' service medical and personnel records. *Comprehensive Psychiatry* 32(5):416-422.

Prigerson, H. G., P. K. Maciejewski, and R. A. Rosenheck. 2001. Combat trauma: Trauma with highest risk of delayed onset and unresolved posttraumatic stress disorder symptoms, unemployment, and abuse among men. *Journal of Nervous and Mental Disease* 189(2):99-108.

Punamaki, R. L., S. R. Qouta, and E. El Sarraj. 2010. Nature of torture, PTSD, and somatic symptoms among political ex-prisoners. *Journal of Traumatic Stress* 23(4):532-536.

Resnick, S. G., and R. A. Rosenheck. 2008. Posttraumatic stress disorder and employment in veterans participating in Veterans Health Administration compensated work therapy. *Journal of Rehabilitation Research & Development* 45(3):427-435.

Roberts, A. L., S. B. Austin, H. L. Corliss, A. K. Vandermorris, and K. C. Koenen. 2010. Pervasive trauma exposure among U.S. sexual orientation minority adults and risk of posttraumatic stress disorder. *American Journal of Public Health* 100(12):2433-2441.

Roberts, A. L., S. E. Gilman, J. Breslau, N. Breslau, and K. C. Koenen. 2011. Race/ethnic differences in exposure to traumatic events, development of post-traumatic stress disorder, and treatment-seeking for post-traumatic stress disorder in the United States. *Psychological Medicine* 41(1):71-83.

Rothbaum, B., E. B. Foa, D. S. Riggs, T. Murdock, and W. Walsh. 1992. A prospective examination of post traumatic stress disorder in rape victims. *Journal of Traumatic Stress* 5(3):455-475.

Sadler, A. G., B. M. Booth, D. Nielson, and B. N. Doebbeling. 2000. Health-related consequences of physical and sexual violence: Women in the military. *Obstetrics and Gynecology* 96(3):473-480.

Sagalyn, D. 2011. *Army general calls for changing name of PTSD*. http://www.pbs.org/newshour/updates/ military/july-dec11/stress_11-04.html (accessed January 30, 2012).

Santiago, P. N., J. E. Wilk, C. S. Milliken, C. A. Castro, C. E. Engel, and C. Hoge. 2010. Screening for alcohol misuse and alcohol-related behaviors among combat veterans. *Psychiatric Services* 61(6):575-581.

Sartor, C. E., V. V. McCutcheon, N. E. Pommer, E. C. Nelson, J. D. Grant, A. E. Duncan, M. Waldron, K. K. Bucholz, P. A. F. Madden, and A. C. Heath. 2011. Common genetic and environmental contributions to post-traumatic stress disorder and alcohol dependence in young women. *Psychological Medicine* 41(7):1497-1505.

Schnurr, P. P., C. A. Lunney, A. Sengupta, and L. C. Waelde. 2003. A descriptive analysis of PTSD chronicity in Vietnam veterans. *Journal of Traumatic Stress* 16(6):545-553.

Seal, K. H., D. Bertenthal, C. R. Miner, S. Sen, and C. Marmar. 2007. Bringing the war back home: Mental health disorders among 103,788 U.S. veterans returning from Iraq and Afghanistan seen at Department of Veterans Affairs facilities. *Archives of Internal Medicine* 167(5):476-482.

Seedat, S., D. J. Stein, and P. D. Carey. 2005. Post-traumatic stress disorder in women: Epidemiological and treatment issues. *CNS Drugs* 19(5):411-427.

Shephard, B. 2000. War, medicine and modernity. *Medical History* 44(2):287-287.

Skinner, K. M., N. Kressin, S. Frayne, T. J. Tripp, C. S. Hankin, D. R. Miller, and L. M. Sullivan. 2000. The prevalence of military sexual assault among female Veterans Administration outpatients. *Journal of Interpersonal Violence* 15(3):291-310.

Smith, T. C., M. A. Ryan, D. L. Wingard, D. J. Slymen, J. F. Sallis, D. Kritz-Silverstein, and The Millennium Cohort Study. 2008. New onset and persistent symptoms of post-traumatic stress disorder self-reported after deployment and combat exposures: Prospective population based U.S. military cohort study. *British Medical Journal* 336(7640):366-371.

Stecker, T., J. Fortney, R. Owen, M. P. McGovern, and S. Williams. 2010. Co-occurring medical, psychiatric, and alcohol-related disorders among veterans returning from Iraq and Afghanistan. *Psychosomatics* 51(6):503-507.

Stein, M. B., J. R. Walker, A. L. Hazen, and D. R. Forde. 1997. Full and partial posttraumatic stress disorder: Findings from a community survey. *American Journal of Psychiatry* 154(8):1114-1119.

Stewart, S. H. 1996. Alcohol abuse in individuals exposed to trauma: A critical review. *Psychological Bulletin* 120(1):83-112.

Storr, C. L., N. S. Ialongo, J. C. Anthony, and N. Breslau. 2007. Childhood antecedents of exposure to traumatic events and posttraumatic stress disorder. *American Journal of Psychiatry* 164(1):119-125.

Suris, A., and L. Lind. 2008. Military sexual trauma—a review of prevalence and associated health consequences in veterans. *Trauma Violence & Abuse* 9(4):250-269.

Suris, A., L. Lind, T. M. Kashner, P. D. Borman, and F. Petty. 2004. Sexual assault in women veterans: An examination of PTSD risk, health care utilization, and cost of care. *Psychosomatic Medicine* 66(5):749-756.

Tanielian, T. L., and L. Jaycox. 2008. *Invisible wounds of war: Psychological and cognitive injuries, their consequences, and services to assist recovery*. Arlington, VA: RAND Corporation.

Tarrier, N., and L. Gregg. 2004. Suicide risk in civilian PTSD patients—predictors of suicidal ideation, planning and attempts. *Social Psychiatry & Psychiatric Epidemiology* 39(8):655-661.

Thomas, J. L., J. E. Wilk, L. A. Riviere, D. McGurk, C. A. Castro, C. W. Hoge. 2010. Prevalence of mental health problems and functional impairment among active component and National Guard soldiers 3 and 12 months following combat in Iraq. *Archives of General Psychiatry* 67(6):614-623.

Tolin, D. F., and E. B. Foa. 2006. Sex differences in trauma and posttraumatic stress disorder: A quantitative review of 25 years of research. *Psychological Bulletin* 132(6):959-992.

Toomey, R., H. K. Kang, J. Karlinsky, D. G. Baker, J. J. Vasterling, R. Alpern, D. J. Reda, W. G. Henderson, F. M. Murphy, and S. A. Eisen. 2007. Mental health of U.S. Gulf War veterans 10 years after the war. *British Journal of Psychiatry* 190:385-393.

True, W. R., J. Rice, S. A. Eisen, A. C. Heath, J. Goldberg, M. J. Lyons, and J. Nowak. 1993. A twin study of genetic and environmental contributions to liability for posttraumatic stress symptoms. *Archives of General Psychiatry* 50(4):257-264.

VA (Department of Veterans Affairs). 2012. *Military sexual trauma*. http://www.ptsd.va.gov/public/pages/military-sexual-trauma-general.asp (accessed January 30, 2012).

VA and DoD. 2010. *VA/DoD clinical practice guideline for management of post-traumatic stress*. Washington, DC: VA and DoD.

Vasterling, J. J., S. P. Proctor, M. J. Friedman, C. W. Hoge, T. Heeren, L. A. King, and D. W. King. 2010. PTSD symptom increases in Iraq-deployed soldiers: Comparison with non-deployed soldiers and associations with baseline symptoms, deployment experiences, and postdeployment stress. *Journal of Traumatic Stress* 23(1):41-51.

Vogt, D., R. Vaughn, M. E. Glickman, M. Schultz, M. Drainoni, R. Elwy, and S. Eisen. 2011. Gender differences in combat-related stressors and their association with postdeployment mental health in a nationally representative sample of U.S. OEF/OIF veterans. *Journal of Abnormal Psychology* 120(4):797-806.

Walker, N., P. McConville, D. Hunter, I. Deary, and L. Whalley. 2002. Childhood mental ability and lifetime psychiatric contact: A 66-year follow-up study of the 1932 Scottish Mental Ability Survey. *Intelligence* 30:233-245.

Warner, C. H., G. N. Appenzeller, T. A. Grieger, S. Belenkly, J. Breitback, J. Parker, C. M. Warner, and C. W. Hoge. 2011. Importance of anonymity to encourage honest reporting in mental health screening after combat deployment. *Archive of General Psychiatry* 68:1065-1071.

Weiss, T., K. Skelton, J. Phifer, T. Jovanovic, C. F. Gillespie, A. Smith, G. Umpierrez, B. Bradley, and K. J. Ressler. 2011. Posttraumatic stress disorder is a risk factor for metabolic syndrome in an impoverished urban population. *General Hospital Psychiatry* 33(2):135-142.

Welke, B. Y. 2001. *Recasting American liberty: Gender, race, law, and the railroad revolution, 1865-1920*. Cambridge, UK: Cambridge University Press.

Wieland, D., M. Hursey, and D. Delgado. 2010. Operation Enduring Freedom (OEF) and Operation Iraqi Freedom (OIF) military mental health issues. Information on the wars' signature wounds: Posttraumatic stress disorder and traumatic brain injury. *Pennsylvania Nurse* 65(3):4-11.

Wilson, J., M. Jones, N. T. Fear, L. Hull, M. Hotopf, S. Wessely, and R. J. Rona. 2009. Is previous psychological health associated with the likelihood of Iraq war deployment? An investigation of the "healthy warrior effect." *American Journal of Epidemiology* 169(11):1362-1369.

Wolf, E. J., M. W. Miller, R. F. Krueger, M. J. Lyons, M. T. Tsuang, and K. C. Koenen. 2010. Posttraumatic stress disorder and the genetic structure of comorbidity. *Journal of Abnormal Psychology* 119(2):320-330.

Xian, H., S. I. Chantarujikapong, J. F. Shrerrer, S. A. Eisen, M. J. Lyons, J. Goldberg, M. Tsuang, and W. True. 2000. Genetic and environmental influences on posttraumatic stress disorder, alcohol, and drug dependence in twin pairs. *Drug and Alcohol Dependence* 61:95-102.

Yaeger, D., N. Himmelfarb, A. Cammack, and J. Mintz. 2006. DSM-IV diagnosed posttraumatic stress disorder in women veterans with and without military sexual trauma. *Journal of General Internal Medicine* 21:S65-S69.

Zatzick, D. F., C. R. Marmar, D. S. Weiss, W. S. Browner, T. J. Metzler, J. M. Golding, A. Stewart, W. E. Schlenger, and K. B. Wells. 1997. Posttraumatic stress disorder and functioning and quality of life outcomes in a nationally representative sample of male Vietnam veterans. *American Journal of Psychiatry* 154(12):1690-1695.

Zlotnick, C., M. Warshaw, M. T. Shea, J. Allsworth, T. Pearlstein, and M. B. Keller. 1999. Chronicity in posttraumatic stress disorder (PTSD) and predictors of course of comorbid PTSD in patients with anxiety disorders. *Journal of Traumatic Stress* 12(1):89-100.

Zlotnick, C., C. L. Franklin, and M. Zimmerman. 2002. Does "subthreshold" posttraumatic stress disorder have any clinical relevance? *Comprehensive Psychiatry* 43(6):413-419.

Zlotnick, C., B. F. Rodriguez, R. B. Weisberg, S. E. Bruce, M. A. Spencer, L. Culpepper, and M. B. Keller. 2004. Chronicity in posttraumatic stress disorder and predictors of the course of posttraumatic stress disorder among primary care patients. *Journal of Nervous and Mental Disease* 192(2):153-159.

3

Neurobiology

This chapter describes the neurobiology of posttraumatic stress disorder (PTSD) and provides a setting for discussing the optimal treatment for PTSD (see Chapter 7). It begins with a discussion of adaptive versus maladaptive stress responses and describes fear conditioning and fear extinction. Models for the development of PTSD are then presented with an overview of the modulators that affect PTSD expression. In particular, in response to the committee's statement of task, physiological markers for PTSD are described (see section on biomarkers) as are brain imaging studies (see section on studies using human subjects) and studies correlating brain region physiology and the diagnosis of PTSD (see section on implications for PTSD prevention, diagnosis, and treatment). The chapter concludes with a discussion of the implications of the neurobiology of PTSD for its prevention, diagnosis, and treatment.

Although some research on the neurobiology of PTSD is funded by the National Institutes of Health, other research on this topic is also sponsored by the Department of Defense (DoD) and the Department of Veterans Affairs (VA) (see Chapter 4). For example, the DoD is funding a study on multimodal neurodiagnostic imaging of traumatic brain imaging (TBI) and PTSD and a study on the neurobiology of tinnitus with PTSD as a secondary outcome, but these studies are ongoing and results are not available. The VA is also funding studies on the neurobiology of PTSD, including examinations of memory and the hippocampus in twins, brain imaging of psychotherapy for PTSD, and neural correlates of cognitive rehabilitation in PTSD.

The etiology of PTSD is linked to a known incident or repeated incidences in which an individual is exposed to a life-threatening event that causes the development of PTSD symptoms. Stimuli present at the time of trauma exposure often become associated with the traumatic event such that subsequent exposure to one or more of those stimuli triggers fear and anxiety. PTSD patients often develop strategies to avoid trauma-associated contexts or cues and develop multiple symptoms, including cognitive and memory impairments and sleep disturbances.

The advent of neuroimaging tools during the past two decades along with the advancement of preclinical research has provided a platform upon which to begin to examine the neurobiology of PTSD, from predisposing factors leading to its development to developing novel strategies to treat the disorder. This chapter reviews some of the models and experimental approaches used in this domain. The committee must emphasize that a comprehensive review of the literature in this area of research is beyond the scope of this report. Moreover, the committee emphasizes there is not a single experimental model that can or will be able to capture every aspect of this complex disorder, and every experimental model (clinical or preclinical) has its advantages and disadvantages (see review by Brewin and Holmes, 2003). With this perspective in mind, the committee uses many references that rely on one or more experimental models or approaches to examine the neurobiology of PTSD, with an objective to build a wealth of information from different approaches that may lead to a comprehensive understanding of the disorder.

ADAPTIVE AND MALADAPTIVE STRESS RESPONSES

The diagnosis of PTSD requires that a person have "experienced, witnessed, or [been] confronted with an event or events that involved actual or threatened death or serious injury, or a threat to the physical integrity of self or others" and that "the person's response involved fear, helplessness or horror" (APA, 2000); see Chapter 2 for the complete diagnostic criteria for PTSD. Research suggests that the term *stress* in relation to disease should be "restricted to conditions where an environmental demand exceeds the natural regulatory capacity of an organism, in particular situations that include unpredictability and uncontrollability" (Koolhaas et al., 2011). Examples of unpredictable and uncontrollable situations include rape, childhood abuse, and military combat (Breslau et al., 1991, 1998; Kessler et al., 1995). Research on PTSD has concentrated on two systems, the sympathetic nervous system and the hypothalamic-pituitary-adrenal (HPA) axis, but there are other neurobiologic systems such as the serotonin system, the opiate system, and sex steroidal systems that have been implicated in pathologic and protective responses to stress (IOM, 2008).

The HPA axis is a neuroendocrine system from which there is successive release of several hormones that leads to the release of cortisol from the adrenal glands. Cortisol circulates to other tissues where it causes an elevation in circulating glucose and, if appropriate, activates immune-cell migration to injured or infected areas of the body. There is some evidence that chronically elevated cortisol concentrations may impair many forms of memory (memory that is dependent on the hippocampus or prefrontal cortex), but such elevated concentrations favor memories that trigger fear (memory that is dependent on the amygdala) (see reviews by McEwen, 2005, 2006; Vanitallie, 2002). This is an important distinction because fear memories depend on the amygdala and extinction memories depend on the hippocampus and prefrontal cortex.

Events that are perceived as uncontrollable and threatening cause a series of reactions via the HPA axis, the locus coeruleus, and the noradrenergic system (Koenen et al., 2009a). These systems have reciprocal connections with limbic structures that mediate fear conditioning and memory consolidation (the amygdala and hippocampus) and prefrontal brain structures that mediate the extinction of fear memories. Structures in the brain initially respond to stress caused by an acute threat through adaptive mechanisms such as energy mobilization, increased vigilance and focus, and the facilitation of memory formation (Charney, 2004). When the body determines there is no longer an acute threat, it attempts to return to homeostasis through an elaborate negative feedback system. Figure 3-1 shows the major pathways that are triggered during a response to stress.

There are some cases where the adaptive response described above becomes persistent and pathologic (Koenen et al., 2009a). When a person is exposed to a traumatic event, sensory stimuli present at the time of exposure become associated with it. Later exposure to one or more of the now-conditioned sensory cues can lead to reactivation of the traumatic memories.

The initial re-exposure to the conditioned cues leads to the expression of intense fear and anxiety in most people. Repeated exposure to those cues in the absence of additional negative reinforcement (that is, without additional traumatic events) will lead to the gradual reduction of emotion associated with the traumatic event (that is, extinction). As stated by Mao et al. (2006), "much evidence indicates that extinction training does not erase memory traces but instead forms inhibitory learning that prevents the expression of the original memory" (see also Quirk, 2002). Reinstatement, renewal, and spontaneous recovery are phenomena that provide direct evidence that fear extinction is new inhibitory learning rather than erasure or forgetting (Archbold et al., 2010; Bouton, 2004; Myers and Davis, 2007). Reinstatement is a phenomenon in which a person or animal undergoes extinction training and is then exposed to an unsignaled unconditioned stimulus (see Box 3-1 for definition), resulting in the reappearance of an ex-

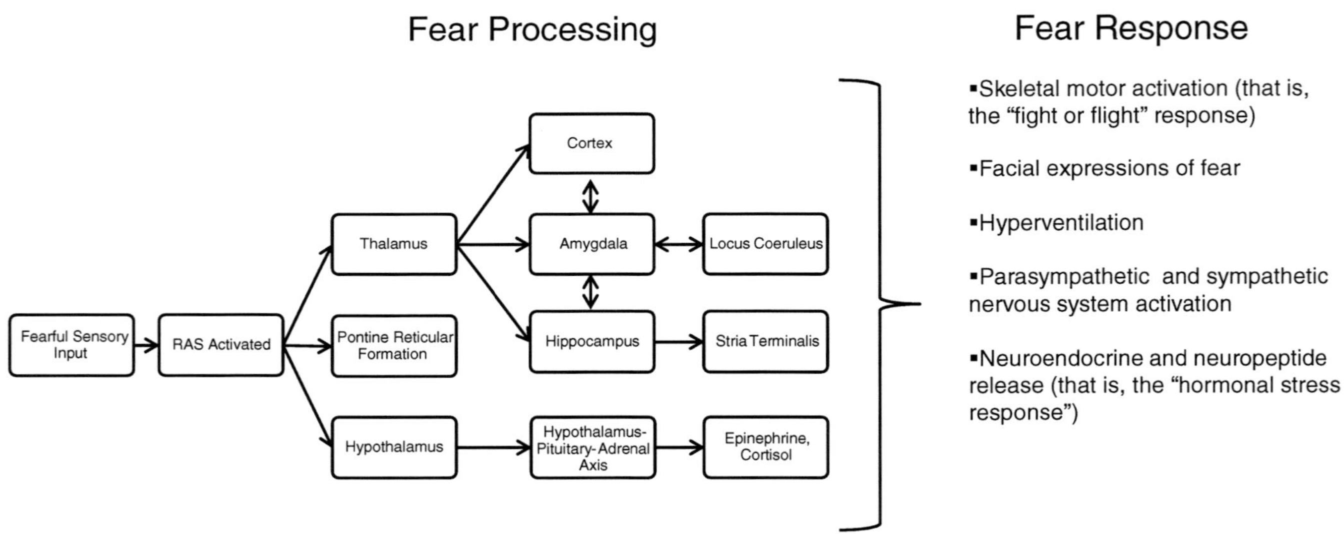

FIGURE 3-1 Depiction of the major pathways triggered during a response to stress. During a normal stress response, the sympathetic nervous system and the reticular activating system (RAS) are activated. The sympathetic nervous system controls the response of internal organs (for example, increasing the heart rate, decreasing digestion activities, and mobilizing energy stores from the liver). The RAS, which is required for a stress response, activates the pontine reticular formation (which induces the startle response), activates the thalamus to stimulate the cortex, and communicates with forebrain structures to activate the hypothalamus, which triggers the HPA axis and the release of epinephrine (IOM, 2008).

tinguished fear response. Renewal occurs when an extinguished conditioned response (see Box 3-1 for definition) reappears in a person or animal in a context that is different from the context in which the extinction training took place. *Spontaneous recovery* is the term used when the extinguished conditioned response reappears after nothing but the passage of time following extinction training.

It has been hypothesized that PTSD may result from a failure to recover from a traumatic experience, which leads to an inability to extinguish the fear and anxiety associated with conditioned sensory cues. For example, a service member might witness a friend being killed while a helicopter is hov-

BOX 3-1
Definitions of Selected Terms Associated with Fear Conditioning and Fear Extinction

Classical conditioning—A process by which previously neutral stimuli acquire meaning to the organism

Unconditioned stimulus (US)—A trigger that produces an automatic, unlearned response

Unconditioned response (UR)—A naturally occurring reaction to a US

Conditioned stimulus (CS)—A neutral trigger that, through classical conditioning, is able to produce a conditioned response

Conditioned response (CR)—The learned reaction and instrumentational actions to a CS

Acquisition—The initial stage of learning, where a neutral stimulus (CS) is associated with a meaningful stimulus (US) and obtains the capacity to elicit a similar response (CR)

Short-term memory—Memory that is held for a short period of time

Long-term memory—Memory that lasts over a long period of time

Consolidation—The process by which short-term memory is converted into long-term memory

Retrieval—Reactivation of the memory trace or expression of a fear memory

Reconsolidation—A process by which a previously consolidated memory, which has been retrieved and becomes labile, undergoes another consolidation

Extinction—The process by which a CS loses the ability to elicit a CR

SOURCE: Adapted from Garakani et al., 2006; reproduced with permission of John Wiley & Sons, Inc.

ering overhead. The service member associates the sounds of the helicopter with the friend's death. Later, when the service member hears a helicopter, he or she may experience the same fear and anxiety that were experienced during the traumatic event. This is a prototypic example of Pavlovian conditioning whereby sounds of the helicopter trigger the service member to prepare for an attack. This reaction would be adaptive in a combat situation but is maladaptive outside of it.

Conditioned fear may also lead to instrumental behaviors that contribute to the development and maintenance of PTSD. Instrumental behaviors often take the form of active and passive avoidance. Such behaviors are exhibited when the organism has control over threats and can minimize exposure to threats and traumas (conditioned and unconditioned stimuli) by virtue of how it responds. For example, a person diagnosed with PTSD may actively avoid reminders of the traumatic event, such as avoiding members of his or her unit because they are reminders of the traumatic experience of combat. A person diagnosed with PTSD may also passively (or involuntarily) avoid reminders of a traumatic situation, such as becoming disengaged. Fear extinction is therefore about learning that the conditioned stimulus no longer predicts the unconditioned stimulus, thus eliminating the need for all defensive responding (such as fear reactions and instrumental responses). Both active and passive avoidance strategies prevent fear reactions and subjective feelings of fear, and they can be adaptive provided they do not interfere with normal activities. Active avoidance mechanisms may even have relevance to active coping strategies that effectively deal with traumatic fear (Cain and LeDoux, 2007).

Fear and anxiety are a normal response to trauma. For the majority of exposed individuals, this fear and anxiety extinguish over time. For a significant minority, they do not. Therefore, it has been hypothesized that PTSD is a disorder of fear extinction (Cohen and Richter-Levin, 2009; Herry et al., 2010; Lang et al., 2000; Rasmusson and Charney, 1997; Rothbaum and Davis, 2003; Siegmund and Wotjak, 2006). The committee recognizes that other models have been proposed, including models for learning and for processing stress, information, memory, and emotion (see reviews by Brewin and Holmes, 2003; Cahill and Foa, 2007; and Ursano et al., 2008). However, it is difficult for one model to capture all aspects of PTSD phenomenology, especially associated symptoms such as shame and guilt, the latter two symptoms are not included in the *Diagnostic and Statistical Maual of Mental Disorders, Fourth Edition* (*DSM-IV*) list of symptoms for the diagnosis of PTSD (APA, 2000).

Box 3-1 defines some terms commonly used in association with fear conditioning and fear extinction. The fear-conditioning model was first described by Pavlov (1927) in a study with dogs. As described by Pitman and Delahanty (2005), a "traumatic event (unconditioned stimulus) over-stimulates endogenous stress hormones (unconditioned response); these mediate an overconsolidation of the event's memory trace; recall of the event in response to reminders (conditioned stimulus) releases further stress hormones (conditioned response); these cause further overconsolidation; and the overconsolidated memory generates PTSD symptoms. Noradrenergic hyperactivity in the basolateral amygdala is hypothesized to mediate this cycle." The three main clusters of PTSD symptoms that result from a persistent pathologic response to uncontrollable stress are re-experiencing or reliving the traumatic event, avoiding reminders of the traumatic event (which prevents extinction of the fear memory) and emotional numbing, and generalized state of hyperarousal or hypervigilance (Koenen et al., 2009a).

In the model of fear extinction, the animal is able to adapt to its environment by dissociating the acquired conditioned fear response from the conditioned stimulus (Cohen and Richter-Levin, 2009). The inability to extinguish a conditioned fear response may play a role in the persistence of PTSD symptoms (Pitman, 1988; Rauch et al., 1998). Of particular interest is whether fear extinction is the result of learning a new response when presented with a conditioned stimulus, unlearning the original fear response when presented with a conditioned stimulus, habituation of the fear response, or a combination of these. As discussed earlier in this section, several reviews point toward the concept that fear extinction is a process more of relearning rather than of removal of a previous memory (Bouton et al., 2011; Cohen and Richter-Levin, 2009; Herry et al., 2010; Maren, 2011; Milad and Quirk, 2012).

Animal studies have shown that the recollection of previously consolidated conditioned fear memories can bring them into a labile state, and these memories then need to go through another phase of reconsolidation. Interrupting this second wave of reconsolidation by using, for example, protein synthesis inhibitors such as anisomycin, has the potential to prevent the restorage of memory (Nader et al., 2000). Reconsolidation blockade has also been shown in humans, and it has been suggested that extinction training may substitute the use of pharmacologic agents to block memory reconsolidation (Schiller et al., 2010). There is, however, some controversy surrounding the relationship between fear extinction and its relationship to fear reconsolidation (that is, memories that have been consolidated have the ability to be altered through retrieval or reactivation) (Myers and Davis, 2007). Differences may be caused by the methods used during studies where deficits were observed in reconsolidation or extinction. These factors may include the amount of time between re-exposure and the previously conditioned cue, protein synthesis in the amygdala and the medial prefrontal cortex, the strength of the conditioned fear memory, and the possibility that the "extinction memory, once firmly established, itself undergoes reconsolidation" (Myers and Davis, 2007).

Neurobiology that supports the animal model of fear conditioning has been much studied. The process is thought to rely heavily on neuronal circuits in the amygdala, prefrontal cortex, hippocampus, and brain stem (Herry et al., 2010; Milad and Quirk, 2012; Ressler, 2010). The neurobiologic processes underlying fear conditioning in animal models and human correlation studies of PTSD are well characterized, and the fear-conditioning model is a guide for the study of the neurobiology of PTSD (Amstadter et al., 2009a; Jovanovic and Ressler, 2010; Lonsdorf and Kalisch, 2011). However, it is important to note that the fear-conditioning model does not capture all features associated with PTSD and is sometimes criticized as too simplistic to explain its pathophysiology. A number of other experimental approaches have been used in both rodents and humans, including symptom-provocation studies, testing of brain responses to the explicit and implicit presentation of fear stimuli in humans, and prolonged-stress exposure models in rodents.

MODELS FOR THE DEVELOPMENT OF PTSD

Numerous experiments have been undertaken in animals and humans to gain a better understanding of the pathophysiology underlying PTSD. The experimental models have benefits and limitations, as will be discussed in the following sections.

Animal Models

Animal models of fear conditioning and extinction have been critical in improving understanding of the neurobiology of PTSD. They are useful because they allow the researcher to manipulate stressors and to control for other variable factors in an experiment. Such models start with a stressor, and the intensity of the stressor (and other determinants) predicts the PTSD. The usual stressors in animals include such conditions as restraint stress, exposure to predators, and underwater foot or tail shocks. Because human PTSD occurs chiefly in the context of life-threatening stressors, the intensity of the stressors used to develop valid animal models need especially careful consideration.

In animal PTSD models, there are complex outcomes that are akin to the variety and severity of PTSD symptoms observed in humans (Kehne and Cain, 2010; Ursano et al., 2009). Animal outcomes include stress, the complementary outcome of fear, and anxiety. Those are sometimes dissociable and indistinct, but all have been characterized in animals (Graham and Milad, 2011; Ressler, 2010; Shin and Liberzon, 2010). Both unconditioned-fear models (for example, experimental models that include an ethologically relevant fear stimulus, elevated plus maze, light–dark test, social interaction, light-enhanced startle, or distress vocalizations) and conditioned-fear models (for example, experimental models that include a conditioned-fear paradigm, conditioned freezing, or fear-potentiated startle) have been developed in animals.

Through the extensive study of animal models of emotional learning and memory (LeDoux, 2000; Maren, 2001), brain regions of interest for PTSD pathology have been described, fear circuits have been defined, and specific molecular outcomes of emotional learning and memory have been identified (Sotres-Bayon et al., 2009). These types of animal models, although they may be incomplete with respect to a full PTSD phenotype, suggest a process for the acquisition and storage of memories, plasticity processes (that is, the ability of pathways in the brain to reorganize structurally and functionally), and molecular markers that might be exploited during the investigation of PTSD resilience, diagnosis, and treatment.

It is important to keep in mind the limitations when evaluating an animal model and its implications for humans. For example, diagnosis of PTSD in humans usually requires a person communicate his or her experiences, thoughts, dreams, and emotions, whereas animal models rely on the observation of behavior. Some of the PTSD phenotypes observed in humans may not be present in animals. Also, the traumatic event that triggers PTSD symptoms in humans may be perceived as life threatening; this perception may cause a type or severity of stress response different from the stress response in an animal after it is restrained or receives a foot shock (Cohen and Richter-Levin, 2009). There are also differences in timing that limit the translation of animal models to human applications. For example, service members may have much longer exposures to traumatic events than animals, and because the average life span of animal models is relatively short, there may not be enough time for PTSD symptoms to develop.

Although no single animal model can capture the complex clinical features of PTSD, a number of models have provided a wealth of information regarding the neural circuits of emotional learning and memory. Examples of animal models for the study of PTSD and PTSD-related phenomena include fear conditioning and extinction models (Cohen and Richter-Levin, 2009), stress-based models (Cohen and Richter-Levin, 2009; Khan and Liberzon, 2004; Yamamoto et al., 2009), fear-potentiated startle models (Davis, 1986; Lang et al., 2000), and learned-helplessness models (Rasmusson and Charney, 1997).

Homologous Brain Structures

Several brain structures and circuits relevant to the fear-learning and fear-extinction processes have been identified in animal models that are homologous to neurologic structures and circuits in humans. For example, the rodent prelimbic cortex increases fear expression and opposes extinction (Vidal-Gonzalez et al., 2006). The human homologue of the rodent prelimbic cortex is the dorsal anterior cingulate cortex (Etkin et al., 2011; Graham and Milad, 2011). The dorsal anterior cingulate cortex has been described as the center for processing cognitive stimuli, error processing and detection, and fear expression (Etkin et al., 2011; Vogt, 2005). The rodent infralimbic subregion plays a key role in inhibiting fear expression and promoting extinction (Milad and Quirk, 2002, 2012; Quirk and Mueller, 2008). The human homologue of the infralimbic subregion appears to be the ventromedial prefrontal cortex, and recent studies show that its structure (Hartley et al., 2011; Milad et al., 2005) and function (Kalisch et al., 2006; Milad et al., 2007; Phelps et al., 2004) correlate with the magnitude of fear extinction. Evidence of the role of the ventromedial prefrontal cortex in the pathophysiology of PTSD comes from a number of recent conditioning and extinction studies in humans (Bremner et al., 2005; Linnman et al., 2012; Milad et al., 2009a).

Studies Using Human Subjects

In humans, the key region involved in fear learning and extinction is the amygdala, which is in the medial temporal lobe (Lang et al., 2000; Rauch et al., 2006). Some evidence suggests that regions of the lateral prefrontal cortex involved in the regulation of cognitive emotion may influence the amygdala (Delgado et al., 2008; Phan et al., 2005; Somerville et al., 2012). Of the 13 amygdala nuclei, 3 (the basal amygdala, lateral amygdala, and central nuclei) are implicated in the brain's response to fear (Amorapanth et al., 2000; Cain and LeDoux, 2008; Garakani et al., 2006; Sah et al., 2003). Functional magnetic resonance imaging (MRI) has limited spatial resolution, and human studies have not yet confirmed the importance of these specific anygdala subnuclei. Other neurologic areas of particular interest include subregions of the medial prefrontal cortex, hippocampus, and the insula. The involvement of these regions has been reported on the basis of resting activity studies that use positron emission tomography, functional MRI studies of patients who were performing a variety of emotional tasks or viewing emotional stimuli, and several structural MRI studies. Some of those findings are reviewed below.

Neuroimaging Studies Using Symptom Provocation

The initial neuroimaging studies of PTSD focused on a paradigm known as symptom provocation. In this paradigm, patients are reminded of their traumatic events while their brains are being scanned. The brain scans are then analyzed for increases and decreases in blood flow in particular regions of the brain. For example, one study reported decreases in medial frontal gyrus blood flow in PTSD participants exposed to reminders of traumatic events compared with trauma-exposed controls who did not have PTSD, and medial frontal gyrus blood flow was inversely correlated with changes in amygdala blood flow (Bremner et al., 1999; Shin et al., 2004). Shin et al. (2004) also reported a positive correlation between changes in amygdala blood flow and symptom severity and a negative correlation between changes in medial frontal gyrus blood flow and symptom severity. Heightened amygdala activity (Rauch et al., 2000; Shin et al., 2004) and diminished ventromedial prefrontal cortex activity (Shin et al., 2005) have also been reported in PTSD subjects who viewed fearful faces during functional MRI compared to trauma-exposed controls who did not have PTSD. The results of those studies reveal critical areas of the brain that play a role in the pathophysiology of PTSD.

Recent studies have also shown that the function of the ventromedial prefrontal cortex and amygdala in patients with PTSD appears to be impaired even in response to the presentation of nontrauma-related stressful cues (Gold et al., 2011; Phan et al., 2006). In addition, functional abnormalities (both resting state and functional reactivation) in the rostral and more dorsal areas of the anterior cingulate cortex have been reported when PTSD patients undergo cognitive tasks (Shin et al., 2009, 2011). Another area that plays a key role in the pathophysiology of PTSD include the insular cortex. This brain region is involved in interoception and the monitoring of internal states and appears to also predict autonomic responses during fear learning (Linnman et al., 2012). People diagnosed with PTSD exhibit exaggerated insula activation in a number of different paradigms, such as during the responses to the presentation of fearful faces, painful stimuli, and traumatic memories (Simmons et al., 2008; Strigo et al., 2010).

Neural Connectivity Studies

More recent studies have used imaging techniques to measure the strength of connectivity between the ventromedial prefrontal cortex and the amygdala and to correlate it with traits that indicate anxiety. For example, when diffusion tensor imaging was used, the strength of the connections between the amygdala and the prefrontal cortex predicted the intensity of a person's anxiety; the weaker the pathway, the greater the intensity of the traits associated with anxiety (Kim and Whalen, 2009). Another study reported that the resting state activity of the amygdala was positively coupled to ventromedial prefrontal cortex activity in subjects who had low levels of anxiety and negatively coupled to ventromedial prefrontal cortex activity in subjects who had high levels of anxiety (Kim et al., 2011a). Together, these studies suggest that a dysfunction in the connection between the ventromedial prefrontal cortex and the amygdala may mediate susceptibility to the anxiety symptoms observed in PTSD. In support of this, recent neuroimaging studies examined the functional connectivity during the resting state in PTSD patients and found dysfunctional connectivity between different nodes of the fear network, including the thalamus, amygdala, insular cortex, hippocampus, and different subregions of the anterior cingulate cortex (Bluhm et al., 2009; Rabinak et al., 2011; Sripada et al., 2012; Yin et al., 2011).

Psychophysiologic and Behavioral Studies

Fear extinction has two components—a learning component (that is, learning to extinguish the fear) and a memory component (that is, recalling a safety memory to block the fear response). One of the hypotheses regarding the psychopathology of PTSD is that people who have PTSD show intact fear learning but impairment in the fear-extinction process. Several studies have directly measured the ability to extinguish fear in anxious populations by using laboratory extinction tasks. In support of that hypothesis, enhanced resistance to extinction has consistently been reported in PTSD populations compared with trauma-exposed controls who did not have PTSD or control groups who did not have PTSD and who had not been exposed to trauma, as indexed by larger differential skin conductive responses to the presence of a conditioned stimulus (Orr et al., 2000), greater heart rate responses (Peri et al., 2000), and stronger online valence and expectancy ratings (Blechert et al., 2007).

Recent studies also show that although learning to extinguish fear may be intact in PTSD, recalling the safety memory (extinction memory) is deficient in PTSD (Milad et al., 2008, 2009a). One of those studies also reported a negative correlation between symptom severity in PTSD and extinction recall (Milad et al., 2009a). In another, enhanced fear conditioning combined with impairments in fear extinction were reported in PTSD subjects compared with trauma-exposed controls who did not have PTSD, and there was a positive correlation between symptom severity and both the enhanced conditioning and the impairment in extinction (Norrholm et al., 2011). Impairment in fear extinction was also reported in PTSD subjects when a model of inhibition that isolates the inhibitory component of extinction was used (Jovanovic et al., 2009); this effect was not detected in a cohort of people who had a diagnosis of depression (Jovanovic and Ressler, 2010).

Neuroimaging Studies of Treatment Outcomes

Another way to examine the relationship between functional brain circuitry and the pathophysiology of a given disorder is to determine whether successful recovery from an adverse health outcome (such as anxiety) correlates with changes in the neural circuitry. Some studies using this approach in PTSD and other anxiety disorders are emerging. For example, one session of intensive exposure therapy has been shown to reduce amygdala, dorsal anterior cingulate cortex, and insula hyperactivation in response to viewing phobia-relevant stimuli in people who have arachnophobia, as measured 2 weeks after exposure (Goossens et al., 2007). Another study reported reduced hyperactivity in the anterior cingulate cortex and insula after cognitive behavioral therapy (CBT) treatment for arachnophobia in comparison with a wait list control group (Straube et al., 2006). Decreases in anterior cingulate cortex blood flow and increases in ventromedial prefrontal cortex blood flow have been reported after CBT for panic disorders (Sakai et al., 2006). Those effects do not appear to be restricted to CBT, as similar neural changes have also been reported after pharmacologic treatment for social phobia (Furmark et al., 2002). The latter study reported a comparable decrease in regional cerebral blood flow in the amygdala and hippocampus after successful treatment with citalopram or CBT. Although those studies are not specific to PTSD, they suggest that successful pharmacologic and psychologic treatments in some cases target the same dysfunction in the neural circuitry that underlies the regulation of emotion.

In a number of recent neuroimaging studies, meditation has appeared to change the structural and functional integrity of several brain regions, including the insula, amygdala, prefrontal cortex, and other regions involved in emotion regulation and empathy (Holzel et al., 2008; Kilpatrick et al., 2011). This could have important implications for PTSD treatment and possibly prevention.

Structural Imaging Studies in PTSD

In addition to function, neuroimaging tools have been used to examine the structural integrity of brain regions implicated in PTSD, with particular emphasis on the hippocampus and prefrontal cortex. Reduced volume in the hippocampus has been reported in a number of studies (Bremner et al., 1995; Kitayama et al., 2005; Stein et al., 1997; Wang et al., 2010a; Woon and Hedges, 2011), and has been proposed to be a predisposing factor for developing PTSD (Gilbertson et al., 2002). However, other studies, including some conducted in children, have failed to replicate the hippocampal reduction in PTSD patients (Bonne et al., 2001; Bremner, 2001; De Bellis et al., 2001; Fennema-Notestine et al., 2002). The cause for this apparent discrepancy regarding hippocampal volume in PTSD is not clear, but it may be related to a number of factors including symptom severity and the chronicity of diagnosis. Structural abnormalities have also been reported in different subregions of the prefrontal cortex (Kasai et al., 2008; Kitayama et al., 2006; Rauch et al., 2003). Unlike the hippocampus, it is proposed that the structural deficits observed in PTSD patients may be the result of having PTSD rather than as a predisposing factor (Kasai et al., 2008).

FACTORS THAT INFLUENCE THE DEVELOPMENT OF PTSD

Exposure to traumatic events is common, particularly for military personnel who may experience multiple deployments. Although exposure to trauma appears to be the rule, the development of PTSD is not. In fact, the majority of service members recover well after trauma without showing signs or symptoms of PTSD (Hoge et al., 2004, 2006; Koenen et al., 2008; Kulka et al., 1990). Those facts have led to the generation of a number of questions: Why is it that some people develop PTSD and others do not? Are there factors that make some people more resilient and others more susceptible to developing PTSD? Could resilience be developed or enhanced, and could the development of PTSD be prevented? Current research efforts in neuroscience, psychology, and psychiatry are trying to answer those questions. In the following sections, the committee summarizes some social and biologic factors that could influence PTSD development and prevention (PTSD prevention is the subject of Chapter 5).

Sex Differences

Emerging evidence from rodent and human imaging studies suggests differences in emotional learning and memory processing between males and females. For example, the network of brain regions that are known to process emotional memory, fear learning, and fear extinction—the amygdala, hippocampus, and prefrontal cortex—is sexually dimorphic (Goldstein et al., 2010). A number of studies show that activation of the amygdala during memory encoding differs between men and women (reviewed in Andreano and Cahill, 2009) and damage to the human ventromedial prefrontal cortex, which is critically involved in fear extinction, differentially affects men and women. Specifically, a unilateral ventromedial prefrontal cortex lesion in the right hemisphere produces severe emotional defects in men, but lesions in the left hemisphere of the same brain region produce no effect (Tranel et al., 2005). The opposite is true in women; a unilateral lesion in the left hemisphere produces severe defects in women, but the same lesion in the right hemisphere has no effects. A study by Bryant and Harvey (2003) of motor vehicle collision survivors examined whether acute stress disorder predicts the development of PTSD (Bryant and Harvey, 2003). The study was based on the idea that "dissociation at the time of trauma results in fragmented encoding of the event, which impedes subsequent emotional processing of the experience and purportedly leads to longer-term psychopathology" (Bryant and Harvey, 2003). Their sample was small, but the authors found that a diagnosis of acute stress disorder was more of a predictor of the development of PTSD in females than in males. Differences in sex can also result in differences in response to PTSD treatments. For example, in a study of PTSD subjects on the effects of treatment with tiagabine, fluoxetine, sertraline alone, and sertraline with CBT, females showed a significantly better response than males (Davidson et al., 2005).

Emerging evidence from experimental human and animal studies indicates that these differences may be influenced by sex hormones. For example, viewing emotionally salient stimuli has been shown to activate the amygdala, the ventromedial prefrontal cortex, and other brain regions involved in the stress-response circuitry differently when a subject is in a high-estrogen state compared to when that subject in a low-estrogen state (Goldstein et al., 2010). Stronger activation of the prefrontal cortex was observed in a go or no-go emotional task in women during the luteal phase (higher estrogen) than during the follicular phase (lower estrogen) (Protopopescu et al., 2005). Activation of the ventromedial prefrontal cortex, the amygdala, and the hippocampus is also increased and associated with facilitated fear inhibition in women in a high-estrogen state (Zeidan et al., 2011). The data suggest that sex hormones (such as estrogen) may be involved in modulating memory formation in women in a way that impacts the control of fear.

Rodent studies have shown direct evidence linking sex hormones (such as estrogen) to synaptic plasticity, activation of molecular machinery involved in learning, and long-term potentiation (for review, see Gillies and McArthur, 2010). Sex hormones also modulate dendritic spine density in the prefrontal cortex (Hao et al., 2006) and modulate the mechanisms by which stress influences the function of the ventromedial prefrontal cortex and the hippocampus (Maeng et al., 2010; Shansky et al., 2010). Recent studies show that in rodents, exogenous estradiol administration facilitates fear inhibition (Chang et al., 2009; Milad et al., 2009b, 2010; Zeidan et al., 2011).

Another important matter to consider in this line of research is oral contraceptives. It has been estimated that 34% of women 18–29 years old in the military are using oral contraceptives (Enewold et al., 2010). If cycling hormones could influence emotional learning and memory, oral contraceptives may influence, modulate, or interfere with these processes. It is known, for example, that most oral contraceptives have an overall effect of reducing cycling estrogens and progesterone in women. A recent study showed that memory formation differed between naturally cycling women and those using oral contraceptives (Nielsen et al., 2011). Thus, future research could be informative in describing the mechanistic differences between the brains of males and females in processing fear extinction. Such research could potentially contribute to an understanding of the relationship between sex and the prevalence of PTSD and to the development of sex-specific treatments for PTSD and other mood and anxiety disorders.

Age

Although trauma exposure of military personnel occurs predominantly during adulthood, it is important to understand how variance in age may influence the formation, consolidation, and retrieval of emotional memories, especially as they are related to fear inhibition in general and to PTSD in particular. A number of studies of fear extinction, for example, have shown that fear-learning and fear-extinction processes differ during the life span. A review by Kim and Richardson (2010) indicates that extinction in preweanling rats is not context dependent—that is, a fear-extinction memory can be expressed in contexts other than the one in which the extinction learning took place. That is a process that does not take place in the adult rat. Moreover, extinction learning and its consolidation in preweanling rats do not require *n*-methyl-d-aspartate (NMDA) receptors (which are important for synaptic plasticity) and do not require the ventromedial prefrontal cortex (Kim and Richardson, 2010). Fear extinction in the adult rat activates the ventromedial prefrontal cortex to inhibit the amygdala, whereas extinction training in early age appears to erase the conditioned fear associations in the amygdala (Gogolla et al., 2009; Kim and Richardson, 2008). During adolescence, extinction learning requires many more training trials (Esmorís-Arranz et al., 2008; Kim et al., 2011b). In the aged rat, fear extinction appears to be impaired and is associated with a shift of excitability from one prefrontal region to another (Kaczorowski et al., 2011). Conclusions from studies of rats imply that fear training in adult rats causes a suppression in fear behavior, whereas in juvenile rats the fear memory is either unlearned or erased (Herry et al., 2010).

A number of neuroimaging studies of humans have shown changes in the amygdala with aging. For example, the response in the amygdala and hippocampus to faces that show emotion compared to faces that have a neutral expression appears to change with age (Iidaka et al., 2002; Wright et al., 2003). A recent study reported that during the encoding of emotionally negative stimuli, the insular and prefrontal cortices are activated to a larger extent in older adults (average age 74.3 years old) than in young adults (average age 24.7 years old). In contrast, greater activation of the amygdala and hippocampus is observed more often in young adults (Fischer et al., 2010). Studies specifically of the neurobiology of fear inhibition in aging have not been conducted. One study, however, reported that older subjects (66–80 years old) exhibit decreased awareness of the association between a neutral cue and an aversive unconditioned stimulus (Labar et al., 2004). Thus, understanding the interaction between age and the function of the network that mediates emotional learning and memory could further the understanding of the etiology of PTSD at different ages and possibly of treatment for PTSD. That is especially important given that recent studies (reviewed above) suggest that such treatments as CBT potentially could change the neural plasticity of the brain regions that mediate fear learning and its extinction.

Cognitive Reserve

Cognitive reserve is related to differences in brain structure (for example, density of neuronal synapses) and function (for example, processing efficiency), and it has been proposed as an important etiologic factor in the development and severity of neuropsychiatric disorders (Barnett et al., 2006; Koenen et al., 2009b). As discussed in Chapter 2, there is evidence from the field of cognitive epidemiology (Deary and Batty, 2007) indicating that intelligence quotient (IQ), a marker of cognitive reserve, is inversely related to a person's risk for being diagnosed with a psychiatric illness (Batty et al., 2005; Walker et al., 2002).

The mechanism of the association between IQ and PTSD is not well understood. Emerging evidence suggests the importance of cognitive processes for the extinction of fear memories. Hoffman and Mathew (2008) argued that the comparable effectiveness of cognitive and exposure therapy for the treatment of fear disorders supports the importance of higher-level cognitive processes in extinction. One hypothesis is that persons with greater cognitive ability are more effective and efficient in engaging in such higher-level cognitive processing and thus more effective in extinguishing fear memories. Given the robust inverse association between cognitive ability and risk of PTSD, a better understanding of the mechanisms underlying this association may be helpful in prevention.

Genetic Factors

Research on the molecular genetics of PTSD is still in its early stages. The first molecular genetic study of PTSD was published in 1991, so this is still a relatively new area of investigation. Chapter 2 discussed family and twin studies that show that PTSD may be heritable and that there is some overlap between the genetic influences on PTSD and genetic influences on other mental disorders (Koenen et al., 2009a). Although there is an extensive literature on PTSD in twins (for example, see Gilbertson et al., 2002; Shin and Liberzon, 2010; Shin et al., 2011), this section focuses on molecular-genetic studies. Recent studies have moved beyond documenting genotype–phenotype associations to identifying epigenetic signatures associated with the disorder (Smith et al., 2011; Uddin et al., 2010) and examining how individual differences in epigenetic programming may modify risk of PTSD in association with exposure to trauma (Koenen et al., 2011). This section provides an overview, not a comprehensive review.

One type of molecular-genetic investigation examines variation in polymorphisms to identify specific genetic variants that may be associated with an increased risk or resilience to the development of a particular phenotype (Amstadter et al., 2009a). By identifying such genes, it may be possible to gain an understanding of the neurobiologic factors that contribute to the development of PTSD or the factors that could be a target for the treatment of the disorder (Amstadter et al., 2009a). Although molecular-genetics research could potentially provide very useful knowledge about the etiology of disorders such as PTSD, it does have limitations, such as the interpretation of research findings or the determination of functional genetic variants (Amstadter et al., 2009a). The committee notes that at the time of this writing, such studies have relied completely on the candidate gene approach. That is, they have selected specific genes posited to be related to PTSD and analyzed variations in those genes in relation to the phenotype. The limitations of this approach and of the field of the genetics of PTSD more broadly have been outlined in detail elsewhere. Specifically, investigators have identified the need for genome-wide association studies of PTSD (Cornelis et al., 2010).

Findings from candidate-gene association studies of PTSD support the observation that many genes associated with PTSD are also related to depression and other anxiety disorders. Table 3-1 is a summary of the results of a systematic literature search for candidate genes for PTSD. The table is not exhaustive but provides an overview of candidate genes that have been the focus of at least one published study in humans (only studies in English were considered). Until recently, most molecular-genetics studies of PTSD focused on the dopaminergic and serotonergic systems, but evidence that PTSD involves dysregulation of other systems has led to increasing interest in genes that play a role in the function of the HPA axis, the locus coeruleus and noradrenergic systems, and neurotrophins. The current evidence of a specific genetic variant that increases vulnerability or resilience to PTSD is not robust. The lack of consistency of associations between specific genetic variants and PTSD may be due to study limitations such as small sample size or substantive differences between studies such as modification of genetic effects by environmental factors that are not accounted for consistently among studies. For example, several candidate-gene studies found significant effects of specific genetic variants only under conditions of extreme traumatic stress (Binder et al., 2008; Kilpatrick et al., 2007).

The environment may also modify genetic effects through molecular mechanisms. DNA methylation is one of the major mechanisms of epigenetic regulation (Bernstein et al., 2007). It involves chemical modifications that regulate DNA accessibility, which in turn alters the transcriptional activity of the surrounding loci. In many cases, increased methylation in specific gene regions (such as the promoter region) is associated with reduced transcriptional activity and therefore with reduced gene expression. Two recent studies of human samples found that those with PTSD were distinguished by methylation profiles that suggest upregulation of immune-system–related genes and relative downregulation of genes involved in neurogenesis and the startle response (Uddin et al., 2010). The upregulation of these genes is indicated by higher concentrations of biomarkers (cytomegalovirus, interlukin-2, interleukin-4, and tumor-necrosis factor-alpha) that are associated with immune system reactivity in participants who have PTSD. Another study showed that SLC6A4 methylation modified the effect that traumatic events had on the development of PTSD when the SLC6A4 genotype was controlled for (Koenen et al., 2011). There was an association between persons who experienced events that were of a more traumatic nature and increased risk for PTSD, but only when lower methylation levels were observed. Persons who experienced events that were of a more traumatic nature appeared to be protected from the development of PTSD when methylation levels were higher. The same interaction was observed regardless of the outcome (PTSD diagnosis, symptom severity, or number of symptoms). The findings described above suggest that gene-specific methylation patterns may be associated with increased risk of and resilience to PTSD (Koenen et al., 2011). The human studies did not, however, demonstrate that the reported PTSD-associated epigenetic differences were associated with downstream differences in gene expression.

A small but growing literature has provided evidence of gene expression patterns that distinguish between those who do and those who do not have PTSD. The majority of these microarray-based studies have assessed gene expression changes in RNA derived from peripheral blood mononuclear cells or whole blood. The earliest work assessed PTSD-associated gene expression signatures in trauma survivors admitted to an emergency room immediately after a traumatic event (Segman et al., 2005). Bioinformatic functional analyses of transcripts that were differentially expressed between those who met *DSM-IV* diagnostic criteria for PTSD at 1 and 4 months, and those who met no PTSD criterion showed reduced expression of transcriptional enhancers, distinct expression signatures of transcripts involved in immune activation, and substantial enrichment of genes that encode neural and endocrine proteins (Segman et al., 2005).

One study used a custom-made "stress/immune" complementary DNA microarray to assess the expression of 384 genes in RNA obtained from whole blood of PTSD-affected and PTSD-unaffected people (Zieker et al., 2007). All the PTSD-affected people had been exposed to the same traumatic event almost 20 years before testing—the Ramstein air show

TABLE 3-1 Overview of Candidate Genes Studied in Relation to Posttraumatic Stress Disorder[a]

Gene	Common name(s)	Location	Published Reports	Significant Findings	Null Findings
RD2 (D2R, D2DR)	Dopamine receptor DR	11q23	6	4 (Comings et al., 1991, 1996; Voisey et al., 2009; Young et al., 2002)	2 (Bailey et al., 2011; Gelernter et al., 1999)
DRD4 (D4DR)	Dopamine receptor D4	11p15.5	1	1 (Dragan and Oniszczenko, 2009)	0
SLC6A3 (DAT1)	Dopamine transporter	5p15.3	4	2 (Drury et al., 2009; Segman et al., 2002; Valente et al., 2011)	2 (Bailey et al., 2011)
DBH	Dopamine beta-hydroxylase	9q34	1	0	1 (Mustapic et al., 2007)
SLC6A4 (HTT, 5HTT, SERT, 5-HTTLPR)	Serotonin transporter	17q11	13	10 (Grabe et al., 2009; Kilpatrick et al., 2007; Koenen et al., 2009c; Kolassa et al., 2010a; Lee et al., 2005; Mercer et al., 2011; Morey et al., 2011; Thakur et al., 2009; Wang et al., 2011; Xie et al., 2009)	3 (Mellman et al., 2009; Sayin et al., 2010; Valente et al., 2011)

HTR2 (5-HT2A)	5-Hydroxytryptamine (serotonin) receptor 2A	13q14-q21	1	1 (Lee et al., 2007)	0
FKBP5	FK506 binding protein 5	6p21	4	4 (Binder et al., 2008; Boscarino et al., 2011; Koenen et al., 2005; Xie et al., 2010)	0
GCCR (NR3C1)	Glucocorticoid receptor	5q31.3	1	0	1 (Bachmann et al., 2005)
CRHR1	Corticotropin-releasing hormone receptor 1	17q12-22	1	1 (Amstadter et al., 2011)	0
RGS2	Regulator of G-protein signaling 2	1q31	1	1 (Amstadter et al., 2009b)	0
CNR1 (CB1, CNR)	Cannabinoid receptor 1 (brain)	6q14-q15	1	0	1 (Lu et al., 2008)
APOE	Apolopoprotein E	19q13	1	1 (Freeman et al., 2005)	0
BDNF	Brain-derived neurotrophic factor	11p13	3	0	3 (Lee et al., 2006; Mustapic et al., 2007; Valente et al., 2011)
NPY	Neuropeptide Y	7p15.1	1	0	1 (Lappalainen et al., 2002)

continued

TABLE 3-1 Continued

Gene	Common name(s)	Location	Published Reports	Significant Findings	Null Findings
GABRA2	$GABA_A$	4p12	1	1 (Nelson et al., 2009)	0
COMT	Catechol-*O*-methyltransferase	22q11	2	2 (Boscarino et al., 2011; Kolassa et al., 2010b)	0
ADCYAP1R1	Receptor for adenylate cyclase-activating polypeptide 1	7p14	2	1 (Ressler et al., 2011)	1 (Chang et al., 2012)
DTNBP1	Dystrobrevin-binding protein 1	6p22	1	1 (Voisey et al., 2010)	0
CRNA5	Cholinergic receptor, neuronal nicotinic, alpha polypeptide 5	15q25.1	1	1 (Boscarino et al., 2011)	0

[a]This list has been updated from Cornelis et al., 2010. Although a systematic literature review was conducted, this list is not exhaustive and includes only human studies published in English.

catastrophe of 1989—and typical PTSD symptoms persisted in this group. Analyses showed a total of 19 differentially expressed transcripts, five and 14 of which were upregulated and downregulated, respectively (Zieker et al., 2007). Most of the downregulated transcripts (which were the focus of the study) were associated with immune functions or with reactive oxygen species.

Most recently, Yehuda et al. (2009) reported levels of expression of whole-blood–derived genes of PTSD-affected and PTSD-unaffected people who were exposed to the attack on New York City on September 11, 2001. Differential expression was detected in 16 genes, several of which are involved in signal transduction, brain and immune cell function, and HPA-axis activity. Although several genes in the study, such as FKBP5 (Binder et al., 2008) and major histone compatibility Class II (Chauhan et al., 2003), had previously been linked to PTSD or other stress-related outcomes, the gene showing the largest difference in expression was mannosidase, alpha, class 2C, member 1 (MAN2C1), a locus that had not previously been linked to PTSD. MAN2C1 distinguishes between those who have and those who do not have PTSD on the basis not only of gene expression (Yehuda et al., 2009) but also of methylation (Uddin et al., 2011).

Collectively, those studies suggest that genotype, methylation, and gene expression differences are promising areas for future research aimed at understanding the etiology of PTSD. However, the committee is not aware of any study that has incorporated all three forms of genetic information into one study, nor are there any definitive findings of any single gene or gene system in the etiology of PTSD.

Sleep

Sleep quality and quantity have been implicated as major factors in the consolidation—that is the conversion of a short-term memory into a long-term memory—of fear-extinction learning. Insomnia and sleep disruptions that affect rapid-eye-movement (REM) sleep are often found in patients who have PTSD, and many studies have investigated the effect of diminished sleep on learning and memory processes. Research has found that the treatment of insomnia may have favorable effects on other pathologic conditions, such as the reduction of co-occurring depressive symptoms (Isaac, 2011). Restoring restful sleep patterns may have the beneficial side effect of reducing the depression symptoms common in PTSD.

Restoring healthy sleep patterns may also preserve REM sleep that contributes to the consolidation of memories associated with fear conditioning and fear extinction. Mohammed et al. (2011) found that REM-sleep deprivation increased the concentration of the neurotransmitters glutamate, glycine, and taurine in the cortex of the rat brain and increased concentrations of glutamate, aspartate, glutamine, and glycine in the hippocampus. Those neurotransmitters affect brain performance, and increased concentrations suggest that REM-sleep deprivation can affect the parts of the brain that are crucial in memory consolidation and motor, sensory, and associative function.

Fear conditioning can decrease REM sleep, but as fear extinction is learned, healthy REM-sleep levels can be restored (Deschaux et al., 2010). Spoormaker et al. (2010) studied REM-sleep disturbances in humans by using functional MRI and skin conductance response measurements. They found that after fear conditioning, REM-deprived participants had "significantly slower decline of [skin-conductance response] and neural activity of the laterodorsal tegmentum." REM sleep not only is implicated as a factor that is fostered by fear learning and supports an appropriate fear response, but when restored in people who have co-occurring depression, it may alleviate depressive symptoms. In contrast, REM-sleep deprivation, which affects concentrations of neurotransmitters in the brain, retards the fear-extinction process.

A recent study reported additional effects of sleep on fear extinction (Pace-Schott et al., 2009). Volunteers underwent a protocol of habituation, conditioning, extinction, and extinction recall. Those phases were carried out in a group that was allowed to get a full night of sleep and a group that had to stay awake during the 12-hour testing period. The authors found that "adequate sleep may promote generalization of extinction memory from specific stimuli treated during exposure therapy to similar stimuli later encountered." Those results are clinically relevant because PTSD patients tend to generalize fear responses to different stimuli. The implication of these results is that adequate sleep could potentially allow generalization of the beneficial effects of therapy to a number of fear-inducing stimuli in PTSD patients.

Chronic Stressors

Chronic stressors can play a role in the development of PTSD by altering brain hormones and receptors that are responsible for fear learning, fear extinction, decision and risk assessment, and mood, thereby increasing vulnerability to fear conditioning. The continual stress faced by service members (such as dangerous environments, fear of attack, intrusive noise and smells, and family distance) leading up to the trigger exposure may also contribute to treatment resistance and overreaction to later fearful stressors. In animal models, Rau et al. (2005) found that "pre-exposure to shock sensitizes conditional fear [in response] to similar less intense stressors," which could explain why the fear response to subtle cues in people who have PTSD may result in more severe fearful responses than would otherwise be merited. They also found the subjects were not as responsive to treatment with NMDA antagonists after sensitization from repeated fear exposures.

Gourley et al. (2009) investigated a cellular mechanism by which chronic stress, in the form of chronic corticosterone exposure, can play a role in the development of PTSD or other psychologic disorders. Exposure to corticosterone over a long period of time, as might be experienced by service members, can lead to a decrease in endogenous corticosterone response to the re-exposure of the fearful context, impair extinction of fear learning, and decrease sucrose preference that is associated with emotional numbing. Chronic corticosterone exposure also decreases the quantity of receptors in the cortex, changing the functioning of the ventromedial prefrontal cortex responsible for processing fear, decision making, and risk taking.

Chronic stress may even affect the long-term genetic expression within the brain that can affect its ability to rebound from fear conditioning. Ponomarev et al. (2010) found that when stress-enhanced fear-learning rats received 15 foot shocks, they "produced robust long-lasting effects on amygdalar transcriptome, which reflected functional and structural changes in neurons and astroglia, which are necessary for plasticity and [stress-enhanced fear-learning]."

IMPLICATIONS FOR PTSD PREVENTION, DIAGNOSIS, AND TREATMENT

Enhancing Resilience

Resilience can be described as a person's ability to "recover or bounce back" (Davidson et al., 2005) from an injury, trauma, insult, or disease (see Chapter 5). There is evidence that some phenotypes or personality attributes increase resilience to stressful situations. They include a person's ability to use coping strategies to deal with stressful situations, the presence of a positive disposition, the ability to reframe a stressful situation in a more positive light, the ability to obtain support from family and friends, and the presence of a moral compass and spirituality in a person's life (Feder et al., 2009). Some of those attributes can be enhanced through psychotherapy or pharmacologic agents.

Resilience in the context of PTSD has been studied relatively little, although the number of studies in the published literature is increasing. Many of the studies have used self-rating scales, such as the Connor-Davidson Resilience Scale, to investigate improvements in resilience after pharmacologic treatment or other experimental protocols (Davidson et al., 2005, 2008; Lavretsky et al., 2010). In addition, although many studies have focused on the adverse effects of stressful situations, Dolbier et al. (2010) suggest that favorable changes can also occur after exposure to a traumatic situation or event (Dolbier et al., 2010; Steinhardt and Dolbier, 2008). These resilience studies and others are discussed in further detail in Chapter 5. These studies are informative, but a better understanding of the neural circuits underlying fear inhibition and extinction is necessary to elucidate the role of resilience in preventing the onset or severity of PTSD symptoms.

Potential Targets for Pharmacologic Treatment of PTSD

Numerous neurotransmitter and neurohormonal systems are involved in the regulation of stress and the dysregulation that characterizes PTSD. Understanding the mechanisms that facilitate the symptoms of PTSD by blocking fear inhibition and extinction is important for the development of pharmacologic targets. Furthermore, having a better understanding of fear reconsolidation may help to identify novel PTSD treatments. Several targets have been identified and are discussed below, but it should be noted that people vary in how they respond to pharmacologic treatments (Narasimhan et al., 2011; Shi et al., 2011; Uher, 2011; Xu et al., 2011a,b).

Glucocorticoids

Glucocorticoids and associated receptors are widely distributed in the central and peripheral nervous systems and play an important role in the body's response to stress (Horvath, 2011). As part of the HPA axis, glucocorticoids play a role in feedback loops of the hippocampal and hypothalamic paraventricular nucleus, in the release of adrenocorticotropin, and in binding to glucocorticoid and mineralocorticoid receptors (Heim and Nemeroff, 2009).

As previously discussed, cortisol is one key glucocorticoid that is involved in the stress response. The mechanisms underlying the function of cortisol are not well known. However, it is thought that low concentrations of cortisol may result in repeated recollections of traumatic memories. Schelling et al. (2004) suggested that administering hydrocortisone reduces the incidence and intensity of traumatic recollections, thereby reducing PTSD symptoms. Putman and Roelofs (2011) reviewed studies that investigated the effects associated with the administration of a single dose of cortisol and concluded that high concentrations of cortisol immediately after a traumatic event may facilitate coping with stress in some individuals. This is supported by a clinical study (using 17 subjects) and a preclinical study (using rats) that were recently undertaken in parallel to investigate the therapeutic effect of hydrocortisone in acutely traumatized participants and the morphologic and molecular alterations in the brain (Zohar et al., 2011). The results suggest that administering a high-dose of hydrocortisone immediately after a traumatic event "may be protective against the subsequent development of PTSD after a traumatic event."

Catecholamines

Catecholamines play an important role in the body's response to stressful situations. Concentrations of these molecules in the blood have been used as markers of stress, and high concentrations indicate that the body is reacting to a stressful situation (Bowirrat et al., 2010). Neurotransmitters that are part of the catecholamine family include epinephrine (adrenaline), norepinephrine (noradrenaline), and dopamine, which are derived from the amino acid tyrosine. In noradrenergic neurons, dopamine is converted into norepinephrine, which then acts as a principal mediator of the central nervous system and autonomic stress responses (Heim and Nemeroff, 2009). Norepinephrine and epinephrine bind to α- and β-adrenergic receptors (Strawn and Geracioti, 2008), and it has been hypothesized that noradrenergic activity increases during traumatic events and results in the enhancement of the coding of a traumatic memory (Debiec et al., 2011). This system has been a target site for several possible therapies for PTSD symptoms.

A drug that targets the adrenergic receptor is yohimbine. Some studies have shown that yohimbine facilitates not only the formation and recall of aversive memories in humans (Cain et al., 2004; Mueller et al., 2009), but also the extinction of cue and contextual fear in rats and mice (Mueller et al., 2009). For example, Cain et al. (2004) administered yohimbine to mice before extinction sessions in several experimental protocols and found that it facilitated long-term extinction learning and extinguished fear faster than controls when tested on the second day of the experimental protocol. The authors suggested that yohimbine might be a useful adjunct to some types of behavior therapy. Morris and Bouton (2007) investigated yohimbine in rats in the context of six different experiments and found that it reduced short-term and long-term freezing caused by the extinguished conditioned stimulus. In contrast, although yohimbine may decrease freezing in rats, there is evidence that it does not strengthen the retention of fear extinction. Mueller et al. (2009) administered yohimbine to rats before extinction training and then tested them the next day without any drugs. They observed a decrease in freezing as described by Cain et al. (2004) and Morris and Bouton (2007), but a second measure of fear expression indicated that "yohimbine failed to enhance long-term retention of extinction" (Mueller et al., 2009). These negative results should be taken with caution because the protocol they used examined fear behavior in conflict with appetitive behavior in hungry rats, which is different than other yohimbine protocols that evaluated fear behavior in isolation.

In humans, there is not yet concrete evidence as to the efficacy and evidence of yohimbine. Based on the animal studies described above and others, Powers et al. (2009) undertook a randomized placebo-controlled clinical trial to test the efficacy of yohimbine to enhance the effects of exposure therapy. Although the study was small (12 participants given the placebo and 12 participants given yohimbine), was composed mostly of students, and was conducted in claustrophobic individuals rather than individuals diagnosed with PTSD, the authors concluded there is some initial evidence in humans that a single dose of yohimbine can increase overall fear reduction, thereby enhancing the clinical outcomes when given to individuals who are undergoing exposure therapy. Based on animal studies, the authors suggested the reduction in fear occurs through the enhancement of extinction memories (Powers et al., 2009). A more recent study in humans failed to detect a yohimbine benefit using extinction-based exposure therapy (Meyerbroeker et al., 2012). In this randomized placebo-controlled trial, 48 participants with a fear of flying completed treatment. These participants were randomized to four sessions of virtual reality exposure therapy combined with yohimbine or four sessions of virtual reality exposure with a placebo. Results indicated that noradrenalin levels were manipulated with yohimbine, but treatment with yohimbine did not appear to enhance exposure therapy. In this study, both the drug and placebo groups showed significant long-term therapy effects, and it is possible that yohimbine may only enhance weak extinction (Cain et al., 2004).

Other adrenergic-blocker drugs that have been investigated include prazosin and propranolol. Several clinical trials have investigated prazosin (Raskind et al., 2003, 2007; Taylor et al., 2006), and results show that treatment with prazosin is more effective than treatment with a placebo. Based on animal studies that show propranolol reduces the consolidation of aversive memories (for example, Rodriguez-Romaguera et al., 2009), research has been conducted on the effectiveness of this drug to prevent PTSD in humans. Most of the results have been negative (Hoge et al., 2012; Pitman et al., 2002; Stein et al., 2007), but there is some evidence that treatment with propranolol may block memory reconsolidation through fear extinction (Schiller et al., 2010). These drugs are discussed in further detail in Chapter 7.

Selective Serotonin Reuptake Inhibitors

Serotonin (5-hydroxytyptamine [5-HT]) is a neurotransmitter that is synthesized from the amino acid tryptophan. It is involved in anxiety, arousal, vigilance, aggression, mood, and impulsivity processes and has been implicated in the pathophysiology of stress and mood disorders (Vermetten and Bremner, 2002). It has been hypothesized that serotonin acts by binding to 5-HT_2 receptors to increase the stress response and by binding to 5-HT_{1A} receptors to facilitate fear extinction (Heim and Nemeroff, 2009). It also affects the stress response by interacting with norepinephrine and corticotrophin-releasing factor. Selective serotonin reuptake inhibitors (SSRIs) are recognized as the primary pharmacologic treatment for PTSD (Norrholm and Jovanovic, 2010). Preventing the reuptake of serotonin results in an increased concentration in the synaptic cleft. SSRIs are discussed further in Chapter 7.

N-methyl-d-aspartate Receptor Agonists and Antagonists

The NMDA receptor binds glutamate and is thought to play a role in memory and learning through synaptic plasticity (Heim and Nemeroff, 2009) and enhanced extinction of the fear response (Graham and Milad, 2011). It is hypothesized that targeting the NMDA receptor can modify or extinguish memories of traumatic events. D-Cycloserine (DCS) is a partial agonist of the NMDA receptor and has been shown to improve the extinction of fear in rodents (Heim and Nemeroff, 2009; Ledgerwood et al., 2005; Myers et al., 2011) when administered in the basolateral amygdala (Norrholm and Jovanovic, 2010). For example, Ledgerwood et al. (2005) investigated the extinction of fear in male rats and the reinstatement of that fear in other contexts. They found that if DCS was administered to a rat immediately after an extinction training exercise and the rat was then re-exposed to the unconditioned stimulus, the conditioned fear would not be reinstated and the rat would not show a fear response. Woods and Bouton (2006) also looked at fear extinction and the renewal of the extinguished fear after administering DCS in female instead of male rats. They reported the fear was extinguished in four trials of DCS dosing, which is confirmed by previous results in animals; however, the facilitated extinction did not have any association with the strength of the renewal effect, so there may still be a potential for relapse. A meta-analysis of English-language journal articles from 1998 to 2007 led to the conclusion that DCS has the ability to enhance fear extinction and exposure therapy if administered immediately before or after extinction training in animals or exposure therapy in humans (Norberg et al., 2008). Limitations of the treatment include nonspecificity to conditioned stimuli and increased tolerance after repeated DCS dosing (Parnas et al., 2005).

Ketamine is hypothesized to ameliorate symptoms of mood and anxiety disorders, including PTSD, by acting as an antagonist at the NMDA receptor (Chambers et al., 1999). It may also reduce the PTSD incidence rate in certain circumstances, although some researchers caution that this association is weak (McGhee et al., 2008). Other modulators of the NMDA receptor are the naturally occurring polyamines spermidine and spermine.

A study in rats showed that intrahippocampal administration of spermidine facilitated the extinction of conditioned fear, probably acting through a subunit of the NMDA receptor (Gomes et al., 2010).

Brain-Derived Neurotrophic Factor

Neurotrophins are involved in the regulation of cell growth and survival, differentiation, apoptosis, and restructuring. Much research has centered around one particular neurotrophin; brain-derived neurotrophic factor (BDNF). Studies of BDNF have shown that it increases the survival of neurons, increases synaptic transmission and plasticity (Kaplan et al., 2010), and blocks or reverses atrophy and neuronal loss caused by stress (Duman and Monteggia, 2006). In a review of the scientific literature, evidence indicates that BDNF is dysregulated in PTSD (Kaplan et al., 2010). The authors also observed that prolonged exposure to glucocorticoids due to chronic stress may reduce BDNF concentrations and may result in retraction, restructuring, and disconnection of dendrites in the hippocampus and ventromedial prefrontal cortex. In another review, Duman and Monteggia (2006) found that hippocampal BDNF was decreased in 11 of 12 animal studies that investigated at stress, but there is limited evidence in humans in the context of PTSD (Duman and Monteggia, 2006; Kaplan et al., 2010). One exception is a study that looked at BDNF plasma concentrations in 18 subjects who had a diagnosis of PTSD and 18 healthy controls (Dell'osso et al., 2009). Results indicated significantly lower blood concentrations in the PTSD patients than in controls, although these results need to be validated by further research. Limitations of the study include the small sample and the lack of a full understanding of how concentrations of BDNF in the blood correlate with concentrations in the brain.

BDNF may play a role in PTSD treatment by promoting neuroplasticity and adaptation to physiologic processes caused by chronic stress. For example, Radecki et al. (2005) performed hippocampal infusions of BDNF in male rats for 14 days. On day 7, the rats were exposed to chronic immobilization stress 2 hours/day for 7 days. The group of 20 rats that received infusion of BDNF and were put under stress was compared with five control groups of 20 rats each: stress treatment and saline infusions, stress treatment with no infusions, saline infusions without stress treatment, nonstressed with no infusions, and BDNF infusions without stress treatments. The authors found that BDNF infusions led to the reversal of stress-induced impairments in spatial learning and memory. Peters et al. (2010) carried out several studies in rats in an effort to investigate the molecular mechanisms underlying extinction-related plasticity. Rats were subjected to auditory fear conditioning and then given infusions of BDNF protein. The results showed that conditioned fear was reduced for up to 48 hours after BDNF infusion even in the absence of extinction training.

In addition to the above studies, treatment with histone deacetylase inhibitors has resulted in an increase in the expression of BDNF in rats and an expansion in the cell populations in the subventricular zone and the hippocampal dentate gyrus (Kim et al., 2009). In a mouse model, treatment with the histone deacetylase inhibitor valproate has been shown to enhance long-term memory for extinction (Bredy et al., 2007). BDNF concentrations and associated proteins necessary for synaptic function have also been found to be increased by exercise. Surgery was performed on 89 male rats to cause lateral fluid-percussion injury (Griesbach et al., 2004). The experimental group and a sham injury group of 72 rats were housed in a cage with or without access to a running wheel at different times after the surgery. The authors saw an increase in endogenous BDNF and enhanced recovery if rats exercised 14–20 days after surgery, but exercise 0–6 days after surgery appeared to disrupt and possibly even delay recovery. In contrast, some negative studies have been associated with BDNF treatment. Rats that had traumatic brain injuries in the parietal cortex were treated with BDNF infusions for 2 weeks and showed no improvements in the measured outcomes of neurologic function, learning, memory, or neuronal loss (Blaha et al., 2000).

BDNF upregulation has been observed with several classes of antidepressant drug treatments (Duman and Monteggia, 2006). Nibuya et al. (1995) investigated the influence of the antidepressant tranylcypromine (a monoamine oxidase inhibitor), desipramine (a tricyclic antidepressant), sertraline (an SSRI), and mianserin (an atypical antidepressant) on the expression of BDNF and its receptor trkB. The authors put male rats through a stress test and compared the antidepressants listed above with several psychotropic drugs (morphine, cocaine, and haloperidol) and saline. The rats were given the pharmacologic agents intraperitoneally in acute and chronic settings. The acute experiment was one dose, and the chronic experiment included dosing once a day for 21 days (except that morphine was administered in a pellet once a day for 5 days). The authors found that BDNF messenger RNA expression was significantly upregulated in the frontal cortex after chronic dosing with tranylcypromine and that BDNF and trkB messenger RNA expression was significantly upregulated in the hippocampus after chronic dosing with all of the antidepressants.

In humans, postmortem samples of the anterior hippocampus were obtained from people who had a diagnosis of major depressive disorder (n = 12), bipolar disorder (n = 11), or schizophrenia (n = 12), and from controls (n = 15) (Chen et al., 2002). The authors used BDNF immunohistochemistry to determine levels of BDNF expression. Although the samples were small, the authors found there were no statistical differences in BDNF expression among the different diagnoses, but BDNF expression in the dentate gyrus, hilus, and supragranular regions of the hippocampus was significantly higher in people who had been treated with antidepressants at the time of death than in those who had not been. Those results, in addition to information in a literature review by D'Sa and Duman (2002), indicate that antidepressant treatments could play a role in treatment of PTSD by promoting neuronal survival and by protecting neurons from stress-induced damage.

Other neurotrophic factors have been linked to the pathophysiology of PTSD, including fibroblast growth factor 2 (FGF2). FGF2 is similar to BDNF in being sensitive to acute stress, particularly in the hippocampal region. Several preliminary studies in rats have shown increases in the expression of FGF2 mRNA in the hippocampus and medial prefrontal cortex after exposure to stress that was uncontrollable (inescapable tail shock) and behaviorally controllable (escapable tail shock) (Bland et al., 2006, 2007). This is a growing field of research that could contribute to the understanding of the pathophysiology of PTSD.

BIOMARKERS

One goal of better understanding the neurobiology of PTSD is to identify biomarkers of the disorder. At least four kinds of biomarkers are of interest. The first are biomarkers that could reliably predict who is at risk for the development of PTSD; such markers may be especially useful in persons—such as service members—who are at high risk for trauma exposure or who have recently been exposed to trauma. The second are biomarkers that could contribute to PTSD diagnosis. Currently, PTSD diagnosis depends completely on self-reporting of symptoms. That is sometimes problematic in military populations because of concerns about stigma, which can lead to an underreporting of symptoms (Corrigan, 2004; Warner et al., 2011), or seeking compensation, which can lead to exaggeration of symptoms (Frueh et al., 1997; IOM, 2007). The third are biomarkers that would be used to match service members to specific evidence-based treatments. The fourth are biomarkers that would be able to predict who is at risk for relapse. These are areas of consideration for moving forward with the prevention, diagnosis, and treatment of PTSD.

It would be beneficial if biomarkers could be used to screen for or diagnose PTSD. For example, peripheral markers, which are found in blood and other bodily fluids, could potentially be used to screen for PTSD. These markers include catecholamine (Yehuda et al., 1992), cortisol (Bremner et al., 2007; de Kloet et al., 2006; Flory et al., 2009; Luo et al., 2012; Vythilingam et al., 2010; Wang et al., 2010b; Yehuda, 2009; Yehuda et al., 2002), dehydroepiandrosterone (Olff et al., 2007; Yehuda et al., 2010),

BDNF (Dell'osso et al., 2009; Frielingsdorf et al., 2010), interleukin-8 (Song et al., 2007), T-cell markers (Lemieux et al., 2008), and peripheral blood mononuclear cells (Segman et al., 2005; Su et al., 2009). Neurologic markers may also be candidates for screening for PTSD. Some that have recently been studied include the difference in activity between certain areas of the brain, such as the dorsolateral prefrontal cortex (Shin et al., 2004, 2006; Pissiota et al., 2002), amygdala (Pissiota et al., 2002; Shin et al., 2004, 2006; Vermetten and Bremner, 2002), and HPA axis (Southwick et al., 1994; Yehuda et al., 1991). Resting metabolism in the brain could potentially also be used to predict autonomic and neuronal responses that are associated with PTSD (Linnman et al., 2012).

PTSD has numerous biologic correlates. In most biologically oriented PTSD research, traditional case–control designs are used to assess whether a given biologic marker is more prevalent in people who have PTSD than in trauma-exposed control subjects that did not develop PTSD. Such studies show whether a biologic factor is a correlate of PTSD; however, research beyond the traditional case–control design is needed to determine whether the biologic factor can be used as a biomarker. To be considered a biomarker of value in predicting risk of PTSD, there must be evidence that the biologic factor was present before trauma exposure, is associated with risk of PTSD, and has predictive validity. To be considered a biomarker of value in diagnosis, a biologic correlate would have to have excellent sensitivity and specificity in distinguishing persons who have and do not have PTSD. Similarly, to be used to match persons who have PTSD with specific treatments, a biomarker would have to be shown to differentiate between those who do and do not respond to specific treatments.

Despite the extensive knowledge of the neurobiology of PTSD, no biologic factors have enough predictive validity to be used at the individual level for any of the purposes described above. For example, C-reactive protein (a marker of inflammation) can be used to identify persons at risk of developing heart disease and distinguish between those who did and did not have a myocardial infarction (Ridker, 2003). No similar biomarkers exist for PTSD. It should also be noted that even if a specific biologic marker of PTSD were identified, such considerations as acceptability, costs, and time would have to be weighed.

SUMMARY

The understanding of the neurobiology of PTSD continues to grow, but there is still much to be learned. A large part of this chapter has focused on studies, both in animals and in humans, that show correlations between a stressor or a risk factor and PTSD symptoms. This work is very important; however, causal studies are necessary to firmly implicate any neurobiologic mechanisms for PTSD risk or resilience, and at present, these studies are lacking. Because many of the required invasive techniques cannot be undertaken in humans, these studies will require animal research on learning and stress systems. Another area of science that could be improved is the understanding of how environmental and biologic factors (such as genetics) contribute to the onset and severity of PTSD symptoms. This research will have important implications for PTSD prevention and treatment. Furthermore, the identification of biomarkers and brain-imaging models for the diagnosis of PTSD would help to reduce the dependence on self-reported symptoms. For the treatment of PTSD, it is important that pharmacologic agents that have the potential to enhance therapy-related learning be investigated further.

This chapter and Chapter 2, which described epidemiologic studies, are intended to set the stage for understanding how science can inform clinical practices in PTSD prevention (Chapter 5), diagnosis (Chapter 6), and treatment (Chapter 7), and for understanding the effects that comorbidities can have on the pathobiology of PTSD (Chapter 8).

REFERENCES

Amorapanth, P., J. E. LeDoux, and K. Nader. 2000. Different lateral amygdala outputs mediate reactions and actions elicited by a fear-arousing stimulus. *Nature Neuroscience* 3:74-79.

Amstadter, A., N. Nugent, and K. Koenen. 2009a. Genetics of PTSD: Fear conditioning as a model for future research. *Psychiatric Annals* 39(6):358-367.

Amstadter, A. B., K. C. Koenen, K. J. Ruggiero, R. Acierno, S. Galea, D. G. Kilpatrick, and J. Gelernter. 2009b. Variant in RGS2 moderates posttraumatic stress symptoms following potentially traumatic event exposure. *Journal of Anxiety Disorders* 23(3):369-373.

Amstadter, A. B., N. R. Nugent, B. Z. Yang, A. Miller, R. Siburian, P. Moorjani, S. Haddad, A. Basu, J. Fagerness, G. Saxe, J. W. Smoller, and K. C. Koenen. 2011. Corticotrophin-releasing hormone type 1 receptor gene (CRHR1) variants predict posttraumatic stress disorder onset and course in pediatric injury patients. *Disease Markers* 30(2-3):89-99.

Andreano, J. M., and L. Cahill. 2009. Sex influences on the neurobiology of learning and memory. *Learning and Memory* 16(4):248-266.

APA (American Psychiatric Association). 2000. *Diagnostic and statistical manual of mental disorders, fourth edition, text revision (DSM-IV-TR)*. Washington, DC: American Psychiatric Association.

Archbold, G. E., M. E. Bouton, and K. Nader. 2010. Evidence for the persistence of contextual fear memories following immediate extinction. *European Journal of Neuroscience* 31(7):1303-1311.

Bachmann, A. W., T. L. Sedgley, R. V. Jackson, J. N. Gibson, R. M. Young, and D. J. Torpy. 2005. Glucocorticoid receptor polymorphisms and post-traumatic stress disorder. *Psychoneuroendocrinology* 30(3):297-306.

Bailey, J. N., A. K. Goenjian, E. P. Noble, D. P. Walling, T. Ritchie, and H. A. Goenjian. 2011. PTSD and dopaminergic genes, DRD2 and DAT, in multigenerational families exposed to the Spitak earthquake. *Psychiatry Research* 178(3):507-510.

Barnett, J. H., C. H. Salmond, P. B. Jones, and B. J. Sahakian. 2006. Cognitive reserve in neuropsychiatry. *Psychological Medicine* 36(8):1053-1064.

Batty, G. D., E. L. Mortensen, and M. Osler. 2005. Childhood IQ in relation to later psychiatric disorder: Evidence from a Danish birth cohort study. *British Journal of Psychiatry* 187:180-181.

Bernstein, B. E., A. Meissner, and E. S. Lander. 2007. The mammalian epigenome. *Cell* 128(4):669-681.

Binder, E. B., R. G. Bradley, W. Liu, M. P. Epstein, T. C. Deveau, K. B. Mercer, Y. Tang, C. F. Gillespie, C. M. Heim, C. B. Nemeroff, A. C. Schwartz, J. F. Cubells, and K. J. Ressler. 2008. Association of FKBP5 polymorphisms and childhood abuse with risk of posttraumatic stress disorder symptoms in adults. *Journal of the American Medical Association* 299(11):1291-1305.

Blaha, G. R., R. Raghupathi, K. E. Saatman, and T. K. McIntosh. 2000. Brain-derived neurotrophic factor administration after traumatic brain injury in the rat does not protect against behavioral or histological deficits. *Neuroscience* 99(3):483-493.

Bland, S. T., M. J. Schmid, B. N. Greenwood, L. R. Watkins, and S. F. Maier. 2006. Behavioral control of the stressor modulates stress-induced changes in neurogenesis and fibroblast growth factor-2. *Neuroreport* 17(6):593-597.

Bland, S. T., J. P. Tamlyn, R. M. Barrientos, B. N. Greenwood, L. R. Watkins, S. Campeau, H. E. Day, and S. F. Maier. 2007. Expression of fibroblast growth factor-2 and brain-derived neurotrophic factor mRNA in the medial prefrontal cortex and hippocampus after uncontrollable or controllable stress. *Neuroscience* 144(4):1219-1228.

Blechert, J., T. Michael, N. Vriends, J. Margraf, and F. H. Wilhelm. 2007. Fear conditioning in posttraumatic stress disorder: Evidence for delayed extinction of autonomic, experiential, and behavioural responses. *Behaviour Research and Therapy* 45(9):2019-2033.

Bluhm, R. L., R. P. Williamson, E. A. Osuch, P. A. Frewen, T. K. Stevens, K. Boksman, R. W. Neurfeld, J. Théberge, and R. A. Lanius. 2009. Alterations in default network connectivity in posttraumatic stress disorder related to early-life trauma. *Journal of Psychiatry and Neuroscience* 34(3):187-194.

Bonne, O., D. Brandes, A. Gilboa, J. M. Gomori, M. E. Shenton, R. K. Pitman, and A. Y. Shalev. 2001. Longitudinal MRI study of hippocampal volume in trauma survivors with PTSD. *American Journal of Psychiatry* 158(8):1284-1251.

Boscarino, J. A., P. M. Erlich, S. N. Hoffman, M. Rukstalis, and W. F. Stewart. 2011. Association of FKBP5, COMT, and CHRNA5 polymorphisms with PTSD among outpatients at risk for PTSD. *Psychiatry Research* 188(1):173-174.

Bouton, M. E. 2004. Context and behavioral processes in extinction. *Learning and Memory* 11(5):485-494.

Bouton, M., T. Todd, D. Vurbic, and N. Winterbauer. 2011. Renewal after the extinction of free operant behavior. *Learning & Behavior* 39(1):57-67.

Bowirrat, A., T. J. Chen, K. Blum, M. Madigan, J. A. Bailey, A. L. Chuan Chen, B. W. Downs, E. R. Braverman, S. Radi, R. L. Waite, M. Kerner, J. Giordano, S. Morse, M. Oscar-Berman, and M. Gold. 2010. Neuro-psychopharmacogenetics and neurological antecedents of posttraumatic stress disorder: Unlocking the mysteries of resilience and vulnerability. *Current Neuropharmacology* 8(4):335-358.

Bredy, T. W., H. Wu, C. Crego, J. Zellhoefer, Y. E. Sun, and M. Barad. 2007. Histone modifications around individual BDNF gene promoters in prefrontal cortex are associated with extinction of conditioned fear. *Learning and Memory* 14:267-276.

Bremner, J. D. 2001. Hypotheses and controversies related to effects of stress on the hippocampus: an argument for stress-induced damage to the hippocampus in patients with posttraumatic stress disorder. *Hippocampus* 11(2):75-81.

Bremner, J. D., P. Randall, T. M. Scott, R. A. Bronen, J. P. Seibyl, S. M. Southwick, R. C. Delaney, G. McCarthy, D. S. Charney, and R. B. Innis. 1995. MRI-based measurement of hippocampal volume in patients with combat-related posttraumatic stress disorder. *American Journal of Psychiatry* 152(7):973-981.

Bremner, J. D., L. H. Staib, D. Kaloupek, S. M. Southwick, R. Soufer, and D. S. Charney. 1999. Neural correlates of exposure to traumatic pictures and sound in Vietnam combat veterans with and without posttraumatic stress disorder: A positron emission tomography study. *Biological Psychiatry* 45(7):806-816.

Bremner, D., E. Vermetten, and M. E. Kelley. 2007. Cortisol, dehydroepiandrosterone, and estradiol measured over 24 hours in women with childhood sexual abuse-related posttraumatic stress disorder. *Journal of Nervous and Mental Disease* 195(11):919-927.

Breslau, N., G. C. Davis, P. Andreski, and E. Peterson. 1991. Traumatic events and posttraumatic stress disorder in an urban population of young adults. *Archives of General Psychiatry* 48:216-222.

Breslau, N., R. Kessler, H. D. Chilcoat, L. R. Schultz, G. C. Davis, and P. Andreski. 1998. Trauma and posttraumatic stress disorder in the community: The 1996 Detroit area survey of trauma. *Archives of General Psychiatry* 55:626-632.

Brewin, C. R., and E. A. Holmes. 2003. Psychological theories of postraumatic stress disorder. *Clinical Psychology Review* 23:339-376.

Bryant, R. A., and A. G. Harvey. 2003. Gender differences in the relationship between acute stress disorder and posttraumatic stress disorder following motor vehicle accidents. *Australian and New Zealand Journal of Psychiatry* 37(2):226-229.

Cahill, S. P., and E. B. Foa. 2007. Chapter 4: Psychological theories of PTSD. In *Handbook of PTSD: Science and Practice*, edited by M. J. Friedman, T. M. Keane, and P. A. Resnick. New York: Guilford Press.

Cain, C. K., and J. E. LeDoux. 2007. Escape from fear: A detailed behavioral analysis of two atypical responses reinforced by CS termination. *Journal of Experimental Psychology. Animal Behavioural Processes* 33(4):451-463.

Cain, C. K., and J. E. Ledoux. 2008. Emotional processing and motivation: In search of brain mechanisms. In *Handbook of Approach and Avoidance Motivation*, edited by A. J. Elliot. New York: Psychology Press. Pp. 17-34.

Cain, C. K., A. M. Blouin, and M. Barad. 2004. Adrenergic transmission facilitates extinction of conditional fear in mice. *Learning & Memory* 11(2):179-187.

Chambers, R. A., J. D. Bremner, B. O. Moghaddam, S. M. Southwick, D. S. Charney, and J. H. Krystal. 1999. Glutamate and post-traumatic stress disorder: Toward a psychobiology of dissociation. *Seminars in Clinical Neuropsychiatry* 4:274-281.

Chang, S. C., P. Xie, R. F. Anton, I. De Vivo, L. A. Farrer, H. R. Kranzler, D. Oslin, S. M. Purcell, A. L. Roberts, J. W. Smoller, M. Uddin, J. Gelernter, and K. C. Koenen. 2012. No association between ADCYAP1R1 and post-traumatic stress disorder in two independent samples. *Molecular Psychiatry* 17(3):239-241.

Chang., Y. J., C. H. Yang, Y. C. Liang, C. M. Yeh, C. C. Huang, and K. S. Hsu. 2009. Estrogen modulates sexually dimorphic contextual fear extinction in rats through estrogen receptor beta. *Hippocampus* 19(11):1142-1150.

Charney, D. S. 2004. Psychobiological mechanisms of resilience and vulnerability: Implications for successful adaptation to extreme stress. *American Journal of Psychiatry* 161(2):195-216.

Chauhan, S., C. H. Leach, S. Kunz, J. W. Bloom, and R. L. Miesfeld. 2003. Glucocorticoid regulation of human eosinophil gene expression. *Journal of Steroid Biochemical Molecular Biology* 84(4):441-452.

Chen, Y., R. P. Sharma, R. H. Costa, E. Costa, and D. R. Grayson. 2002. On the epigenetic regulation of the human reelin promoter. *Nucleic Acids Research* 30(13):2930-2939.

Cohen, H., and G. Richter-Levin. 2009. Toward animal models of post-traumatic stress disorder. In *Post-traumatic stress disorder: Basic science and clinical practice*. New York: Humana Press.

Comings, D. E., B. G. Comings, D. Muhleman, G. Dietz, B. Shabbahrami, and D. Tast. 1991. The dopamine D2 receptor locus as a modifying gene in neuropsychiatric disorder. *Journal of the American Medical Association* 266:1793-1800.

Comings, D. E., D. Muhleman, and R. Gysin. 1996. Dopamine D2 receptor (DRD2) gene and susceptibility to posttraumatic stress disorder: A study and replication. *Biological Psychiatry* 40:368-372.

Cornelis, M. C., N. R. Nugent, A. B. Amstadter, and K. C. Koenen. 2010. Genetics of post-traumatic stress disorder: Review and recommendations for genome-wide association studies. *Current Psychiatry Report* 12(4):313-326.

Corrigan, P. 2004. How stigma interferes with mental health care. *American Psychologist* 59(7):614-625.

Davidson, J. R., V. M. Payne, K. M. Connor, E. B. Foa, B. O. Rothbaum, M. A. Hertzberg, and R. H. Weisler. 2005. Trauma, resilience and saliostasis: Effects of treatment in post-traumatic stress disorder. *International Clinical Psychopharmacology* 20(1):43-48.

Davidson, J., D. S. Baldwin, D. J. Stein, R. Pedersen, S. Ahmed, J. Musgnung, I. Benattia, and B. O. Rothbaum. 2008. Effects of venlafaxine extended release on resilience in post-traumatic stress disorder: An item analysis of the Connor-Davidson Resilience Scale. *International Clinical Psychopharmacology* 23(5):299-303.

Davis, M. 1986. Pharmacological and anatomical analysis of fear conditioning using the fear-potentiated startle paradigm. *Behavioural Neuroscience* 100(6):814-824.

De Bellis, M. D., J. Hall, A. M. Boring, K. Frustaci, and G. Moritz. 2001. A pilot longitudinal study of hippocampal volumes in pediatric maltreatment-related posttraumatic stress disorder. *Biological Psychiatry* 50(4):305-309.

de Kloet, C. S., E. Vermetten, E. Geuze, A. Kavelaars, C. J. Heijnen, and H. G. M. Westenberg. 2006. Assessment of HPA-axis function in posttraumatic stress disorder: Pharmacological and non-pharmacological challenge tests, a review. *Journal of Psychiatric Research* 40(6):550-567.

Deary, I. J., and G. D. Batty. 2007. Cognitive epidemiology. *Journal of Epidemiology and Community Health* 61(5):378-384.

Debiec, J., D. E. A. Bush, and J. E. LeDoux. 2011. Noradrenergic enhancement of reconsolidation in the amygdala impairs extinction of conditioned fear in rats—a possible mechanism for the persistence of traumatic memories in PTSD. *Depression and Anxiety* 28(3):186-193.

Delgado, M. R., K. I. Nearing, J. E. LeDoux, and E. A. Phelps. 2008. Neural circuitry underlying the regulation of conditioned fear and its relation to extinction. *Neuron* 59(5):829-838.

Dell'osso, L., C. Carmassi, A. Del Debbio, M. C. Dell'osso, C. Bianchi, E. da Pozzo, N. Origlia, L. Domenici, G. Massimetti, D. Marazziti, and A. Piccinni. 2009. Brain-derived neurotrophic factor plasma levels in patients suffering from post-traumatic stress disorder. *Progress in Neuro-Psychopharmacology & Biological Psychiatry* 33(5):899-902.

Deschaux, O., A. Thevenet, G. Spennato, C. Arnaud, J. L. Moreau, and R. Garcia. 2010. Low-frequency stimulation of the hippocampus following fear extinction impairs both restoration of rapid eye movement sleep and retrieval of extinction memory. *Neuroscience* 170(1):92-98.

Dolbier, C. L., S. S. Jaggars, and M. A. Steinhardt. 2010. Stress-related growth: Pre-intervention correlates and change following a resilience intervention. *Stress and Health* 26(2):135-147.

Dragan, W. L., and W. Ç. Oniszczenko. 2009. The association between dopamine D4 receptor exon III polymorphism and intensity of PTSD symptoms among flood survivors. *Anxiety, Stress & Coping: An International Journal* 22(5):483-495.

Drury, S. S., K. P. Theall, B. J. Keats, and M. Scheeringa. 2009. The role of the dopamine transporter (DAT) in the development of PTSD in preschool children. *Journal of Traumatic Stress* 22(6):534-539.

D'Sa, C., and R. S. Duman. 2002. Antidepressants and neuroplasticity. *Bipolar Disorders* 4(3):183-194.

Duman, R. S., and L. M. Monteggia. 2006. A neurotrophic model for stress-related mood disorders. *Biological Psychiatry* 59(12):1116-1127.

Enewold, L., L. A. Brinton, K. A. McGlynn, S. H. Zahm, J. F. Potter, and K. Zhu. 2010. Oral contraceptive use among women in the military and the general U.S. population. *Journal of Women's Health* 19(5):839-845.

Esmorís-Arranz, F. J., C. Méndez, and N. W. Spear. 2008. Contextual fear conditioning differs for infant, adolescent, and adult rats. *Behavioural Processes* 78(3):340-350.

Etkin, A., T. Egner, and R. Kalisch. 2011. Emotional processing in anterior cingulate and medial prefrontal cortex. *Trends in Cognitive Sciences* 15(2):85-93.

Feder, A., E. J. Nestler, and D. S. Charney. 2009. Psychobiology and molecular genetics of resilience. *Nature Reviews Neuroscience* 10(6):446-457.

Fennema-Notestine, C., M. B. Stein, C. M. Kennedy, S. L. Archibald, and T. L. Jernigan. 2002. Brain morphometry in female victims of intimate partner violence with and without posttraumatic stress disorder. *Biological Psychiatry* 52(11):1089-1101.

Fischer, H., L. Nyberg, and L. Backman. 2010. Age-related differences in brain regions supporting successful encoding of emotional faces. *Cortex* 46(4):490-497.

Flory, J. D., R. Yehuda, R. Grossman, A. S. New, V. Mitropoulou, and L. J. Siever. 2009. Childhood trauma and basal cortisol in people with personality disorders. *Comprehensive Psychiatry* 50(1):34-37.

Freeman, T., V. Roca, F. Guggenheim, T. Kimbrell, and W. S. Griffin. 2005. Neuropsychiatric associations of apolipoprotein E alleles in subjects with combat-related posttraumatic stress disorder. *Journal of Neuropsychiatry and Clinical Neurosciences* 17(4):541-543.

Frielingsdorf, H., K. G. Bath, F. Soliman, J. Difede, B. J. Casey, and F. S. Lee. 2010. Variant brain-derived neurotrophic factor VAL66MET endophenotypes: Implications for posttraumatic stress disorder. *Annals of the New York Academy of Sciences* 1208:150-157.

Frueh, B. C., P. B. Gold, and M. A. de Arellano. 1997. Symptom overreporting in combat veterans evaluated for PTSD: Differentiation on the basis of compensation seeking status. *Journal of Personality Assessment* 68(2):369-384.

Furmark, T., M. Tillfors, I. Marteinsdottir, H. Fischer, A. Pissiota, B. Langstrom, and M. Fredrikson. 2002. Common changes in cerebral blood flow in patients with social phobia treated with citalopram or cognitive-behavioral therapy. *Archive of General Psychiatry* 59(5):425-433.

Garakani, A., S. J. Mathew, and D. S. Charney. 2006. Neurobiology of anxiety disorders and implications for treatment. *Mount Sinai Journal of Medicine* 73(7):941-949.

Gelernter, J., S. Southwick, S. Goodson, A. Morgan, L. Nagy, and D. S. Charney. 1999. No association between D2 dopamine receptor (DRD2) 'A' system alleles, or DRD2 haplotypes, and posttraumatic stress disorder. *Biological Psychiatry* 45:620-625.

Gilbertson, M. W., M. E. Shenton, A. Ciszewski, K. Kasai, N. B. Lasko, S. P. Orr, and R. K. Pitman. 2002. Smaller hippocampal volume predicts pathologic vulnerability to psychological trauma. *Nature Neuroscience* 5:1242-1247.

Gillies, G. E., and S. McArthur. 2010. Estrogen actions in the brain and the basis for differential action in men and women: a case for sex-specific medicines. *Pharmacologic Reviews* 62(2):155-198.

Gogolla, N., P. Caroni, A. Lüthi, and C. Herry. 2009. Perineuronal nets protect fear memories from erasure. *Science* 325(5945)1258-1261.

Gold, A. L., L. M. Shin, S. P. Orr, M. A. Carson, S. L. Rauch, M. L. Macklin, N. B. Lasko, L. J. Metzger, D. D. Dougherty, N. M. Alpert, A. J. Fischman, and R. K. Pitman. 2011. Decreased regional cerebral blood flow in medial prefrontal cortex during trauma-unrelated stressful imagery in Vietnam veterans with post-traumatic stress disorder. *Psychological Medicine* 41(12):2563-2572.

Goldstein, J. M., M. Jerram, B. Abbs, S. Whitfield-Gabrieli, and N. Makris. 2010. Sex differences in stress response circuitry activation dependent on female hormonal cycle. *Journal of Neuroscience* 30(2):431-438.

Gomes, G. M., C. F. Mellow, M. M. da Rosa, G. V. Bochi, J. Ferreira, S. Barron, and M. A. Rubin. 2010. Polyaminergic agents modulate contextual fear extinction in rats. *Neurobiology of Learning and Memory* 93(4):589 595.

Goossens, L., S. Sunaert, R. Peeters, E. J. L. Griez, and K. R. J. Schruers. 2007. Amygdala hyperfunction in phobic fear normalizes after exposure. *Biological Psychiatry* 62(10): 1119-1125.

Gourley, S. L., A. T. Kedves, P. Olausson, and J. R. Taylor. 2009. A history of corticosterone exposure regulates fear extinction and cortical NR2B, GLUR2/3, and BDNF. *Neuropsychopharmacology* 34(3):707-716.

Grabe, H. J., C. Spitzer, C. Schwahn, A. Marcinek, A. Frahnow, S. Barnow, M. Lucht, H. J. Freyberger, U. John, H. Wallaschofski, H. Volzke, and D. Rosskopf. 2009. Serotonin transporter gene (SLC6A4) promoter polymorphisms and the susceptibility to posttraumatic stress disorder in the general population. *American Journal of Psychiatry* 166(8):926-933.

Graham, B. M., and M. R. Milad. 2011. Translational research in the neuroscience of fear extinction: Implications for anxiety disorders. *American Journal of Psychiatry* 168(12): 1255-1265.

Griesbach, G. S., D. A. Hovda, R. Molteni, A. Wu, and F. Gomez-Pinilla. 2004. Voluntary exercise following traumatic brain injury: Brain-derived neurotrophic factor upregulation and recovery of function. *Neuroscience* 125(1):129-139.

Hao, J., P. R. Rapp, A. E. Leffler, S. R. Leffler, W. G. Janssen, W. Lou, H. McKay, J. A. Roberts, S. L. Wearne, P. R. Hof, and J. H. Morrison. 2006. Estrogen alters spine number and morphology in prefrontal cortex of aged female rhesus moneys. *Journal of Neuroscience* 26(9):2571-2578.

Hartley, C. A., B. Fischl, and E. A. Phelps. 2011. Brain structure correlates of individual differences in the acquisition and inhibition of conditioned fear. *Cereberal Cortex* 21(9):1954-1962.

Heim, C., and C. B. Nemeroff. 2009. Neurobiology of posttraumatic stress disorder. *CNS Spectrums* 14(1):13-24.

Herry, C., F. Ferraguti, N. Singewald, J. J. Letzkus, I. Ehrlich, and A. Luthi. 2010. Neuronal circuits of fear extinction. *European Journal of Neuroscience* 31(4):599-612.

Hoffman, E. J., and S. J. Mathew. 2008. Anxiety disorders: A comprehensive review of pharmacotherapies. *Mount Sinai Journal of Medicine* 75(3):248-262.

Hoge, C. W., C. A. Castro, S. C. Messer, D. McGurk, D. I. Cotting, and R. L. Koffman. 2004. Combat duty in Iraq and Afghanistan, mental health problems, and barriers to care. *New England Journal of Medicine* 351(1):13-22.

Hoge, C. W., J. L. Auchterlonie, and C. S. Milliken. 2006. Mental health problems, use of mental health services, and attrition from military service after returning from deployment to Iraq or Afghanistan. *Journal of the American Medical Association* 295(9):1023-1032.

Hoge, E. A., J. J. Worthington, J. T. Nagurney, Y. Chang, E. B. Kay, C. M. Geterowski, A. R. Katzman, J. M. Goetz, M. L. Rosasco, N. B. Lasko, R. M. Zusman, M. H. Pollack, S. P. Orr, and R. K. Pitman. 2012. Effect of acute posttrauma propranolol on PTSD outcome and physiological responses during script-driven imagery. *CNS Neuroscience and Therapeutics* 18(1):21-27.

Holzel, B. K., U. Ott, T. Gard, H. Hempel, M. Weygandt, K. Morgen, and D. Vaitl. 2008. Investigation of mindfulness meditation practitioners with voxel-based morphometry. *Social Cognitive and Affective Neuroscience* 3(1):55-61.

Horvath, G. 2011. Neurochemistry of endogenous antinociception. *Advances in Neurobiology* 1:118.

Iidaka, T., T. Okada, T. Murata, M. Omori, H. Kosaka, N. Sadato, and Y. Yonekura. 2002. Age-related differences in the medial temporal lobe responses to emotional faces as revealed by fMRI. *Hippocampus* 12(3):352-362.

IOM (Institute of Medicine). 2007. *PTSD compensation and military service*. Washington, DC: The National Academies Press.

IOM. 2008. *Gulf War and health: Physiologic, psychologic, and psychosocial effects of deployment-related stress*. Washington, DC: The National Academies Press.

Isaac, F. 2011. The relationship between insomnia and depressive symptoms: Genuine or artifact? *Neuropsychiatric Disease and Treatment* 7:57-63.

Jovanovic, T., and K. J. Ressler. 2010. How the neurocircuitry and genetics of fear inhibition may inform our understanding of PTSD. *American Journal of Psychiatry* 167(6):648-662.

Jovanovic, T., S. D. Norrholm, J. E. Fennell, M. Keyes, A. M. Fiallos, K. M. Myers, M. Davis, and E. J. Duncan. 2009. Posttraumatic stress disorder may be associated with impaired fear inhibition: Relation to symptom severity. *Psychiatry Research* 167(1-2):151-160.

Kaczorowski, C. C., S. J. Davis, and J. R. Moyer, Jr. 2011. Aging redistributes medial prefrontal neuronal excitability and impedes extinction of trace fear conditioning. *Neurobiology of Aging* April 30 [Epub ahead of print].

Kalisch, R., E. Korenfeld, K. E. Stephan, N. Weiskopf, B. Seymour, and R. J. Dolan. 2006. Context-dependent human extinction memory is mediated by a ventromedial prefrontal and hippocampal network. *Journal of Neuroscience* 26(37):9503-9511.

Kaplan, G. B., J. J. Vasterling, and P. C. Vedak. 2010. Brain-derived neurotrophic factor in traumatic brain injury, post-traumatic stress disorder, and their comorbid conditions: Role in pathogenesis and treatment. *Behavioural Pharmacology* 21(5-6):427-437.

Kasai, K., H. Yamasue, M. W. Gilbertson, M. E. Shenton, S. L. Rauch, and R. K. Pitman. 2008. Evidence for acquired pregenual anterior vingulate gray matter loss from a twin study of combat-related posttraumatic stress disorder. *Biological Psychiatry* 63(6):550-556.

Kehne, J. H., and C. K. Cain. 2010. Therapeutic utility of non-peptidic CRF1 receptor antagonists in anxiety, depression, and stress-related disorders: Evidence from animal models. *Pharmacology & Therapeutics* 128(3):460-487.

Kessler, R. C., A. Sonnega, E. Bromet, M. Hughes, and C. B. Nelson. 1995. Posttraumatic stress disorder in the national comorbidity survey. *Archives of General Psychiatry* 52:1048-1060.

Khan, S., and I. Liberzon. 2004. Topiramate attenuates exaggerated acoustic startle in an animal model of PTSD. *Psychopharmacology* 172(2):225-229.

Kilpatrick, D. G., K. C. Koenen, K. J. Ruggiero, R. Acierno, S. Galea, H. S. Resnick, J. Roitzsch, J. Boyle, and J. Gelernter. 2007. The serotonin transporter genotype and social support and moderation of posttraumatic stress disorder and depression in hurricane-exposed adults. *American Journal of Psychiatry* 164(11):1693-1699.

Kilpatrick, L. A., B. Y. Suyenobu, S. R. Smith, J. A. Bueller, T. Goodman, J. D. Creswell, K. Tillisch, E. A. Mayer, and B. D. Naliboff. 2011. Impact of mindfulness-based stress reduction training on intrinsic brain connectivity. *Neuroimage* 56(1):290-298.

Kim, H. J., P. Leeds, and D. M. Chuang. 2009. The HDAC inhibitor, sodium butyrate, stimulates neurogenesis in the ischemic brain. *Journal of Neurochemistry* 110(4):1226-1240.

Kim, J. H., S. Li, and R. Richardson. 2011b. Immunohistochemical analyses of long-term extinction of conditioned fear in adolescent rats. *Cerebral Cortex* 23(3):530-538.

Kim, J. H., and R. Richardson. 2008. The effect of temporary amgydala inactivation on extinction and reextinction of fear in the developing rat: Unlearning as a potential mechanism for extinction early in development. *Journal of Neuroscience* 28(6):1282-1290.

Kim, J. H., and R. Richardson. 2010. Extinction in preweanling rats does not involve NMDA receptors. *Neurobiology of Learning and Memory* 94(2):176-182.

Kim, M. J., and P. J. Whalen. 2009. The structural integrity of an amygdala-prefrontal pathway predicts trait anxiety. *Journal of Neuroscience* 29(37):11614-11618.

Kim, M. J., D. G. Gee, R. A. Loucks, F. C. Davis, and P. J. Whalen. 2011a. Anxiety dissociates dorsal and ventral medial prefrontal cortex functional connectivity with the amygdala at rest. *Cerebral Cortex* 21(7):1667-1673.

Kitayama, N., V. Vaccarino, M. Kutner, P. Weiss, and J. D. Bremner. 2005. Magnetic resonance imaging (MRI) measurement of hippocampal volume in posttraumatic stress disorder: A meta-analysis. *Journal of Affective Disorders* 88(1):79-86.

Kitayama, N. S. Quinn, and J. D. Bremner. 2006. Smaller volume of anterior cingulate cortex in abuse-related posstraumatic stress disorder. *Journal of Affective Disorders* 90(2-3):171-174.

Koenen, K. C., G. Saxe, S. Purcell, J. W. Smoller, D. Bartholomew, A. Miller, E. Hall, J. Kaplow, M. Bosquet, S. Moulton, and C. Baldwin. 2005. Polymorphisms in FKBP5 are associated with peritraumatic dissociation in medically injured children. *Molecular Psychiatry* 10(12):1058-1059.

Koenen, K. C., S. D. Stellman, J. F. Sommer, Jr., and J. M. Stellman. 2008. Persisting posttraumatic stress disorder symptoms and their relationship to functioning in Vietnam veterans: A 14-year follow-up. *Journal of Traumatic Stress* 21(1):49-57.

Koenen, K. C., I. De Vivo, J. Rich-Edwards, J. W. Smoller, R. J. Wright, and S. M. Purcell. 2009a. Protocol for investigating genetic determinants of posttraumatic stress disorder in women from the Nurses' Health Study II. *BMC Pyschiatry* 9:29.

Koenen, K. C., T. E. Moffitt, A. L. Roberts, L. T. Martin, L. Kubzansky, H. Harrington, R. Poulton, and A. Caspi. 2009b. Childhood IQ and adult mental disorders: A test of the cognitive reserve hypothesis. *American Journal of Psychiatry* 166(1):50-57.

Koenen, K. C., A. Aiello, E. Bakshis, A. B. Amstadter, K. J. Ruggiero, R. Acierno, D. G. Kilpatrick, J. Gelernter, and S. Galea. 2009c. County-level social environment modifies the association between serotonin transporter genotype and risk of post-traumatic stress disorder in adults. *American Journal of Epidemiology* 169(6):704-711.

Koenen, K. C., M. Uddin, S. C. Chang, A. E. Aiello, D. E. Wildman, E. Goldmann, and S. Galea. 2011. Slc6a4 methylation modifies the effect of the number of traumatic events on risk for posttraumatic stress disorder. *Depression and Anxiety* 28(8):639-647.

Kolassa, I. T., V. Ertl, C. Eckart, F. Glockner, S. Kolassa, A. Papassotiropoulos, D. J. de Quervain, and T. Elbert. 2010a. Association study of trauma load and SLC6A4 promoter polymorphism in posttraumatic stress disorder: Evidence from survivors of the Rwandan genocide. *Journal of Clinical Psychiatry* 71(5):543-547.

Kolassa, I. T., S. Kolassa, V. Ertl, A. Papassotiropoulos, and D. J. De Quervain. 2010b. The risk of posttraumatic stress disorder after trauma depends on traumatic load and the catechol-O-methyltransferase val(158)met polymorphism. *Biological Psychiatry* 67(4): 304-308.

Koolhaas, J. M., A. Bartolomucci, B. Buwalda, S. F. de Boer, G. Flugge, S. M. Korte, P. Meerlo, R. Murison, B. Olivier, P. Palanza, G. Richter-Levin, A. Sgoifo, T. Steimer, O. Stiedl, G. van Dijk, M. Wohr, and E. Fuchs. 2011. Stress revisited: A critical evaluation of the stress concept. *Neuroscience and Biobehavioral Reviews* 35(5):1291-1301.

Kulka, R. A., W. E. Schlenger, J. A. Fairbank, R. L. Hough, B. K. Jordan, C. R. Marmar, and D. S. Weiss. 1990. *Trauma and the Vietnam War generation: Report of findings from the National Vietnam Veterans Readjustment Study*. New York: Bruner/Mazel.

Labar, K. S., C. A. Cook, D. C. Torpey, and K. A. Welsh-Bohmer. 2004. Impact of healthy aging on awareness and fear conditioning. *Behavioural Neuroscience* 118(5):905-915.

Lang, P. J., M. Davis, and A. Ohman. 2000. Fear and anxiety: Animal models and human cognitive psychophysiology. *Journal of Affective Disorders* 61(3):137-159.

Lappalainen, J., H. R. Kranzler, R. Malison, L. H. Price, D. Van Dyck, J. H. Krystal, and J. Gelernter. 2002. A functional neuropeptide Y *leu7pro* polymorphism associated with alcohol dependence in a large population sample from the United States. *Archives of General Psychiatry* 59:825-831.

Lavretsky, H., P. Siddarth, and M. R. Irwin. 2010. Improving depression and enhancing resilience in family dementia caregivers: A pilot randomized placebo-controlled trial of escitalopram. *American Journal of Geriatric Psychiatry* 18(2):154-162.

Ledgerwood, L., R. Richardson, and J. Cranney. 2005. D-cycloserine facilitates extinction of learned fear: Effects on reacquisition and generalized extinction. *Biological Psychiatry* 57(8):841-847.

LeDoux, J. E. 2000. Emotion circuits in the brain. *Annual Review of Neuroscience* 23:155-184.

Lee, H. J., M. S. Lee, R. H. Kang, H. Kim, S. D. Kim, B. S. Kee, Y. H. Kim, Y. K. Kim, J. B. Kim, B. K. Yeon, K. S. Oh, B. H. Oh, J. S. Yoon, C. Lee, H. Y. Jung, I. S. Chee, and I. H. Paik. 2005. Influence of the serotonin transporter promoter gene polymorphism on susceptibility to posttraumatic stress disorder. *Depression and Anxiety* 21(3):135-139.

Lee, H., R. Kang, S. Lim, J. Paik, M. Coi, and M. Lee. 2006. No association between the brain-derived nurotrophic factor gene val66met polymorphism and post-traumatic stress disorder. *Stress and Health* 22(2):115-119.

Lee, H., S. Kwak, J. Paik, R. Kang, and M. Lee. 2007. Association between serotonin 2a receptor gene polymorphism and posttraumatic stress disorder. *Psychiatry Investigations* 4(2):104-108.

Lemieux, A., C. L. Coe, and M. Carnes. 2008. Symptom severity predicts degree of T cell activation in adult women following childhood maltreatment. *Brain, Behavior, and Immunity* 22(6):994-1003.

Linnman, C., M. A. Zeidan, R. K. Pitman, and M. R. Milad. 2012. Resting cerebral metabolism correlates with skin conductance and functional brain activation during fear conditioning. *Biological Psychology* 89(2):450-459.

Lonsdorf, T. B., and R. Kalisch. 2011. A review on experimental and clinical genetic association studies on fear contitioning, extinction and cognitive-behavioral treatment. *Translational Psychiatric* 1(9):e41.

Lu, A. T., M. N. Ogdie, M. Jarvelin, I. K. Moilanen, S. K. Loo, J. T. McCracken, J. J. McGough, M. H. Yang, L. Peltonen, S. F. Nelson, R. M. Cantor, and S. L. Smalley. 2008. Association of the cannabinoid receptor gene (CNR1) with ADHD and post-traumatic stress disorder. *American Journal of Medical Genetics Part B: Neuropsychiatric Genetics* 147B(8):1488-1494.

Luo, H., X. Hu, X. Liu, X. Ma, W. Guo, C. Qiu, Y. Wang, Q. Wang, X. Zhang, W. Zhang, G. Hannum, K. Zhang, X. Liu, and T. Li. 2012. Hair cortisol level as a biomarker for altered hypothalamic-pituitary-adrenal activity in female adolescents with posttraumatic stress disorder after the 2008 Wenchuan earthquake. *Biological Psychiatry* Feb 1 [Epub ahead of print].

Maeng, L. Y., J. Waddell, and T. J. Shors. 2010. The prefrontal corex communicates with the amygdala to impair learning after acute stress in females but not in males. *Journal of Neuroscience* 30(48):16188-16196.

Mao, S. C., Y. H. Hsiao, and P. W. Gean. 2006. Extinction training in conjunction with a partial agonist of the glycine site on the NMDA receptor erases memory trace. *Journal of Neuroscience* 26(35):8892-8899.

Maren, S. 2001. Neurobiology of Pavlovian fear conditioning. *Annual Review of Neuroscience* 24:897-931.

Maren, S. 2011. Seeking a spotless mind: Extinction, deconsolidation, and erasure of fear memory. *Neuron* 70(5):830-845.

McEwen, B. S. 2005. Glucocorticoids, depression, and mood disorders: Structural remodeling in the brain. *Metabolism Clinical and Experimental* 54(Suppl 1):20-23.

McEwen, B. S. 2006. Protective and damaging effects of stress mediators: Central role of the brain. *Dialogues in Clinical Neuroscience* 8(4):367-381.

McGhee, L. L., C. V. Maani, T. H. Garza, K. M. Gaylord, and I. H. Black. 2008. The correlation between ketamine and posttraumatic stress disorder in burned service members. *Journal of Trauma* 64:S195-S198; Discussion S197-S198.

Mellman, T. A., T. Alim, D. D. Brown, E. Gorodetsky, B. Buzas, W. B. Lawson, D. Goldman, and D. S. Charney. 2009. Serotonin polymorphisms and posttraumatic stress disorder in a trauma exposed African American population. *Depression and Anxiety* 26(11):993-997.

Mercer, K. B., H. K. Orcutt, J. F. Quinn, C. A. Fitzgerald, K. N. Conneely, R. T. Barfield, C. F. Gillespie, and K. J. Ressler. 2011. Acute and posttraumatic stress symptoms in a prospective gene X environment study of a university campus shooting. *Archives of General Psychiatry* 69(1):89-97.

Meyerbroeker, K., M. B. Powers, A. van Stegeren, and P. M. Emmelkamp. 2012. Does yohimbine hydrochloride facilitate fear extinction in virtual reality treatment of fear of flying? A randomized placebo-controlled trial. *Psychotherapy and Psychosomantics* 81(1):29-37.

Milad, M. R., and G. J. Quirk. 2002. Neurons in medial prefrontal cortex signal memory for fear extinction. *Nature* 420(6911):70-74.

Milad, M. R., and G. J. Quirk. 2012. Fear extinction as a model for translational neuroscience: Ten years of progress. *Annual Review of Psychology* 63:129-151.

Milad, M. R., S. P. Orr, R. K. Pitman, and S. L. Rauch. 2005. Context modulation of memory for fear extinction in humans. *Psychophysiology* 42(4):456-464.

Milad, M. R., C. I. Wright, S. P. Orr, R. K. Pitman, G. J. Quirk, and S. L. Rauch. 2007. Recall of fear extinction in humans activates the ventromedial prefrontal cortex and hippocampus in concert. *Biological Psychiatry* 62(5):446-454.

Milad, M. R., S. P. Orr, N. B. Lasko, Y. C. Chang, S. L. Rauch, and R. K. Pitman. 2008. Presence and acquired origin of reduced recall for fear extinction in PTSD: Results of a twin study. *Journal of Psychiatric Research* 42(7):515-520.

Milad, M. R., S. A. Igoe, K. Lebron-Milad, and J. E. Novales. 2009a. Estrous cycle phase and gonadal hormones influence conditioned fear extinction. *Neuroscience* 164(3):887-895.

Milad, M. R., R. K. Pitman, C. B. Ellis, A. L. Gold, L. M. Shin, N. B. Lasko, M. A. Zeidan, K. Handwerger, S. P. Orr, and S. L. Rauch. 2009b. Neurobiological basis of failure to recall extinction memory in posttraumatic stress disorder. *Biological Psychiatry* 66(12):1075-1082.

Milad, M. R., M. A. Zeidan, A. Contero, R. K. Pitman, A. Klibanski, S. L. Rauch, and J. M. Goldstein. 2010. The influence of gonadal hormones on conditioned fear extinction in healthy humans. *Neuroscience* 168(3):652-658.

Mohammed, H. S., H. S. A. Ezz, Y. A. Khadrawy, and N. A. Noor. 2011. Neurochemical and electrophysiological changes induced by paradoxical sleep deprivation in rats. *Behavioural Brain Research* 225(1):39-46.

Morey, R. A., A. R. Hariri, A. L. Gold, M. A. Hauser, H. J. Munger, F. Dolcos, and G. McCarthy. 2011. Serotonin transporter gene polymorphisms and brain function during emotional distraction from cognitive processing in posttraumatic stress disorder. *BioMed Central Psychiatry* 11:76.

Morris, R. W., and M. E. Bouton. 2007. The effect of yohimbine on the extinction of conditioned fear: A role for context. *Behavioral Neuroscience* 121(3):501-514.

Mueller, D., L. A. Olivera-Figueroa, D. S. Pine, and G. J. Quirk. 2009. The effects of yohimbine and amphetamine on fear expression and extinction in rats. *Psychopharmacology* 204(4):599-606.

Mustapic, M., N. Pivac, D. Kozaric-Kovacic, M. Dezeljin, J. F. Cubells, and D. Muck-Seler. 2007. Dopamine beta-hydroxylase (DBH) activity and -1021c/t polymorphism of DBH gene in combat-related posttraumatic stress disorder. *American Journal of Medical Genetics Part B: Neuropsychiatric Genetics* 144B:1087-1089.

Myers, K. M., and M. Davis. 2007. Mechanisms of fear extinction. *Molecular Psychiatry* 12(2):120-150.

Myers, K. M., W. A. Carlezon, Jr., and M. Davis. 2011. Glutamate receptors in extinction and extinction-based therapies for psychiatric illness. *Neuropsychopharmacology* 36(1):274-293.

Nader, K., G. E. Schafe, and J. E. LeDoux. 2000. Fear memories require protein synthesis in the amygdala for reconsolidation after retrieval. *Nature* 406(6797):722-726.

Narasimhan, S., T. D. Aquino, R. Hodge, K. Rickels, and F. W. Lohoff. 2011. Association analysis between the val66met polymorphism in the brain-derived neurotrophic factor (BDNF) gene and treatment response to venlafaxine xr in generalized anxiety disorder. *Neuroscience Letters* 503(3):200-202.

Nelson, E. C., A. Agrawal, M. L. Pergadia, M. T. Lynskey, A. A. Todorov, J. C. Wang, R. D. Todd, N. G. Martin, A. C. Heath, A. M. Goate, G. W. Montgomery, and P. A. F. Madden. 2009. Association of childhood trauma exposure and GABRA2 polymorphisms with risk of posttraumatic stress disorder in adults. *Molecular Psychiatry* 14:234-238.

Nibuya, M., S. Morinobu, and R. S. Duman. 1995. Regulation of BDNF and TRKB mRNA in rat brain by chronic electroconvulsive seizure and antidepressant drug treatments. *Journal of Neuroscience* 15(11):7539-7547.

Nielsen, S. E., N. Ertman, Y. S. Lakhani, and L. Cahill. 2011. Hormonal contraception usage is associated with altered memory for an emotional story. *Neurobiology of Learning and Memory* 96(2):378-384.

Norberg, M. M., J. H. Krystal, and D. F. Tolin. 2008. A meta-analysis of D-cycloserine and the facilitation of fear extinction and exposure therapy. *Biological Psychiatry* 63(12): 1118-1126.

Norrholm, S. D., and T. Jovanovic. 2010. Tailoring therapeutic strategies for treating posttraumatic stress disorder symptom clusters. *Neuropsychiatric Disease and Treatment* 6:517-532.

Norrholm, S. D., T. Jovanovic, I. W. Olin, L. A. Sands, I. Karapanou, B. Bradley, and K. J. Ressler. 2011. Fear extinction in traumatized civilians with posttraumatic stress disorder: Relation to symptom severity. *Biological Psychiatry* 69(6):556-563.

Olff, M., G. J. de Vries, Y. Guzelcan, J. Assies, and B. P. R. Gersons. 2007. Changes in cortisol and DHEA plasma levels after psychotherapy for PTSD. *Psychoneuroendocrinology* 32(6):619-626.

Orr, S. P., L. J. Metzger, N. B. Lasko, M. L. Macklin, T. Peri, and R. K. Pitman. 2000. De novo conditioning in trauma-exposed individuals with and without posttraumatic stress disorder. *Journal of Abnormal Psychology* 109(2):290-298.

Pace-Schott, E. F., M. R. Milad, S. P. Orr, S. L. Rauch, R. Stickgold, and R. K. Pitman. 2009. Sleep promotes generalization of extinction of conditioned fear. *Sleep* 32(1):19-26.

Parnas, A. S., M. Weber, and R. Richardson. 2005. Effects of multiple exposures to D-cycloserine on extinction of conditioned fear in rats. *Neurobiology of Learning and Memory* 83(3):224-231.

Pavlov, I. P. 1927. *Conditioned reflexes: An investigation of the physiological activity of the cerebral cortex*. London, UK: Oxford University Press.

Peri, T., G. Ben-Shakhar, S. P. Orr, and A. Y. Shalev. 2000. Psychophysiologic assessment of aversive conditioning in posttraumatic stress disorder. *Biological Psychiatry* 47(6): 512-519.

Peters, J., L. M. Dieppa-Perea, L. M. Melendez, and G. J. Quirk. 2010. Induction of fear extinction with hippocampal-infralimbic BDNF. *Science* 328(5983):1288-1290.

Phan, K. L., D. A. Fitzgerald, P. J. Nathan, G. J. Moore, T. W. Uhde, and M. E. Tancer. 2005. Neural substrates for voluntary suppression of negative affect: A functional magnetic resonance imaging study. *Biological Psychiatry* 57(3):210-219.

Phan, K. L., J. C. Britton, S. F. Taylor, L. M. Fig, and I. Liberzon. 2006. Corticolimbic blood flow during nontraumatic emotional processing in posttraumatic stress disorder. *Archives of General Psychiatry* 63(2):184-192.

Phelps, E. A., M. R. Delgado, K. I. Nearing, and J. E. LeDoux. 2004. Extinction learning in humans: Role of the amygdala and VMPFC. *Neuron* 43(6):897-905.

Pissiota, A., O. Frans, M. Fernandez, L. von Knorring, H. Fischer, and M. Fredrikson. 2002. Neurofunctional correlates of posttraumatic stress disorder: A PET symptom provocation study. *European Archives of Psychiatry and Clinical Neuroscience* 252(2):68-75.

Pitman, R. K. 1988. Post-traumatic stress disorder, conditioning, and network theory. *Psychiatric Annals* 18(3):182-189.

Pitman, R. K., and D. L. Delahanty. 2005. Conceptually driven pharmacologic approaches to acute trauma. *CNS Spectrums* 10(2):99-106.

Pitman, R. K., K. M. Sanders, R. M. Zusman, A. R. Healy, F. Cheema, N. B. Lasko, L. Cahill, and S. P. Orr. 2002. Pilot study of secondary prevention of posttraumatic stress disorder with propranolol. *Biological Psychiatry* 51(2):189-192.

Ponomarev, I., V. Rau, E. I. Eger, R. A. Harris, and M. S. Fanselow. 2010. Amygdala transcriptome and cellular mechanisms underlying stress-enhanced fear learning in a rat model of posttraumatic stress disorder. *Neuropsychopharmacology* 35(6):1402-1411.

Powers, M. B., J. A. Smits, M. W. Otto, C. Sanders, and P. M. Emmelkamp. 2009. Facilitation of fear extinction in phobic participants with a novel cognitive enhancer: A randomized placebo controlled trial of yohimbine augmentation. *Journal of Anxiety Disorders* 23(3):350-356.

Protopopescu, X., H. Pan, M. Altemus, O. Tuescher, M. Polanecsky, B. McEwen, D. Silbersweig, and E. Stern. 2005. Orbitofrontal cortex activity related to emotional processing changes across the menstrual cycle. *Proceedings of the National Academy of Sciences of the United States of America* 102(44):16060-16065.

Putman, P., and K. Roelofs. 2011. Effects of single cortisol administrations on human affect reviewed: Coping with stress through adaptive regulatoin of automatic cognitive processing. *Psychoneuroendocrinology* 36(4):439-448.

Quirk, G. J. 2002. Memory for extinction of conditioned fear is long-lasting and persists following spontaneous recovery. *Learning & Memory* 9(6):402-407.

Quirk, G. J., and D. Mueller. 2008. Neural mechanisms of extinction learning and retrieval. *Neuropsychopharmacology* 33(1):56-72.

Rabinak, C. A., M. Angstadt, R. C. Welsh, A. E. Kenndy, M. Lyubkin, B. Martis, and K. L. Phan. 2011. Altered amygdala resting-state function connectivity in post-traumatic stress disorder. *Frontiers in Psychiatry* 2:62.

Radecki, D. T., L. M. Brown, J. Martinez, and T. J. Teyler. 2005. BDNF protects against stress-induced impairments in spatial learning and memory and LTP. *Hippocampus* 15(2):246-253.

Raskind, M. A., E. R. Peskind, E. D. Kanter, E. C. Petrie, A. Radant, C. E. Thompson, D. J. Dobie, D. Hoff, R. J. Rein, K. Straits-Troster, R. G. Thomas, and M. M. McFall. 2003. Reduction of nightmares and other PTSD symptoms in combat veterans by prazosin: A placebo-controlled study. *American Journal of Psychiatry* 160(2):371-373.

Raskind, M. A., E. R. Peskind, D. J. Hoff, K. L. Hart, H. A. Holmes, D. Warren, J. Shofer, J. O'Connell, F. Taylor, C. Gross, K. Rohde, and M. E. McFall. 2007. A parallel group placebo controlled study of prazosin for trauma nightmares and sleep disturbance in combat veterans with post-traumatic stress disorder. *Biological Psychiatry* 61(8):928-934.

Rasmusson, A. M., and D. S. Charney. 1997. Animal models of relevance to PTSD. *Annals of the New York Academy of Science* 821:332-351.

Rau, V., J. P. DeCola, and M. S. Fanselow. 2005. Stress-induced enhancement of fear learning: An animal model of posttraumatic stress disorder. *Neuroscience and Biobehavioral Reviews* 29(8):1207-1223.

Rauch, S., L. M. Shin, P. J. Whalen, and R. K. Pitman. 1998. Neuroimaging and the neuroanatomy of PTSD. *CNS Spectrums* 3(Suppl. 2):30-41.

Rauch, S. L., P. J. Whalen, L. M. Shin, S. C. McInerney, M. L. Macklin, N. B. Lasko, S. P. Orr, and R. K. Pitman. 2000. Exaggerated amygdala response to masked facial stimuli in posttraumatic stress disorder: A functional MRI study. *Biological Psychiatry* 47(9):769-776.

Rauch, S. L., L. M. Shin, E. Segal, R. K. Pitman, M. A. Carson, K. McMullin, P. J. Whalen, and N. Makris. 2003. Selectively reduced regional cortical volumes inpost-traumatic stress disorder. *Neuroreport* 14(7):913-916.

Rauch, S. L., L. M. Shin, and E. A. Phelps. 2006. Neurocircuitry models of posttraumatic stress disorder and extinction: Human neuroimaging research—past, present, and future. *Biological Psychiatry* 60(4):376-382.

Ressler, K. J. 2010. Amygdala activity, fear, and anxiety: Modulation by stress. *Biological Psychiatry* 67(12):1117-1119.

Ressler, K. J., K. B. Mercer, B. Bradley, T. Jovanovic, A. Mahan, K. Kerley, S. D. Norrholm, V. Kilaru, A. K. Smith, A. J. Myers, M. Ramirez, A. Engel, S. E. Hammack, D. Toufexis, K. M. Braas, E. B. Binder, and V. May. 2011. Post-traumatic stress disorder is associated with PACAP and the PAC1 receptor. *Nature* 470(7335):492-497.

Ridker, P. M. 2003. Clinical application of C-reactive protein for cardiovascular disease detection and prevention. *Circulation* 107(3):363-369.

Rodriguez-Romaguera, J., F. Sotres-Bayon, D. Mueller, and G. J. Quirk. 2009. Systemic propranolol acts centrally to reduce conditioned fear in rats without impairing extinction. *Biological Psychiatry* 65(10):887-892.

Rothbaum, B. O., and M. Davis. 2003. Applying learning principles to the treatment of post-trauma reactions. *Annals of the New York Academy of Sciences* 1008:112-121.

Sah, P., E. S. Faber, M. Lopez De Armentia, and J. Power. 2003. The amygdaloid complex: Anatomy and physiology. *Physiological Reviews* 83(3):803-834.

Sakai, Y., H. Kumano, M. Nishikawa, Y. Sakano, H. Kaiya, E. Imabayashi, T. Ohnishi, H. Matsuda, A. Yasuda, A. Sato, M. Diksic, and T. Kuboki. 2006. Changes in cerebral glucose utilization in patients with panic disorder treated with cognitive-behavioral therapy. *Neuroimage* 33(1):218-226.

Sayin, A., S. Kucukyildirim, T. Akar, Z. Bakkaloglu, A. Demircan, G. Kurtoglu, B. Demirel, S. Candansayar, and H. Mergen. 2010. A prospective study of serotonin transporter gene promoter (5-HTT gene linked polymorphic region) and intron 2 (variable number of tandem repeats) polymorphisms as predictors of trauma response to mild physical injury. *DNA and Cell Biology* 29(2):71-77.

Schelling, G., E. Kilger, B. Roozendaal, D. J. de Quervain, J. Briegel, A. Dagge, H. B. Rothenhausler, T. Krauseneck, G. Nollert, and H. P. Kapfhammer. 2004. Stress doses of hydrocortisone, traumatic memories, and symptoms of posttraumatic stress disorder in patients after cardiac surgery: A randomized study. *Biological Psychiatry* 55(6):627-633.

Schiller, D., M. H. Monfils, C. M. Raio, D. C. Johnson, J. E. Ledoux, and E. A. Phelps. 2010. Preventing the return of fear in humans using reconsolidation update mechanisms. *Nature* 463:49-53.

Segman, R. H., R. Cooper-Kazaz, F. Macciardi, T. Goltser, Y. Halfon, T. Dobroborski, and A. Y. Shalev. 2002. Association between the dopamine transporter gene and posttraumatic stress disorder. *Molecular Psychiatry* 7:903-907.

Segman, R. H., N. Shefi, T. Goltser-Dubner, N. Friedman, N. Kaminski, and A. Y. Shalev. 2005. Peripheral blood mononuclear cell gene expression profiles identify emergent posttraumatic stress disorder among trauma survivors. *Molecular Psychiatry* 10(5):500-513, 425.

Shansky, R. M., C. Hamo, P. R. Hof, W. Lou, B. S. McEwen, and J. H. Morrison. 2010. Estrogen promotes stress sensitivity in a prefrontal cortex-amygdala pathway. *Cerebral Cortex* 20(11):2560-2567.

Shi, Y., Y. Yuan, Z. Xu, M. Pu, C. Wang, Y. Zhang, Z. Liu, L. Li, and Z. Zhang. 2011. Genetic variation in the calcium/calmodulin-dependent protein kinase (CAMK) pathway is associated with antidepressant response in females. *Journal of Affective Disorders* 136(3):558-566.

Shin, L. M., and I. Liberzon. 2010. The neurocircuitry of fear, stress, and anxiety disorders. *Neuropsychopharmacology* 35(1):169-191.

Shin, L. M., S. P. Orr, M. A. Carson, S. L. Rauch, M. L. Macklin, N. B. Lasko, P. M. Peters, L. J. Metzger, D. D. Dougherty, P. A. Cannistraro, N. M. Alpert, A. J. Fischman, and R. K. Pitman. 2004. Regional cerebral blood flow in the amygdala and medial prefrontal cortex during traumatic imagery in male and female Vietnam veterans with PTSD. *Archives of General Psychiatry* 61(2):168-176.

Shin, L. M., C. I. Wright, P. A. Cannistraro, M. M. Wedig, K. McMullin, B. Martis, M. L. Macklin, N. B. Lasko, S. R. Cavanagh, T. S. Krangel, S. P. Orr, R. K. Pitman, P. J. Whalen, and S. L. Rauch. 2005. A functional magnetic resonance imaging study of amygdala and medial prefrontal cortex responses to overtly presented fearful faces in posttraumatic stress disorder. *Archives of General Psychiatry* 62(3):273-281.

Shin, L. M., S. L. Rauch, and R. K. Pitman. 2006. Amygdala, medial prefrontal cortex, and hippocampal function in PTSD. *Psychobiology of Posttraumatic Stress Disorder: A Decade of Progress* 1071:67-79.

Shin, K. M., N. B. Lasko, M. L. Macklin, R. D. Karpf, M. R. Milad, S. P. Orr, J. M. Goetz, A. J. Fischman, S. L. Rauch, and R. K. Pitman. 2009. Resting metabolic activity in the cingulate cortex and vulnerability to posttraumatic stress disorder. *Archives of General Psychiatry* 66(10):1099-1107.

Shin, L. M., G. Bush, M. R. Milad, N. B. Lasko, K. H. Brohawn, K. C. Hughes, M. L. Macklin, A. L. Gold, R. D. Karpf, S. P. Orr, S. L. Rauch, and R. K. Pitman. 2011. Exaggerated activation of dorsal anterior cingulate cortex during cognitive interference: A monozygotic twin study of posttraumatic stress disorder. *American Journal of Psychiatry* 168(9):979-985.

Siegmund, A., and C. T. Wotjak. 2006. Toward an animal model of posttraumatic stress disorder. *Annals of the New York Academy of Sciences* 1071:324-334.

Simmons, A. N., M. P. Paulus, S. R. Thorp, S. C. Matthews, S. B. Norman, and M. B. Stein. 2008. Functional activation and neural networks in women with posttraumatic stress disorder related to intimate partner violence. *Biological Psychiatry* 64(8):681-690.

Smith, A. K., K. N. Conneely, V. Kilaru, K. B. Mercer, T. E. Weiss, B. Bradley, Y. Tang, C. F. Gillespie, J. F. Cubells, and K. J. Ressler. 2011. Differential immune system DNA methylation and cytokine regulation in post-traumatic stress disorder. *American Journal of Medical Genetics Part B, Neuropsychiatric Genetics* 156(6):700-708.

Somerville, L. H., D. D. Wagner, G. S. Wig, J. M. Moran, P. J. Whalen, and W. M. Kelley. 2012. Interactions between transient and sustained neural signals support the generation and regulation of anxious emotion. *Cerebral Cortex* Jan 16 [Epub ahead of print].

Song, Y., D. Zhou, Z. Guan, and X. Wang. 2007. Disturbance of serum interleukin-2 and interleukin-8 levels in posttraumatic and non-posttraumatic stress disorder earthquake survivors in northern China. *Neuroimmunomodulation* 14(5):248-254.

Sotres-Bayon, F., L. Diaz-Mataix, D. E. Bush, and J. E. LeDoux. 2009. Dissociable roles for the ventromedial prefrontal cortex and amygdala in fear extinction: NR2B contribution. *Cerebral Cortex* 19(2):474-482.

Southwick, S. M., D. Bremner, J. H. Krystal, and D. S. Charney. 1994. Psychobiologic research in post-traumatic stress disorder. *Psychiatric Clinics of North America* 17(2):251-264.

Spoormaker, V. I., A. Sturm, K. C. Andrade, M. S. Schroter, R. Goya-Maldonado, F. Holsboer, T. C. Wetter, P. C. Samann, and M. Czisch. 2010. The neural correlates and temporal sequence of the relationship between shock exposure, disturbed sleep and impaired consolidation of fear extinction. *Journal of Psychiatric Research* 44(16):1121-1128.

Sripada, R. K., A. P. King, S. N. Garfinkel, X. Wang, C. S. Sripada, R. C. Welsh, and I. Liberzon. 2012. Altered resting-state amygdala functional connectivity in men with posttraumatic stress disorder. *Journal of Psychiatry and Neuroscience* 37(2):110069 [Epub ahead of print].

Stein, M. B., C. Koverola, C. Hanna, M. G. Torchia, and B. McClarty. 1997. Hippocampal volume in women victimized by childhood sexual abuse. *Psychological Medicine* 27(4):951-959.

Stein, M. B., C. Kerridge, J. E. Dimsdale, and D. B. Hoyt. 2007. Pharmacotherapy to prevent PTSD: Results from a randomized controlled proof-of-concept trial in physically injured patients. *Journal of Traumatic Stress* 20(6):923-932.

Steinhardt, M., and C. Dolbier. 2008. Evaluation of a resilience intervention to enhance coping strategies and protective factors and decrease symptomatology. *Journal of American College Health* 56(4):445-453.

Straube, T., H. J. Mentzel, and W. H. R. Miltner. 2006. Neural mechanisms of automatic and direct processing of phobogenic stimuli in specific phobia. *Biological Psychiatry* 59(2):162-170.

Strawn, J. R., and T. D. Geracioti, Jr. 2008. Noradrenergic dysfunction and the psychopharmacology of posttraumatic stress disorder. *Depression & Anxiety* 25(3):260-271.

Strigo, I. A., A. N. Simmons, S. C. Matthews, E. M. Grimes, C. B. Allard, L. E. Reinhardt, M. P. Paulus, and M. B. Stein. 2010. Neural correlates of altered pain response in women with posstraumatic stress disorder from intimate parner violence. *Biological Psychiatry* 65(5):442-450.

Su, T. P., L. Zhang, M. Y. Chung, Y. S. Chen, Y. M. Bi, Y. H. Chou, J. L. Barker, J. E. Barrett, D. Maric, X. X. Li, H. Li, M. J. Webster, D. Benedek, J. R. Carlton, and R. Ursano. 2009. Levels of the potential biomarker p11 in peripheral blood cells distinguish patients with PTSD from those with other major psychiatric disorders. *Journal of Psychiatric Research* 43(13):1078-1085.

Taylor, F. B., K. Lowe, C. Thompson, M. M. McFall, E. R. Peskind, E. D. Kanter, N. Allison, J. Williams, P. Martin, and M. A. Raskind. 2006. Daytime prazosin reduces psychological distress to trauma-specific cues in civilian trauma posttraumatic stress disorder. *Biological Psychiatry* 59(7):577-581.

Thakur, G. A., R. Joober, and A. Brunet. 2009. Development and persistence of posttraumatic stress disorder and the 5-HTTLPR polymorphism. *Journal of Traumatic Stress* 22(3):240-243.

Tranel, D., H. Damasio, N. L. Denburg, and A. Bechara. 2005. Does gender play a role in functional asymmetry of ventromedial prefrontal cortex? *Brain: A Journal of Neurology* 128(Pt 12):2872-2881.

Uddin, M., A. E. Aiello, D. E. Wildman, K. C. Koenen, G. Pawelec, R. de Los Santos, E. Goldmann, and S. Galea. 2010. Epigenetic and immune function profiles associated with posttraumatic stress disorder. *Proceedings of the National Academy of Sciences of the United States of America* 107(20):9470-9475.

Uddin, M., S. Galea, S. C. Chang, A. E. Aiello, D. E. Wildman, R. de los Santos, and K. C. Koenen. 2011. Gene expression and methylation signatures of MAN2C1 are associated with PTSD. *Disease Markers* 30(2-3):111-121.

Uher, R. 2011. Genes, environment, and individual differences in responding to treatment for depression. *Harvard Review of Psychiatry* 19(3):109-124.

Ursano, R. J., L. H. Zhang, C. J. Hough, C. S. Fullerton, D. M. Benedek, T. A. Grieger, and H. C. Holloway. 2008. Models of PTSD and traumatic stress: the importance of research "from bedside to bench to bedside." *Progress in Brain Research* 167:203-215.

Ursano, R. J., L. Zhang, H. Li, L. Johnson, J. Carlton, C. S. Fullerton, and D. M. Benedek. 2009. PTSD and traumatic stress from gene to community and bench to bedside. *Brain Research* 1293:2-12.

Valente, N. L., H. Vallada, Q. Cordeiro, K. Miguita, R. A. Bressan, S. B. Andreoli, J. J. Mari, and M. F. Mello. 2011. Candidate-gene approach in posttraumatic stress disorder after urban violence: Association analysis of the genes encoding serotonin transporter, dopamine transporter, and BDNF. *Journal of Molecular Neuroscience* 44(1):59-67.

Vanitallie, T. B. 2002. Stress: A risk factor for serious illness. *Metabolism* 51(6 Suppl 1):40-45.

Vermetten, E., and J. D. Bremner. 2002. Circuits and systems in stress. II. Applications to neurobiology and treatment in posttraumatic stress disorder. *Depression and Anxiety* 16(1):14-38.

Vidal-Gonzalez, I., B. Vidal-Gonzalez, S. L. Rauch, and G. J. Quirk. 2006. Microstimulation reveals opposing influences of prelimbic and infralimbic cortex on the expression of conditioned fear. *Learning & Memory* 13(6):728-733.

Vogt, B. A. 2005. Pain and emotion interactions in subregions of the cingulate gyrus. *Nature Reviews Neuroscience* 6(7):533-544.

Voisey, J., C. D. Swagell, I. P. Hughes, P. Morris, A. van Daal, E. P. Nobel, B. Kann, K. A. Heslop, R. M. Young, and B. R. Lawford. 2009. The DRD2 gene 957c>t polymorphism is associated with posttraumatic stress disorder in war veterans. *Depression and Anxiety* 26(1):28-33.

Voisey, J., C. D. Swagell, I. P. Hughes, J. P. Connor, B. R. Lawford, R. M. Young, and C. P. Morris. 2010. A polymorphism in the dysbindin gene (DTNBP1) associated with multiple psychiatric disorders including schizophrenia. *Behavioral and Brain Functions* 6:41.

Vythilingam, M., J. M. Gill, D. A. Luckenbaugh, P. W. Gold, C. Collin, O. Bonne, K. Plumb, E. Polignano, K. West, and D. Charney. 2010. Low early morning plasma cortisol in posttraumatic stress disorder is associated with co-morbid depression but not with enhanced glucocorticoid feedback inhibition. *Psychoneuroendocrinology* 35(3):442-450.

Walker, N., P. McConville, D. Hunter, I. J. Deary, and L. J. Whalley. 2002. Childhood mental ability and lifetime psychiatric contact: A 66-year follow-up study of the 1932 Scottish mental ability survey. *Intelligence* 30:233-245.

Wang, Z., T. C. Neylan, S. G. Mueller, M. Lenoci, D. Truran, C. R. Marmar, M. W. Weiner, and N. Schuff. 2010a. Magnetic resonance imaging of hippocampal subfields in posttraumatic stress disorder. *Archives of General Psychiatry* 67(3):296-303.

Wang, H. H., Z. J. Zhang, Q. R. Tan, H. Yin, Y. C. Chen, H. N. Wang, R. G. Zhang, Z. Z. Wang, L. Guo, L. H. Tang, and L. J. Li. 2010b. Psychopathological, biological, and neuroimaging characterization of posttraumatic stress disorder in survivors of a severe coalmining disaster in China. *Journal of Psychiatric Research* 44(6):385-392.

Wang, Z., D. G. Baker, J. Harrer, M. Hamner, M. Price, and A. Amstadter. 2011. The relationship between combat-related posttraumatic stress disorder and the 5-HTTLPR/RS25531 polymorphism. *Depression and Anxiety* 28(12):1067-1073.

Warner, C. H., G. N. Appenzeller, T. A. Grieger, S. Belenkly, J. Breitback, J. Parker, C. M. Warner, and C. W. Hoge. 2011. Importance of anonymity to encourage honest reporting in mental health screening after combat deployment. *Archives of General Psychiatry* 68:1065-1071.

Woods, A. M., and M. E. Bouton. 2006. D-cycloserine facilitates extinction but does not eliminate renewal of the conditioned emotional response. *Behavioral Neuroscience* 120(5): 1159-1162.

Woon, F., and D. W. Hedges. 2011. Gender does not moderate hippocampal volume deficits in adults with posttraumatic stress disorder: A meta-analysis. *Hippocampus* 31(3):243-252.

Wright, C. I., B. Martis, K. McMullin, L. M. Shin, and S. L. Rauch. 2003. Amygdala and insular responses to emotionally valenced human faces in small animal-specific phobia. *Biological Psychiatry* 54(10):1067-1076.

Xie, P., H. R. Kranzler, J. Poling, M. B. Stein, R. F. Anton, K. Brady, R. D. Weiss, L. Farrer, and J. Gelernter. 2009. Interactive effect of stressful life events and the serotonin transporter 5-HTTLPR genotype on posttraumatic stress disorder diagnosis in 2 independent populations. *Archives of General Psychiatry* 66(11):1201-1209.

Xie, P., H. R. Kranzler, J. Poling, M. B. Stein, R. F. Anton, L. A. Farrer, and J. Gelernter. 2010. Interaction of FKBP5 with childhood adversity on risk for post-traumatic stress disorder. *Neuropsychopharmacology* 35(8):1684-1692.

Xu, Z., Z. Zhang, Y. Shi, M. Pu, Y. Yuan, X. Zhang, and L. Li. 2011a. Influence and interaction of genetic polymorphisms in catecholamine neurotransmitter systems and early life stress on antidepressant drug response. *Journal of Affective Disorders* 133(1-2):165-173.

Xu, Z., Z. Zhang, Y. Shi, M. Pu, Y. Yuan, X. Zhang, L. Li, and G. P. Reynolds. 2011b. Influence and interaction of genetic polymorphisms in the serotonin system and life stress on antidepressant drug response. *Journal of Psychopharmacology* 133(1-2):165-173.

Yamamoto, S., S. Morinobu, S. Takei, M. Fuchikami, A. Matsuki, S. Yamawaki, and I. Liberzon. 2009. Single prolonged stress: Toward an animal model of posttraumatic stress disorder. *Depression & Anxiety* 26(12):1110-1117.

Yehuda, R. 2009. Status of glucocorticoid alterations in post-traumatic stress disorder. *Glucocorticoids and Mood Clinical Manifestations, Risk Factors, and Molecular Mechanisms* 1179:56-69.

Yehuda, R., E. L. Giller, S. M. Southwick, M. T. Lowy, and J. W. Mason. 1991. Hypothalamic pituitary-adrenal dysfunction in posttraumatic-stress-disorder. *Biological Psychiatry* 30(10):1031-1048.

Yehuda, R., S. Southwick, E. L. Giller, X. Ma, and J. W. Mason. 1992. Urinary catecholamine excretion and severity of PTSD symptoms in Vietnam combat veterans. *Journal of Nervous and Mental Disease* 180(5):321-325.

Yehuda, R., S. L. Halligan, R. Grossman, J. A. Golier, and C. Wong. 2002. The cortisol and glucocorticoid receptor response to low dose dexamethasone administration in aging combat veterans and holocaust survivors with and without posttraumatic stress disorder. *Biological Psychiatry* 52(5):393-403.

Yehuda, R., G. Cai, J. A. Golier, C. Sarapas, S. Galea, M. Ising, T. Rein, J. Schmeidler, B. Muller-Myhsok, F. Holsboer, and J. D. Buxbaum. 2009. Gene expression patterns associated with posttraumatic stress disorder following exposure to the World Trade Center attacks. *Biological Psychiatry* 66(7):708-711.

Yehuda, R., L. M. Bierer, L. C. Pratchett, and M. Pelcovitz. 2010. Using biological markers to inform a clinically meaningful treatment response. *Annals of the New York Academy of Sciences* 1208:158-163.

Yin, Y., L. Li, C. Jin, X. Hu, L. Duan, L. T. Eyler, Q. Gong, M. Song, T. Jiang, M. Liao, Y. Zhang, and W. Li. 2011. Abnormal baseline brain activity in posttraumatic stress disorder: a resting-state functional magnetic resonance imaging study. *Neuroscience Letters* 498(3):185-189.

Young, B. R., B. R. Lawford, E. P. Noble, B. Kanin, A. Wilkie, T. Ritchie, L. Arnold, and S. Shadforth. 2002. Harmful drinking in military veterans with posttraumatic stress disorder: Association with the D2 dopamine receptor a1 allele. *Alcohol and Alcoholism* 37(5):451-456.

Zeidan, M. A., S. A. Igoe, C. Linnman, A. Vitalo, J. B. Levine, A. Klibanski, J. M. Goldstein, and M. R. Milad. 2011. Estradiol modulates medial prefrontal cortex and amygdala activity during fear extinction in women and female rats. *Biological Psychiatry* 70(10): 920-927.

Zieker, J., D. Zieker, A. Jatzko, J. Dietzsch, K. Nieselt, A. Schmitt, T. Bertsch, K. Fassbender, R. Spanagel, H. Northoff, and P. J. Gebicke-Haerter. 2007. Differential gene expression in peripheral blood of patients suffering from post-traumatic stress disorder. *Molecular Psychiatry* 12(2):116-118.

Zohar, J., H. Yahalom, N. Kozlovsky, S. Cwikel-Hamzany, M. A. Matar, Z. Kaplan, R. Yehuda, and H. Cohen. 2011. High dose hydrocortisone immediately after trauma may alter the trajectory of PTSD: Interplay between clinical and animal studies. *European Neuropsychopharmacology* 21(11):796-809.

4

Programs and Services for PTSD in the Department of Defense and the Department of Veterans Affairs

This chapter introduces the programs and services provided by the Department of Defense (DoD) and the Department of Veterans Affairs (VA) health care systems with a special emphasis on care of those who have posttraumatic stress disorder (PTSD). The two health care systems are distinct entities that serve different, but at times overlapping, populations. Together they cover the many stages of a military career, including service on multiple bases, service in the theater of war, the transition from the DoD to the VA, and being a veteran (see Figure 4-1).

The chapter first provides an introduction to the DoD health care system, a summary of current PTSD programs for prevention or resilience, screening, diagnosis, and treatment in the DoD (including on base, off base, and in the theater of war); and a brief discussion of training opportunities for PTSD treatment. It then focuses on the transition between the DoD and the VA health care systems before providing an introduction to the VA health care system; a summary of current PTSD programs for resilience, screening, diagnosis, and treatment in the VA; and a discussion of training in evidence-based PTSD treatments. The chapter ends with a short discussion of current and future research directions and cost considerations for mental health care.

THE DEPARTMENT OF DEFENSE HEALTH CARE SYSTEM

The DoD is tasked with providing "the military forces needed to deter war and to protect the security of our country" (DoD, 2012). Its mission is carried out by more than 1.4 million active-duty personnel and 1.1 mil-

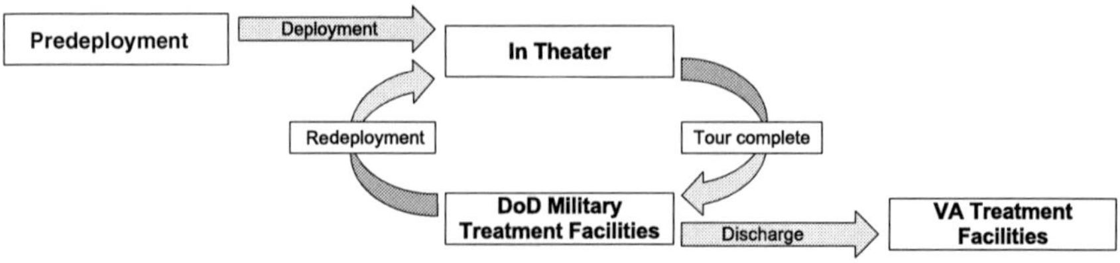

FIGURE 4-1 Potential points of mental health contact for service members during their careers.

lion reservists who serve domestically and internationally for a variety of purposes, from fighting wars to humanitarian and peace-keeping missions (DoD, 2012). The military consists of three departments—the Army, the Navy (which includes the Marine Corps), and the Air Force. Although all branches have a reserve component, only the Army and the Air Force have a National Guard component. Active-duty service members are employed full-time in the military, but members of the National Guard and reserve components serve in the military on a part-time basis. In general, they are required to work one weekend each month and serve a 2-week active-duty tour each year. The National Guard is under state jurisdiction unless federally activated. National Guard and reservists live in the civilian community (not on bases), work in civilian jobs, and do not have continuous access to DoD sources of health care (unless they are on active duty). The availability of health care for National Guard and Reservists is discussed in more detail later in this chapter.

The Military Health System (MHS) provides many health programs and services in an effort to keep active service members, retired personnel, and their families healthy. Overseen by the Office of the Assistant Secretary of Defense for Health Affairs, the MHS is responsible for maintaining the readiness of military personnel by promoting physical and mental fitness, providing emergency and long-term casualty care, and ensuring the delivery of health care to all service members, retirees, and their families through coordinated efforts of the medical departments of the Army, Navy (includes the Marine Corps), and Air Force; the joint chiefs of staff, the combatant command surgeons; and private-sector health care providers, hospitals, and pharmacies (IOM, 2010a). Figure 4-2 shows the organizational structure of the major health care services provided by the DoD. In addition to several offices and programs, the MHS provides health care services through several military-wide organizations: Force Health Protection and Readiness, Defense Centers of Excellence for Psychological Health and Traumatic Brain Injury (DCoE), Uniformed Services University of the Health Sciences

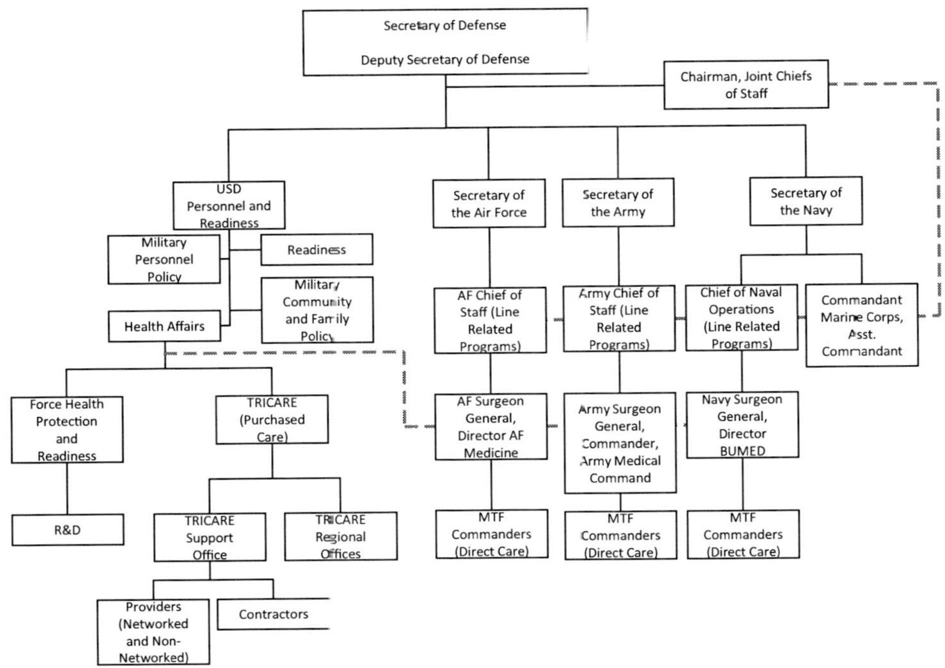

FIGURE 4-2 Organization of health care services provided by the DoD. The Office of the Assistant Secretary of Defense for Health Affairs oversees Force Health Protection and Readiness programs and the purchased portion of TRICARE, and it has an administrative and policy relationship to the military treatment facilities (MTFs) (as indicated by the dotted line).
NOTE: BUMED = Bureau of Medicine and Surgery, R&D = Research and Development, USD = Undersecretary of Defense.
SOURCE: Glover et al., 2011.

(USUHS), and TRICARE (DoD, 2012). A description of each of those organizations is in Table 4-1.

Although TRICARE is sometimes used to describe only purchased care, its network of services and programs is far reaching. The present committee uses the term *TRICARE* in a broader sense: as a wide-reaching health care provider for service members, retirees, and their families that delivers *direct care* through military treatment facilities (MTFs) and *purchased care* through network and non-network civilian health professionals, hospitals, and pharmacies (TRICARE, 2011). The relationship between TRICARE and MTFs is shown in Figure 4-2. The purchased care portion of TRICARE offers three primary plans: TRICARE Standard, TRICARE Extra, and TRICARE Prime (see TRICARE, 2011, for details of these three primary plans). To enroll in any TRICARE plan, service members, their families, and retirees must first establish eligibility through the Defense Enrollment Eligibility Reporting System. Active-duty service members, veterans, and reservists who have been activated for at least 30 consecutive days are automatically enrolled, but service members must register family members and update their status.

In FY 2011, about 9.7 million beneficiaries were eligible for DoD medical care, and 5.5 million beneficiaries were enrolled in TRICARE. Care of beneficiaries was provided through a network of 59 hospitals and medical centers and 363 health clinics in the direct-care system, and almost 380,000 individual providers and more than 3,000 network acute-care hospitals in the purchased-care system. There has been an increase in the number of TRICARE enrollees (particularly retirees) assigned to civilian primary-care managers because of a continued lack of resources and capacity in MTFs. Of the 9.7 million beneficiaries in the United States, about 34% were retirees and family members under 65 years old, 21% were retirees and family members 65 years old or older, 21% were active-duty family members, 14% were active-duty service members, 6% were National Guard or reserve family members, and 4% were members of the National Guard or reserves (TRICARE, 2011).

MENTAL HEALTH CARE IN THE DEPARTMENT OF DEFENSE

TRICARE authorizes a wide spectrum of practitioners to provide mental health care to its beneficiaries, including "psychiatrists and other physicians, clinical psychologists, certified psychiatric nurse specialists, clinical social workers, certified marriage and family therapists, pastoral counselors, and mental health counselors" (IOM, 2010b). The authorized practitioners may deliver inpatient or outpatient care (including mental health care, such as psychotherapy, psychoanalysis, testing, and medication

TABLE 4-1 Mental Health Components of the Military Health System

MHS Component Organizations	Descriptions
TRICARE	TRICARE is a "health care plan using military health care as the main delivery system." It is "augmented by a civilian network of providers and facilities" and provides services to the "uniformed services, activated National Guard and Reserve, retired military, and their families worldwide" (TRICARE, 2012).
Force Health Protection and Readiness	"The Deputy Assistant Secretary of Defense (DASD) for Force Health Protection and Readiness (FHP&R) is the principal staff assistant and advisor to the Assistant Secretary of Defense (Health Affairs) for all medically related Department of Defense policies, programs, and activities. The office is responsible for deployment medicine, force health protection, medical readiness, international health agreements, deployment related health policy, theater information systems, humanitarian and health missions, and national disaster support" (FHP&R, 2012).
Defense Centers of Excellence for Psychological Health and Traumatic Brain Injury	DCoE "assesses, validates, oversees and facilitates prevention, resilience, identification, treatment, outreach, rehabilitation, and reintegration programs for psychological health (PH) and traumatic brain injury (TBI) to ensure the Department of Defense meets the needs of the nation's military communities, warriors and families" (DCoE, 2012a).
Uniformed Services University of the Health Sciences	The USUHS is the nation's federal health sciences university. It is focused on education, research, service, and consultation specifically as they are related to military medicine, disaster medicine, military medical readiness, and public health during peace and war (USUHS, 2012).
Surgeons general of each service	The organization of the MHS includes the surgeons general of the Army, Navy, Air Force, and Coast Guard. In the Army and Navy, these three-star generals also have command of their medical personnel, clinics, and hospitals. In all branches, the surgeons general have overall responsibility for the medical operations within their specific branches.
MHS offices and programs	MHS offices and programs include • Chief Human Capital Office • Clinical and Program Policy • Council of Review Boards • Defense Health Board • Information Management • Innovation Investment Process • inTransition • Office of Strategy Management • Patient Safety Program • Physical Disability Board of Review

management), acute care, psychiatric partial hospitalization, and residential treatment center care.

Mental health care can also be described in terms of preclinical and clinical care. Preclinical care is commonly called *counseling*, and the several types of counseling are usually loosely defined. For example, service members and their families have the opportunity to seek counseling from chaplains, unit-embedded mental health care providers, community service programs (Tanielian and Jaycox, 2008) and from such facilities as Marine Corps counseling centers. The more formal route for clinical care is generally through MTFs in outpatient clinic or inpatient psychiatric-ward settings (Tanielian and Jaycox, 2008). Costs of intensive outpatient programs for mental health care that have become common in the private sector and the VA may not be reimbursed under TRICARE. Instead, patients may need to be referred to residential or inpatient care, which can be much more expensive and farther away from home (DoD, 2007).

In response to previous reports that noted particular problems with the education on and implementation of evidence-based practice guidelines (DoD, 2007; IOM, 2006), the MHS has worked to improve in these respects. On the basis of recommendations from the DoD Task Force on Mental Health (DoD, 2007), the MHS is pursuing implementation of evidence-based practices, training and education, quality measures, and monitoring (IOM, 2010a). The MHS has resolved to improve primary care for mental health conditions by 2016. It also aims to make improvements by increasing the number of providers that accept the purchased-care portion of TRICARE by "bridging cultural differences between military and civilian providers" and by increasing outreach to civilian providers (TRICARE, 2011).

The DoD is also concerned with mental health care in the theater of war and has undertaken research to try to gain a better understanding of this topic. Since 2003, mental health advisory teams (MHATs) have been assembled annually in Iraq and, beginning in 2007, in Afghanistan to obtain information on symptoms of PTSD, anxiety, and depression; on barriers to care (including stigma); and on other mental health care issues in the theater of war. The first three MHATs were sponsored by the U.S. Army surgeon general and focused solely on Army soldiers. Starting with MHAT IV in 2006, both soldiers and marines were sampled. In 2010, the MHAT team included representation of the Army, Navy, and Air Force. It collected anonymous survey results from soldiers and marines and from behavioral health personnel in an effort to assess theater-wide mental health and well-being, to examine the delivery of behavioral health care, and to provide recommendations for sustainment and improvement of mental health care (MHAT VII, 2011). It was found that about 20% of service members reported symptoms of acute stress (PTSD), depression, or anxiety; that higher rates of psychologic problems and lower morale are associated with longer deployments, multiple deployments, and greater time away from base camp; and that good leadership provides the support necessary to promote positive mental health and well-being in the deployed (MHAT VII, 2011).

Services and Programs for PTSD

This section gives some examples of PTSD services and programs that are commonly used in the DoD and provides an overview of the pathways through which a service member is screened for PTSD, a diagnosis is made, and treatment is instituted; it is not a catalog of all PTSD services and programs provided by the DoD. It should be noted that no single source within the DoD or any of the service branches maintains a complete list of such programs, tracks the development of new or emerging programs, or has appropriate resources in place to direct service members to programs that may best meet their individual needs. However, a recent review by Weinick et al. (2011) includes a list of DoD programs that address psychologic health and traumatic brain injury. Of the 211 programs identified in the review, 103 were PTSD-related programs for service members, veterans, civilians, and their families. See Appendix C for a list of the PTSD-specific programs offered in the DoD. (For a list of all programs in the DoD that address psychologic health [including PTSD] and traumatic brain injury of U.S. service members, veterans, and their families, see Appendixes A.1, A.2, A.3, and A.4 of Weinick et al. [2011].)

Resilience Programs

DoD resilience programs help to prepare service members for stressful encounters and traumatic events while they serve on military missions. The goal of such programs is to reduce the number of service members who develop mental health problems and to keep all service members as physically and mentally fit as possible during deployment. DoD Directive 6490.05 implemented combat and operational stress control (COSC) programs for all services. Directive 6490.05 was reissued as Instruction 6490.05 (November 22, 2011) *Maintenance of Psychological Health in Military Operations* "to enhance readiness, contribute to combat effectiveness, enhance the physical and mental health of military personnel, and prevent or minimize adverse effects associated with combat and operational stress" (DoD, 2011a). It included principles for COSC, procedures for COSC-specific education programs, guidance for military leaders (including a command that leaders ensure access to mental health services without stigma), a model for delivering COSC programs, and guidance on surveillance and monitoring. In addition, the instruction established specific requirements for the early detection and management of any "physical, emotional, cognitive or behavioral reactions, adverse consequences, or psychological injuries of service members who have been exposed to stressful or traumatic events in combat or military operations" (DoD, 2011a).

The Navy and Marine Corps have a strong COSC program called Operational Stress Control and Readiness (OSCAR), which has two specific goals: to maintain an active force and to promote the health of service members and their family members. The program works through mentors who try to identify and assist fellow service members who have combat and operational stress problems, extenders who are nonmental health clinicians or chaplains, and embedded mental health personnel (Meredith et al., 2011; U.S. Marine Corps, 2012). One resource through which Navy and Marine Corps members can find assistance for mental health concerns is the Naval Center for Combat and Operational Stress Control, which is part of the Navy Bureau of Medicine and Surgery. The center promotes psychologic resilience, recommends best practices for the diagnosis of and treatment for PTSD, seeks to reduce stigma for service members who are looking for or receiving mental health care, and provides support for family members.

In the Air Force, traumatic stress response teams have been established to provide support to service members that are expected to be exposed to traumatic situations (U.S. Air Force, 2006). The teams provide pre-exposure consultations to units and communities and implement combat stress control programs.

The Army has a long history of COSC and other resilience programs and services that target prevention of PTSD and other stress reactions. It is working to integrate a program called Comprehensive Soldier Fitness into basic training. Comprehensive Soldier Fitness is "a structured, long-term assessment and development program to build the resilience and enhance the performance of every Soldier, Family member, and [Department of the Army] civilian" (U.S. Army, 2012a). The program, which began in 2009, focuses on positive psychology and building resilience. It includes an assessment tool that provides a baseline for a soldier's emotional, social, spiritual, and family strengths. Specific resilience modules include institutional (life-cycle) resilience training that is specific to the different phases of a soldier's career; operational (deployment-cycle) resilience training that prepares a soldier for deployment; and family resilience training that prepares a soldier and his or her family for the transition back from deployment. There has been some controversy over the Comprehensive Soldier Fitness model. Brunwasser et al. (2009) completed a meta-analysis to evaluate the effectiveness of the Penn Resiliency Program, the program on which Comprehensive Soldier Fitness was based, for alleviating symptoms of depression in youth; they concluded that the program showed modest and inconsistent results. The Comprehensive Soldier Fitness program is not a research program, but there are concerns that it was launched without pilot testing, that it was based on a model that was developed for a different population, and that there are few data to indicate whether it promotes resilience (Eidelson, 2011; Quick, 2011). Some of the concerns have been addressed by the Office of Comprehensive Soldier Fitness, as described by Seligman (2011). (See Chapter 5 for further discussion on prevention programs in the DoD.)

Screening and Diagnosis

The DoD has implemented a series of screenings and assessments during the deployment cycle—the pre-deployment health assessment, the post-deployment health assessment (PDHA), and the post-deployment health reassessment (PDHRA). The pre-deployment health assessment was initiated in 1998 and is administered within 60 days before deployment. It documents general health information on each service member. A health care provider reviews the service member's responses and may refer him or her for further evaluation if a health concern that may potentially affect the service member's ability to deploy is identified. However, there is only one mental health question: "During the past year, have you sought counseling or care for your mental health?" This question is of limited usefulness for the assessment of predeployment mental health concerns (see Chapter 6 for more discussion of predeployment screening). An affirmative response to the question results in referral for an interview by a trained medical provider who may then sign a form indicating medical readiness for deployment.

During the 1990–1991 Gulf War, no system or screen was in place to document exposure to environmental toxicants and therefore no records to indicate exposures in the case of later claims of "Gulf War syndrome." To try to prevent that type of problem in the future, the PDHA was created and implemented in 1998. The assessment is given to service members within 30 days after they leave their assigned posts or after their return from deployment. It documents exposure to toxic substances, such as petroleum and chemical weapons, and questions on PTSD, depression, and suicide were added in later iterations (GAO, 2008b). The PTSD questions (questions 10–14 on the screen) were drawn from standardized scales for PTSD and depression with input from civilian and military subject-matter experts. A service member completes the assessment independently, and a health care provider then reviews the form, interviews the service member about any identified deployment-related concerns, and makes referrals for further evaluation if it is appropriate (GAO, 2008b).

In 2003, discussions regarding people who had various symptoms that emerged months after they returned from deployment took place. To capture the population, the DoD developed the PDHRA and began its implementation in 2005. Standard PTSD and depression questions were added in later updates (questions 11, 12a–d, and 14a–b on the screen). The assessment is administered 3–6 months after deployment and focuses on latent health concerns of service members that have emerged after deployment. Like the pre-deployment health assessment and the PDHA, the PDHRA is first completed by the service member, who is then interviewed by a health care provider about any deployment-related health concerns. If it is appropriate, the service member is referred for further evaluation. The PDHRA was first fielded in the Army in 2005 and is now administered in all the services, including the National Guard and reserve components. Because many service members have had repeat deployments, many have multiple forms on file. Information from these screening instruments is centralized in a database maintained by the Armed Forces Surveillance Center, which allows researchers and health care providers to review them on a population basis and individually.

About one-fourth of those deployed to Iraq and Afghanistan have been National Guard and reservists (IOM, 2010b). Like active-duty service members, National Guard and reserve service members are required to complete the predeployment and postdeployment health assessments. Because the PDHRA is administered 3–6 months after return from deployment and National Guard and reserve service members may have returned to their civilian roles by that time, the PDHRA may be administered on drill weekends or by telephone.

In 2006, the Periodic Health Assessment (PHA) was initiated for all active-duty and selected reserve service members (DoD, 2004, 2006). Those "who are not TRICARE beneficiaries and not eligible for services under any DoD program, but who require further evaluations, treatments, care, or clinical preventive services should be referred to their civilian health care providers" (DoD, 2006). Reservists who are not part of the selected group are given a similar periodic examination, the Reserve Component Periodic Health Assessment. Both health assessments are annual screens to assess changes in health status and medical readiness, especially changes in health that may affect a service member's ability to perform military duties. The PHA and the Reserve Component Periodic Health Assessment are given by a health care provider and include information about current and previous medical conditions, laboratory tests and other screening results (for example, tests for cholesterol and triglycerides, vision, hearing, and dental conditions), immunizations, and health behaviors (for example, tobacco use, alcohol and substance dependence, occupational stresses, suicidal ideation, and other mental health concerns). The health care provider reviews the medical record and makes referrals for additional care or evaluation as necessary (GAO, 2008a). The benefit of the annual screen for all service members is that it identifies changes in health status in people who have not been recently deployed.

The committee heard during its open sessions about the controversy associated with receiving a diagnosis of PTSD during deployment. In combat settings, military mental health providers assess fitness for duty and work with commanders who are focused on maintaining readiness, combat power, and unit cohesion (Warner et al., 2011). Although traumatic-event management—whose purpose is to decrease the effect of the potentially traumatic event and prevent long-term adverse consequences—is provided to individuals and units after an incident, military mental health providers may be hesitant to diagnosis acute stress disorder (ASD) or PTSD in a war zone. The committee heard that some possible explanations for this reluctance include providers believing or being taught that PTSD cannot be diagnosed in the theater of war because the trauma is still ongoing, although the termination of potential trauma exposure is not part of the *Diagnostic and Statistical Manual of Mental Disorders, Fourth Edition* (*DSM-IV*) diagnostic criteria (APA, 2000); some providers may feel pressure to evacuate people who have PTSD from the theater of war, potentially adversely affecting unit cohesion and readiness; and providers are encouraged to use another less stigmatizing term for PTSD, such as combat stress reaction or adjustment reaction, to explain symptoms of ASD or PTSD. In some cases, the use of those terms might be accurate, but a potential consequence of not diagnosing ASD or PTSD is the subsequent failure to then use appropriate evidence-based treatments for these disorders. For example, combat stress reaction is treated through the use of the BICEPS model—brevity, immediacy, centrality or contact, expectancy, proximity, and simplicity. However, the BICEPS model does not include a recommendation for the use of evidence-based cognitive behavioral treatments for ASD or PTSD, and therefore, may result in the DoD overlooking or avoiding the use of treatments that appear to have the strongest evidence for their efficacy for the treatment of these disorders. Some mental health providers related concerns from service members who believed that focusing on their trauma while deployed would result in a loss of their ability to remain mission ready, and some mental health providers thought that effective treatments in combat settings would require hospitalization or aeromedical evacuation out of the theater of war, and that some treatments for ASD and PTSD might increase a service member's risk for suicide. However, mental health providers do not express the same reservations about the use of psychotropic and sleep medications by a deployed service member as they did about the use of cognitive behavioral therapy (CBT) in combat settings.

Screening for PTSD in the DoD most commonly uses questions from the Primary Care PTSD (PC-PTSD) screen that are incorporated into longer surveys (such as the PDHA and the PDHRA) or the PTSD Checklist.

However, committee expertise and interviews during the committee's visit to Fort Hood indicated that many patients who show symptoms of PTSD are not identified through screens but through a family care physician, self-referral, or referral from a family member, work colleague, or friend. After a service member screens positive for PTSD, whether through a screen or through an interview with a primary care provider, the service member is often referred to a mental health professional for evaluation. Patients who have been referred are to receive an initial evaluation within 24 hours and a full evaluation within 14 days after referral. The diagnosis of PTSD can be made only after a careful and comprehensive clinical evaluation performed by a qualified professional, such as a psychologist or psychiatrist. The interviewer should obtain details of chief complaints, lifetime history of exposures to trauma, frequency and severity of symptoms of PTSD and other morbidity, level of function (disability), quality of life, medical history and present health, family and supports, recreation, personal strengths and vulnerabilities, styles of coping with stress, and experiences in the military.

Many service members are returning from deployment in Operation Enduring Freedom (OEF) and Operation Iraqi Freedom (OIF), and a small percentage of them are returning with PTSD and mental health concerns. That is supported by data from a large population-based study of Army and Marine Corps service members after deployment (Hoge et al., 2006). The total study sample was made up of 16,318 OEF service members and 222,620 who served in OIF. The service members who screened positive for PTSD on the PDHA (two or more affirmative responses to the four questions) made up 4.7% of those deployed to Afghanistan and 9.8% of those deployed to Iraq (Hoge et al., 2006). In addition, data presented to the committee showed that although the percentage of service members who screen positive for PTSD on the PDHA or PDHRA has remained roughly constant over the last year (about 10% of service members returning from deployment report symptoms of PTSD), the number of referrals for additional evaluation or treatment increased from 20% in 2005 to 40% in 2009 (Dinneen, 2011). It should be noted that not everyone who is given a referral seeks treatment; 32% of those who are referred by MTFs for outpatient mental health care do not activate the referral. As of the first quarter of 2010, data indicate treatment rates are about 65% of those referred (Dinneen, 2011).

Treatment

Service members can be treated for PTSD in numerous services, programs, and settings, including counseling centers, general inpatient and outpatient mental health services, and specialized treatment programs. As previously mentioned, the committee did not create a catalog of all the services, programs, and settings. However, a recent review of programs and services for psychologic health in the DoD shows that 98 DoD programs are specific to PTSD care for service members (Weinick et al., 2011). They include programs that are DoD-wide and programs that are specific to the Army, Air Force, Navy, Marine Corps, reserves, or National Guard. Treatment for PTSD in the DoD is performed by a variety of health professionals, in the theater of war and in other settings on and off base. Many service members who have a diagnosis of PTSD receive counseling, medication, or both at an outpatient setting through a mental health department (DCoE, 2012b; VA, 2012a). Figure 4-3 illustrates the different treatment pathways available to service members who seek treatment for PTSD, and the pathways are discussed below.

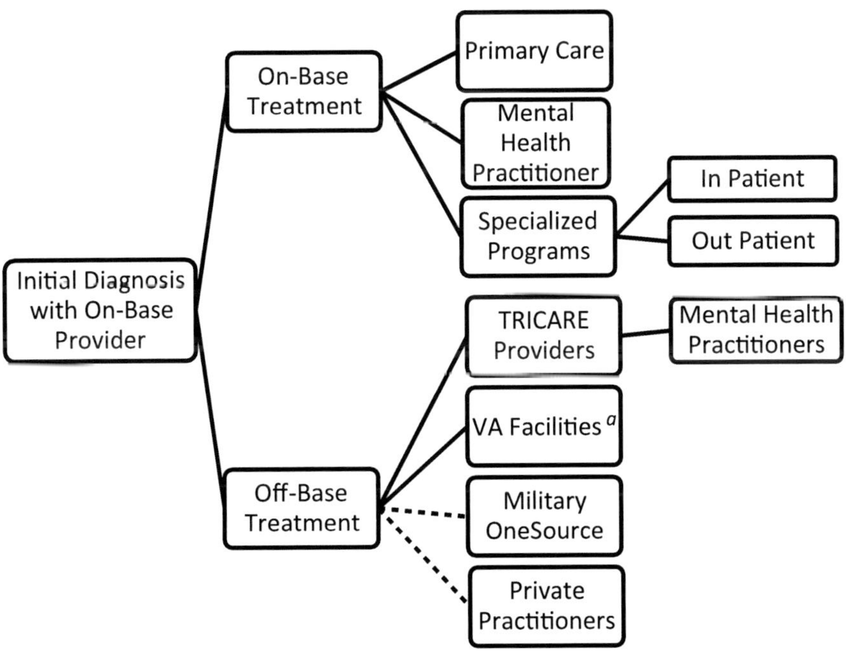

FIGURE 4-3 PTSD treatment pathways available in the DoD. Military OneSource and care through private practitioners is available off base, but these treatment options do not originate from an initial diagnosis and referral from an on-base provider. To distinguish these two treatment options from treatment through TRICARE providers or VA facilities, a dotted line has been used to differentiate the different treatment pathways.
[a] Treatment for service members in VA facilities is rare, but it is an option.

Additionally, an increasing number of programs and individual service members use some form of complementary and alternative medicine (CAM) to treat symptoms of anxiety, depression, and pain. McPherson and Schwenka (2004) found that of 291 soldiers, retirees, and spouses who were surveyed, 81% used one or more forms of CAM therapy. Of the respondents who used CAM therapy, 16% used it for anxiety and 14% used it for depression (PTSD was not specified as a condition to be treated). A larger study of 1,305 active-duty and reserve Navy and Marine Corps personnel found that 37% has used at least one CAM therapy in the preceding year, with herbal therapies being the most commonly used therapy (16%) (Smith et al., 2007). Fifty percent of those using a CAM treatment reported moderate or severe body pain; other medical conditions treated by CAM therapies were not identified. The types of CAM treatments and therapies are diverse and may include nutrition supplements and herbal supplements, yoga, massage, or meditation alone or in combination. White et al. (2011) using data from the Millennium Cohort Study found that of 44,287 military participants, 39% reported using at least one CAM therapy, and that those who used CAM therapies had more physician-based medical services (hospitalizations and outpatient care) than those who did not use CAM therapies, possibly because they report more health conditions and symptoms.

On Base

Service members can receive PTSD treatment on base from a primary care provider, through referrals to mental health specialists or social workers, and in both inpatient and outpatient treatment settings. The VA and the DoD created a clinical practice guideline in 2010 to provide health care professionals with algorithms and evidence-based practice recommendations to guide their provision of PTSD treatment (VA and DoD, 2010). Although the guideline does not have the same enforcement capabilities as policies, it is expected that clinicians will adhere to this guideline in accordance with their own clinical experience.

Primary care. Service members who seek help for PTSD symptoms are not limited to on-base treatment through mental health professionals. In fact, about 90% of service members who receive a diagnosis of a mental health illness are seen in primary care settings (VA and DoD, 2010). The *Clinical Practice Guideline for Management of Post-Traumatic Stress* suggests that "Primary Care providers who identify patients with possible PTSD should consider referral to a Mental Health or PTSD clinic" (VA and DoD, 2010). The provider should consider a patient's desire and preferences for the referral, the patient's mental health status, and the severity of the mental health symptoms and could consider initiating and monitoring such treatments as pharmacotherapy or supportive counseling. The guideline also suggests that a multidisciplinary approach be taken that includes the patient's primary care provider.

The U.S. Army Medical Command has implemented a three-component treatment model called RESPECT-Mil for the management of PTSD by primary care clinicians. The training manual for the model follows the clinical guideline described above (VA and DoD, 2010). In the RESPECT-Mil treatment model, the primary care clinician is responsible for the recognition, diagnosis, and management of PTSD in the patient; is supported by the work of care facilitators; and is responsible for continued support and monitoring of the patient and communication with the patient and a behavioral specialist (Oxman et al., 2008). As part of the RESPECT-Mil initiative, primary care practices are working to include behavioral health consultants in the clinical staff. The consultants provide in-clinic consultations and focused interventions for service members who need support. After diagnosis and assessment, the primary care clinician presents a variety of treatment options—counseling, medication, or a combination of both—and considers patient preferences when drawing up a treatment plan. When a treatment plan has been established, the primary care clinician will explain the role of the care facilitator and offer continued services to coordinate and monitor care (Oxman et al., 2008).

As of Fall 2011, RESPECT-Mil had been implemented in 32 of 37 Army sites and in 84 primary care clinics. In the clinics where RESPECT-Mil had been implemented, providers screened service members for PTSD and other mental illness in more than 1.1 million separate clinical visits (DoD, 2011b). About 13% of the visits resulted in a positive screen for PTSD or depression, and about 73% of those who screened positive received one or more mental health diagnoses. As the DoD phases in its primary care model of the patient-centered medical home—that is, a health care setting model with goals of providing comprehensive primary care for all family members and facilitating partnerships between the patient, his or her physician, and members of his or her family (if appropriate) (Patient-Centered Primary Care Collaborative, 2007)—it plans to use RESPECT-Mil as the basis of its mental health care delivery (DoD, 2011b).

The Air Force has developed the Behavioral Health Optimization Program (BHOP), which integrates mental health and primary care services (U.S. Air Force, 2011). That has resulted in increased availability of mental health services for service members and their families, and the program has reduced stigma by making mental health care a routine part of primary medical care. In surveys of BHOP patients, 97% indicated that they were satisfied or very satisfied with their care. In addition to substantial reductions in psychologic distress, fewer than 10% of the patients had to be referred to more intensive, specialty care services, and this suggests that integrated providers are able to manage the needs of most mental health patients within the primary care setting (U.S. Air Force, 2011). A small study by Cigrang et al. (2011) found that evidence-based treatments can be delivered successfully in military primary care settings using the behavioral health consultant model developed by the Air Force. Patients were referred to the psychologist by primary care providers in an integrated primary care and mental health clinic.

The Navy has also integrated mental health and primary care services through deployment health clinics. Staff at the clinics include primary care providers, psychologists, psychiatrists, social workers, and certified medical assistants (Koffman, 2007). The clinics have been implemented at several installations and provide several deployment-related services, including care for PTSD and other mental health problems (Tanielian and Jaycox, 2008). The Navy has also piloted the Behavioral Health Integration Project, whose purpose is to ensure continuity of care by placing mental health service providers in primary care facilities. Mental health service providers work as consultants to the primary care providers and "provide sailors with short, focused assessments, brief interventions, skill training, and behavioral change plans" (Meredith et al., 2011).

Mental health practitioners. Service members who screen positive for PTSD symptoms on the PDHA or the PDHRA are referred to mental health practitioners after a health assessment interview with a DoD health care professional (GAO, 2006). The DoD employs psychiatrists, psychologists, social workers, and other mental health professionals to diagnose conditions in and treat service members who receive mental health referrals. Service members can also be referred to services through case managers, mental health triage, or buddy referral or by seeking care at the on-base military behavioral health care clinic.

As previously mentioned, a recommended treatment algorithm is detailed in the *Clinical Practice Guideline for Management of Post-Traumatic Stress* (VA and DoD, 2010). Once treatment options have been discussed and the patient and provider agree upon goals and expectations for treatment, the mental health professional should determine the optimal setting for the care and treatment plan. Beginning with the first-line treatment of psychotherapeutic interventions, pharmacotherapy, or both, the clinician is directed by the treatment algorithm to reassess the patient's symptoms in order to appropriately modulate the level of care being provided based on symptom severity. Qualified mental health professionals are encouraged to adhere to evidence-based treatment guidelines such as CBT. For a detailed description of psychotherapy treatment options, see Chapter 7. Personal specialization and training often dictate the treatment options provided by each clinician. Psychiatrists are incorporated into the treatment plan when psychiatric medications are a part of the treatment plan, though they too are capable of delivering psychotherapy and counseling as part of a service member's treatment plan. Social workers also provide treatment through individual, group, and family counseling; triage of symptom severity; and fit-for-duty assessments of service members.

Specialized PTSD treatment programs. On some bases, service members may be referred to specialized PTSD programs. These programs include inpatient and outpatient services, depending on severity of the case. Hospitals with psychiatric wards are able to provide inpatient psychiatric acute treatment to patients not on active duty and patients who have TRICARE Prime coverage. That is accomplished through teams of psychiatrists, nurses, case managers, and other relevant professionals who provide counseling and pharmacotherapy to stabilize the patient's condition. At Fort Hood, for example, services include diagnostic evaluations, psychotherapy, pharmacotherapy, occupational and physical training, and medical referrals as needed (U.S. Army, 2012b).

For service members who need longer-term facilitated medical support in an inpatient setting, the Warrior Transition Unit was created by the Army in 2007 to help transition the service member either back to active duty or out of the military. Nurse case managers coordinate medical appointments and treatment, including pharmacotherapy, cognitive therapy, and CAM treatments (Saito, 2011).

Several other treatment programs are available on base or on an installation. The National Intrepid Center of Excellence, a clinic on the campus of the Naval Support Activity in Bethesda, Maryland, supports patients who have traumatic brain injury and associated psychologic health conditions such as PTSD (Miller, 2011). It uses an interdisciplinary approach that includes several types of services, such as counseling, medication, physical rehabilitation, CAM treatments, nutrition, art therapy, and spiritual consultation. Specialized care programs for PTSD and trauma spectrum symptoms are offered through the Deployment Health Clinical Center and consist of a 3-week, intensive, integrative program that uses CBT and iRest yoga nidra meditation techniques—a manualized multistage treatment protocol developed specifically for combat veterans (Carnes, 2011). The restoration and resilience program at Fort Bliss is a 6-month program that focuses on retaining soldiers who would otherwise receive medical discharges (TRICARE, 2008). Because it is a 6-month program, it has been both criticized for its length and applauded for its comprehensiveness, but it has proved very hard to export to other installations. The South Texas Research Organizational Network Guiding Studies on Trauma and Resilience (STRONG STAR)—funded by the DoD's Psychological Health and Traumatic Brain Injury Research Program—is working toward early interventions that can be used for the detection and prevention or treatment for PTSD (STRONG STAR, 2012a). The consortium of STRONG STAR experts is using clinical trials, exploratory and preclinical studies, and two evidence-based therapies (prolonged exposure [PE] and cognitive processing therapy [CPT]) to treat people for PTSD. The studies are being carried out in several locations, primarily in San Antonio and Fort Hood (STRONG STAR, 2012b).

Military bases may also offer outpatient treatment facilities that specialize in PTSD care with a focus on diverse kinds of treatments. Many programs use aspects of the evidence-based psychotherapy treatments recommended by an established clinical guideline (VA and DoD, 2010), but many integrate CAM. Anecdotal evidence is often supportive; however, few programs are consistent among service branches or at military bases of the same branch and many lack evaluation or grounding in randomized controlled trials. During a site visit to Fort Hood in September 2011, the committee learned that the waiting lists for on-base specialized treatment programs can be long; this indicates a need for these programs to meet the treatment preferences for service members and an imperative to assess the programs in an effort to ensure the treatment regimens are evidence based and effective.

Off Base

Off-base treatment for PTSD is usually coordinated by on-base case managers. The managers ensure a continuum of care by providing oversight of off-base appointments and by keeping informed of treatments that a service member receives from contracted TRICARE providers or at VA facilities. Service members may also seek care through mental health practitioners in a private practice setting or through Military OneSource, but these services are not reported to the case managers and do not become a part of the DoD mental health record.

TRICARE network providers. TRICARE network providers include psychologists, psychiatrists, counselors, and social workers. Treatment availability depends on the population of mental health professionals who are practicing in the area around each military base. Service members must receive a referral from their primary care manager or behavioral health care clinic for approval to receive treatment from network providers. Care and appointments are organized by the network case managers. TRICARE reimburses providers for a variety of treatment options that are consistent with the VA/DoD guideline (VA and DoD, 2010), including psychotherapy and medication management; however, the treatment options provided to the service member depend on the individual practice and experience of the providers. Thus, it is difficult to establish whether the clinicians are practicing evidence-based treatment, and, if they are, whether the treatment is effective. Communication between on-base case managers and off-base TRICARE providers is limited by patient confidentiality concerns and the reporting habits of individual providers, and this makes it difficult to coordinate care between the two treatment sites and to ensure patients receive the best available care.

Treatment for service members in VA facilities. In some cases, active-duty service members are referred to VA treatment facilities for their PTSD care. These facilities generally provide a focus that local DoD facilities lack. For example, the Women's Trauma Recovery Program in Palo Alto, California, is a resource for women who have experienced military sexual trauma and have PTSD. An active-duty service member may also use a VA facility if the facility has available bed space in specialized intensive PTSD programs to handle DoD overflow. TRICARE pays for treatment of active-duty service members at these facilities.

Military OneSource. Military OneSource is an Internet-based and in-person resource that offers assistance with a broad array of issues, such as money management, employment, education, child care, family relationships, relocation, and deployment. For active-duty service members who do not wish to receive counseling from military mental health professionals or TRICARE contractors, Military OneSource can provide up to 12 complimentary face-to-face counseling sessions for each service member per specific problem. Counseling options are also available online and by telephone. Because this is a confidential service, care coordination between Military OneSource and other off-base or on-base providers depends on the information shared by the service member.

Private practitioners. Another option for service members who do not wish to receive treatment from DoD-affiliated programs or clinicians is to seek mental health care from private practitioners. As civilians who are not contracted by TRICARE or employed by the DoD, these mental health practitioners are not bound by the established VA and DoD guideline (VA and DoD, 2010). TRICARE will not cover treatment by private practitioners, and the practitioners are not expected to report diagnosis or treatment progress to the DoD.

In the Theater of War

A stakeholder report from the MHS states that "each quarter, approximately 5,000 deployed service members receive about 14,000 mental health encounters while in the theater of operations" (MHS, 2012). Mental health care in each of the services is provided in the combat theater by embedded psychiatrists, psychologists, social workers, mental health specialists, psychiatric nurse practitioners, occupational therapists and technicians, and general-practice doctors and clinicians. Chaplains are unique in that they train and deploy with the military unit to which they are assigned; they may provide informal counseling and routinely refer service members to more formal mental health resources and treatment facilities in deployed settings (Tanielian and Jaycox, 2008).

Most embedded mental health providers are deployed as part of COSC teams. For the Navy and Marine Corps, mental health teams are integrated at the regiment level as part of the OSCAR program. The Army uses a dual-provider structure; each division has a psychiatrist and a senior noncommissioned officer, supported by a unit-embedded behavioral health officer and an enlisted mental health specialist (Tanielian and Jaycox, 2008). Air Force behavioral health personnel may attach to and deploy with Army units to supplement and support personnel. In support of OEF in-theater mental health services, the Air Force provided 62% of mental health assets and the Army and the Navy 35% and 3%, respectively (MHAT VII, 2011). A combined total of 147 mental health providers from all services were deployed during the joint-MHAT VII assessment, for an overall staffing ratio of one mental health provider to 646 service members (MHAT VII, 2011). Although the ratio varied by service—for example, the Army mental health care model indicated the ratio was about one mental health provider to every 700–800 soldiers—this staffing ratio was found to be adequate. Findings from the latest joint MHAT indicate mental health personnel have provided more mental health services to service members outside the combat-stress control unit location than in previous years, but substantial barriers remain for both providers and users regarding acceptance and implementation of telehealth technologies (MHAT VII, 2011). Research is ongoing to improve understanding of the characteristics of mental health encounters in the theater of war.

Theater Mental Health Encounter Data is a pilot program developed and implemented by the integrated mental health practitioners who were part of the 1st Marine Division OSCAR team deployed in Iraq from January 2006 to January 2007. Overall, the 9 psychiatrists and 10 psychologists in the embedded team documented 3,180 encounters with 1,336 service members (Conway et al., 2011). Larson et al. (2011) used Theater Mental Health Encounter Data to investigate the incidence and types of mental disorders that service members presented with in theater. They found that 82 of the 1,078 service members who had been seen by a division psychiatrist or one of the mental health providers were given an initial diagnosis of PTSD while in theater.

Provider Training

Training military and civilian mental health care providers to give excellent PTSD care is an important goal of the DoD. Training includes educating providers in the nuances of military terminology and culture so treatment is oriented toward the experiences of service members and their families. Below are some examples of training opportunities in the DoD. Some of the barriers to training are discussed in Chapter 9.

In 2010, the Office of the Assistant Secretary of Defense issued a memorandum to the surgeons general of the Army, Navy, and Air Force, the director of the Marine Corps Staff, and the director of Health and Safety of the U.S. Coast Guard (DoD, 2010). The memorandum provided guidance on training regarding PTSD and acute stress disorders. The key recommendation is that all mental health providers have formal training in evidence-based psychotherapies that is consistent with the *VA/DoD Clinical Practice Guideline for Management of Post-Traumatic Stress* (2010); however, no instructions were provided on how to track the training or to whom this would be reported. It also suggested objectives for the implementation of treatment and guidance for achieving military culture competence, for obtaining clinical consultation after training, and for continuing education opportunities (for example, through training events offered by DCoE).

Specific training in evidence-based care for PTSD is available through several sources. The USUHS Center for Deployment Psychology conducts workshops and courses and issues certifications to military and civilian health care providers. Training modules include the assessment of PTSD, the etiology of PTSD, and an overview of evidence-based treatments for PTSD. In collaboration with Widener University, they also offer a 6- to 12-month post-master's degree certificate program that aims to give health care providers knowledge of best clinical practices for addressing the behavioral health needs of service members, veterans, and their families. Training seminars and courses are provided through other platforms. The DCoE posts information on training events for specific PTSD therapies (such as PE, CPT, and virtual reality exposure therapy) that are geared to mental health care providers (DCoE, 2012c). DoD providers can access an Internet-based curriculum offered by the VA called PTSD 101 (VA, 2012b). This online course covers such topics as background and assessment of PTSD, clinical practice guidelines, treatments, specific traumas that increase risk of PTSD and other mental health problems, consideration of special populations, and general health care information. DoD and VA health care providers can earn continuing education credits for several of these modules. A series of training conferences that are geared specifically to chaplains and clergy have been developed. The goal of these conferences is to train chaplains and clergy to recognize PTSD symptoms and other service-related mental health conditions so they can refer personnel to appropriate care (GAO, 2011a).

Training for TRICARE contractors is variable. There are optional conferences, workshops, and Internet-based training options, but none is mandated. A recent Institute of Medicine (IOM, 2010a) report, *Provision of Mental Health Counseling Services Under TRICARE*, recommended that TRICARE implement a mental health quality monitoring and management system. The system would require TRICARE mental health counselors to meet several criteria—including minimum education, licensure, and clinical experience requirements—and would involve "a systematic process for continued professional education and training to ensure continuing improvement in the clinical evidence base and accommodation of the changing needs of the TRICARE population" (IOM, 2010a).

TRANSITIONING BETWEEN THE DEPARTMENT OF DEFENSE AND THE DEPARTMENT OF VETERANS AFFAIRS HEALTH CARE SYSTEMS

An estimated 2.6 million service members were deployed in OEF and OIF from October 2001 through September 20, 2011 (GAO, 2011a); as of 2008, at least 868,000 OEF and OIF service members (including National Guard and reservists) had left active duty (IOM, 2010b). Generally, those who are eligible to receive care through the VA have either been discharged from active duty in the armed forces (see Box 4-1 for eligibility) and tran-

BOX 4-1
Eligibility for Department of Veterans Affairs Health Care

Veterans who may qualify for health care benefits offered through the VA include those who served under active-duty military service in the Army, Navy, Air Force, Marines, or Coast Guard (or Merchant Marines during World War II) and reservists and National Guard members who were called to active duty by a Federal Executive Order. Benefits depend on the veteran's priority status, which is based on a number of factors including service-connected disability, income, or other special status. All veterans who have served in a theater of combat operations within the past 5 years from the date they apply for VA health care are eligible. Other factors that qualify include separation from the service for medical reasons or hardship, discharge from the service due to disability, former prisoners of war, Purple Heart Medal recipient, receiving a VA pension or disability benefits, and receiving state Medicaid benefits. A person who has been discharged under dishonorable conditions is not eligible for benefits through the VA.

SOURCE: VA, 2012b.

sition to the VA only once, or return from activated deployment with the National Guard or reserves and are immediately eligible for VA care. In select cases multiple transitions between DoD and VA health care occur. That particularly affects National Guard and reserve members who have been activated and deactivated more than once. Some retirees may also choose to receive portions of their care from the DoD (through purchased TRICARE services), from the VA, or in the private sector if they have other medical coverage with Medicare or employer-provided plans.

Veterans who are enrolled in the VA have access to a comprehensive medical benefits package that includes a range of outpatient and inpatient services. Once enrolled, the veteran remains enrolled and is able to access health care at any VA facility in the United States.

A service member's transition from active duty to the VA is supported in several ways. In recent years, the VA has expanded its efforts to reach out to veterans transitioning from service in OIF and OEF. Special OIF and OEF outreach teams have been funded and established in every VA facility. The teams work with staff from VA's community-based readjustment counseling service centers (usually called Vet Centers) to seek out veterans recently discharged from active-duty status, including those in reserve components. A VA facility near a military base may also assign VA staff at an MTF to facilitate the transfer of injured service members to VA care as they are discharged.

VA personnel are present during the administration of the PDHRA to National Guard and reserve service members so that the service members can get information about eligibility for VA benefits and make follow-up appointments at VA facilities. The VA coordinates with the DoD to receive dates and locations of PDHRA administration, the number of service members referred to VA facilities, and copies of the PDHRA for people who access VA health care (GAO, 2008b). If a service member completes the PDHRA through a telephone interview, a VA benefits brochure, a copy of the PDRHA, and contact information of a VA liaison is mailed out after the interview (GAO, 2008b).

The Federal Recovery Coordination Program was originally conceived as an effort to ensure care coordination for severely wounded and ill OEF and OIF service members, who will most likely be separated from the military because of their conditions (including PTSD). The program, housed in the VA, has provided services to only a very small number of separating service members and veterans (about 2,000), but its goal is to use federal recovery coordinators as the points of contact for patient case managers in the DoD, the VA, and any other case management programs to monitor and coordinate both the clinical and nonclinical services needed by program enrollees (GAO, 2011b). Two Government Accountability Office (GAO) reports (2011c,d) cited challenges in program enrollment, staffing needs, caseloads, and placement locations. The reports indicated there were substantial coordination problems with other DoD and VA programs that could result in duplication of effort, inefficiency, and confusion of enrollees. A third GAO report (2011c) on integrating DoD and VA care coordination programs was also critical of the lack of collaboration between the two departments in terms of case management and care coordination. The committee notes that the Federal Recovery Coordination Program only serves a very small number of service members and veterans. Such efforts need to be carefully scrutinized as to their effectiveness before they are more widely implemented; the lack of such effective programs means that many service members and veterans are underserved.

THE DEPARTMENT OF VETERANS AFFAIRS HEALTH CARE SYSTEM

Treatment for PTSD and other mental health conditions is an important part of the VA's mission of providing medical care to eligible veterans. In FY 2010, an estimated 790,000 veterans were identified as having a service-connected mental health disorder (GAO, 2011a). During FY 2010, 438,091 veterans (includes those service-connected for PTSD and those not service-connected for PTSD) were treated for the disorder in the VA health care system (NEPEC, 2011a). The latter made up 8.4% of all users of VA health care services, and the number was more than double the number treated for PTSD in FY 2002 (NEPEC, 2011a). That increase is directly related to the influx of veterans returning from deployments in OIF and OEF. During FY 2010, 82,239 veterans of OIF and OEF are known to have received PTSD services through the VA health care system; they amounted to 24.6% of all OIF and OEF veterans using the system (NEPEC, 2011a), although this underestimates the actual number because reporting from the Vet Centers is incomplete. Many of the 191,501 veterans who were reported to have used the Vet Centers received care for PTSD, but many of them are not included in the previously cited figures (see the discussion of Vet Centers later in this chapter). Data are not available on the number of people who use Vet Center services and have received a diagnosis of PTSD. Although the VA has built a system of specialized programs focused on treatment for PTSD, most of PTSD-related services are offered in general mental health and medical settings.

Organization

The VA is the second largest cabinet-level department in the federal government (the DoD is the largest) and has, in the aggregate, the largest health care system in the United States. Like other federal departments, the VA accomplishes its mission through subcabinet agencies. The three primary subcabinet agencies in the VA are the Veterans Health Administration (VHA), the Veterans Benefits Administration (VBA), and the National Cemetery Administration (see Figure 4-4).

The VHA has about 239,000 full-time employees—more than 80% of the VA's staff—and 53,000 independent licensed health care practitioners (VA, 2012c). The VHA accounts for about half of VA expenditures. The VHA provides health care services for enrolled eligible veterans through a fully integrated system of health care delivery assets. Those assets include 152 VA medical centers that typically are composed of an acute-care hospi-

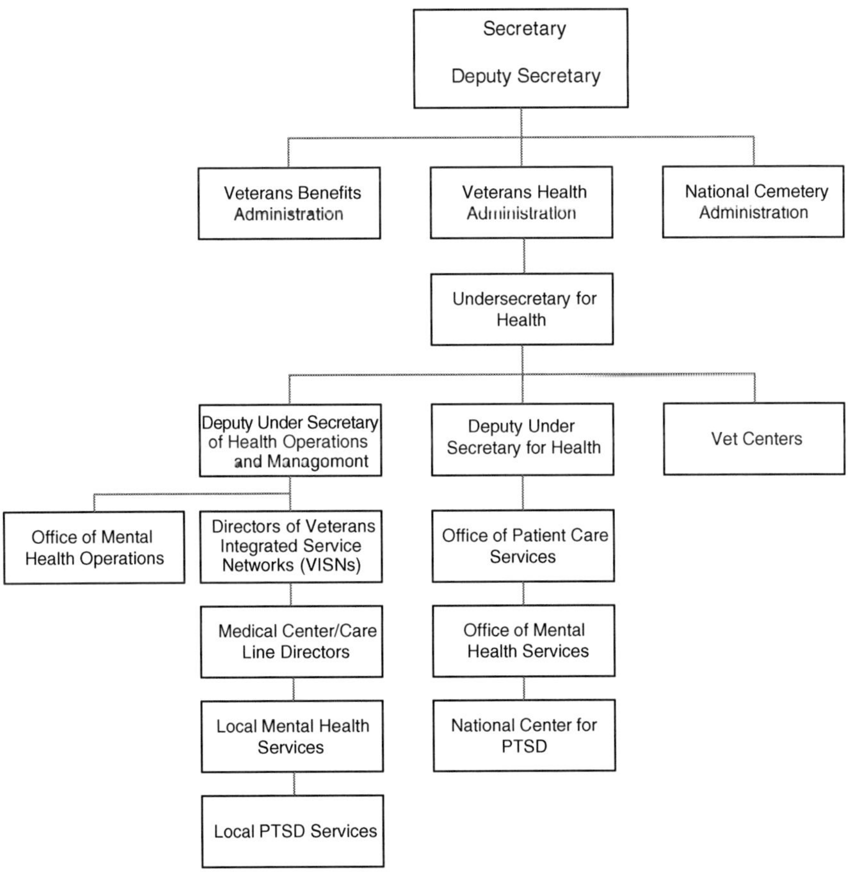

FIGURE 4-4 A partial representation of the Department of Veterans Affairs organization (only selected offices and services are depicted).

tal, an array of hospital-based clinics, a community living center (a skilled nursing facility), and various rehabilitation or other specialized treatment facilities (VA, 2012d). The VHA also manages more than 40 domiciliaries (residential care facilities) for veterans who have mental health or other long-term care needs, nearly 1,400 associated community-based outpatient clinics (VA, 2012d), and about 300 Vet Centers (VA, 2012e). A substantial amount of mental health care is provided in hospital-based primary care clinics and the community-based outpatient clinics, as well as the Vet Centers.

The VBA manages an array of programs that provide financial, educational, and employment assistance, and other services, such as compensation, pension, and survivors' benefits, home loan guaranties, and life insurance coverage. The National Cemetery Administration is responsible for operating the 131 national cemeteries and providing oversight and management of the 33 soldiers' lots, confederate cemeteries, and monument sites in the United States (VA, 2010a).

The VA health care system is organized into 21 veterans integrated service networks (VISNs) (Kizer and Dudley, 2009). The VISNs are the system's basic operating units. Each VISN is responsible for the care of the population of veterans living in a defined geographic area of the United States and its possessions. The VISNs provide health services through their component VA medical centers, community-based outpatient clinics, and other care delivery assets, including an array of contractual relationships and partnership with private health care providers. Administrative and budgetary authority for the provision of services in the VHA rests with the VISN directors. The medical centers also oversee and distribute payments for contractual health care services provided to veterans.

An initiative to establish the community-based outpatient clinics was launched in the middle 1990s to increase access to care by establishing clinics in locations that were more geographically convenient for veterans than the large VA medical centers. The community-based outpatient clinics now provide both primary care and mental health care in most locations. Each community-based outpatient clinic is administratively and financially linked to a VA medical center where there is generally an integrated mental health care service or a set of clinical services (for example, psychiatry, psychology, social work, and nursing) that collaborate to provide and manage mental health services. The local mental health service manages and provides most of the treatment services for PTSD. The VA health care system uses a system-wide electronic health record, the VistA–Computerized Patient Record System, and a common comprehensive administrative database in which all medical contacts are documented (for example, outpatient encounters, inpatient stays, and residential stays).

As of September 30, 2011, there were about 22.2 million living U.S.

veterans, 8.3 million (37%) of whom were enrolled in the VA health care system (VA, 2011a); of these, about 5.2 million were treated by the VA during FY 2010 (GAO, 2011a). More than 80% of enrolled veterans over 65 years old are Medicare beneficiaries, and more than 25% of VA health care enrollees are beneficiaries of two or more non-VA federal health plans (such as Medicare, Medicaid, TRICARE, and the Indian Health Service) (Kizer, 2012). Relatively few VA health care beneficiaries are also enrolled in employer-provided health plans or have other private health insurance coverage. Thus, not every VA health care enrollee receives treatment in a VA facility every year, but over the course of 3 years, most do use VA services at some point. Unlike TRICARE for military retirees, spouses, and dependents, any dependents of veterans are not covered for health care services by the VA health care system except when services (such as marriage and family counseling) are a necessary part of treatment for a veteran and in a few other special situations (for example, spina bifida care for children of Vietnam veterans exposed to Agent Orange). The VHA's Vet Centers provide some care for PTSD, but other mental health services are generally not provided in these counseling centers, although a VA staff psychiatrist may go to the center to see patients. VA medical center clinical staff who see patients at the Vet Center enter data on the encounters into the VA medical record.

Vet Centers

As previously discussed, the VHA provides services through about 300 Vet Centers located throughout the United States and its possessions. The Vet Centers were formally established by an act of Congress in 1979, and were, by design, not aligned under the management of local VA medical centers (as shown in Figure 4-4). The intent was that they would be perceived as community centers where veterans could get "help without hassles" and not be stigmatized by receiving counseling or behavioral health services. They were originally targeted to serve only Vietnam veterans, many of whom had PTSD or other readjustment issues, but they have expanded their mission to include veterans of all conflicts.

Vet Centers are designed to assist in the continuing and successful readjustment of veterans to civilian life. That includes counseling, assessment, and rehabilitation services for veterans and, in some cases, family members. Vet Centers maintain records that are different from those of the medical system, and data cannot be combined across the VA medical and Vet Center systems. A separate Vet Center central office is responsible for oversight and evaluation, which includes developing policy and planning, and has administrative and budgetary authority over the Vet Centers. During FY 2010, 191,508 veterans and family members made 1,273,035 visits to Vet

Centers (VA, 2012e). Reportedly, 39% of Vet Center service recipients do not use VA medical services (Batres, 2011).

The VHA and Vet Centers have different policies with regard to PTSD treatment. Although VHA mental health services are seldom carried out in Vet Centers, each Vet Center must have an external clinical consultant who is required to perform at least 4 hours of clinical consultation each month. Providers in Vet Centers include social workers, clinical psychologists, mental health counselors, professionally trained counselors, and counseling therapists (VA, 2011b). Counseling services provided in these venues focus on assisting combat veterans in readjusting from military to civilian life (GAO, 2011a). Specifically, to ensure that providers are performing high-quality counseling, it is Vet Center policy for team leaders or clinical coordinators to conduct monthly reviews of randomly selected patient clinical records for each full-time provider (VA, 2002b). Vet Center policy also requires providers to review patient treatment plans (including type and estimated duration of counseling or therapy and expected outcomes) during the first five visits and then at least once every 6 months thereafter (VA, 2002a). Of the randomized sample, nearly 90% of records had a current treatment plan.

Most Vet Centers reported using the *DSM* or a combination of the *DSM* and validated instruments such as the PC-PTSD screen and the PTSD Checklist, to screen for PTSD. Although VHA policy mandates that all veterans who have PTSD must have access to CPT or PE in VHA facilities (VA, 2008), Vet Centers are not required to have these therapies available, although many of them do. In a survey of 27 Vet Centers, 21 had provided one or more forms of evidence-based therapy (VA, 2011b).

In FY 2010, an estimated 41% of veterans who were enrolled in the VA health care system were living in rural areas (GAO, 2011a). To support veterans and their families who live in these areas in the contiguous 48 states, Hawaii, and Puerto Rico, the VA has a fleet of 70 mobile Vet Centers. The mobile units increase access to readjustment counseling and other services and are equipped with satellite dishes, audio-visual equipment, multiple telephone lines, dedicated fax lines, laptop computers, encrypted computer lines, and wireless Internet (Tyson and VA, 2009). The interior of a mobile unit is divided into private counseling rooms that can be used for individual or small-group counseling sessions (VA, 2012f).

MENTAL HEALTH CARE IN THE DEPARTMENT OF VETERANS AFFAIRS

In FY 2011, the VA employed an estimated 21,000 mental health care providers (GAO, 2011a). The VHA offers a broad array of services, including all the primary and specialized medical and mental health services that are commonly offered through comprehensive health care systems in the United States. It also offers vocational rehabilitation services; services that address homelessness; prevention, screening, diagnosis, treatment, and rehabilitation services for veterans who have PTSD; and comprehensive evaluations of veterans who are applying for compensation because of PTSD that was caused or aggravated by their time in service. The comprehensive PTSD evaluations are used to support the efforts of the VBA to adjudicate claims for service connection of veterans' PTSD. Most of these services are provided by VHA staff, but occasionally local VA medical centers contract with community providers to provide services. In 2007, to increase the availability of mental health services, the VA required its mental health clinics to provide information about regular hours of service, such as early morning, evening, and weekend appointments.

From 2006 through 2010, an estimated 2.1 million veterans received mental health care from the VA, 10% of whom were OEF and OIF veterans (GAO, 2011a); of all OEF and OIF veterans receiving any health care during this 5-year period, 38% received mental health care (GAO, 2011a). In FY 2010, the five most common mental health diagnostic categories were adjustment reaction (including PTSD), depressive disorder, episodic mood disorder, neurotic disorder, and substance abuse disorder. Some veterans may have received a diagnosis of more than one mental health disorder.

Policy expectations for PTSD services are detailed in the VHA handbook *Programs for Veterans with Post-Traumatic Stress Disorder (PTSD)* (VA, 2010b). The VA funds several national evaluation centers that are responsible for, among other tasks, evaluations for specific categories of mental health services and programs, including some PTSD programs. In addition, the VA National Center for PTSD (discussed below) sponsors and promotes research on associated factors and treatments, training, and education; participates in the development of clinical practice guidelines; and disseminates information to the public on PTSD. Vet Center representatives collaborate with the National Center for PTSD and have participated in the development of clinical practice guidelines.

Whereas the VHA is responsible for providing care and services to veterans for PTSD, the VBA evaluates and adjudicates all claims for PTSD service connection and pays pensions awarded to veterans whose PTSD is found to be service connected. The VBA also provides rehabilitation services for those who are substantially impaired by PTSD that is service connected. That includes evaluation services, educational and vocational training services, vocational rehabilitation services, and other supportive services necessary to rehabilitate veterans who have service-connected PTSD and maintain them at the highest possible functional level. VBA staff provides some of the initial evaluation services and act as case managers in the rehabilitation process. Most services are provided through payments by the VBA to educational, vocational, and rehabilitation institutions or service providers. The VBA also provides additional services for patients who have PTSD, such as loans, non–service-connected pensions, and GI Bill educational benefits. Those services are available for all veterans with PTSD, regardless of whether their PTSD has been adjudicated as being service-connected.

In July 2011, the VHA announced a reorganization of mental health support in the VHA Central Office in Washington, DC. The VA realigned the VHA to enhance effective oversight and to improve support of the VA's health care programs, including mental health programs (Schoenhard, 2011). The Office of Mental Health Operations (OMHO) in the Office of the Deputy Undersecretary for Health for Operations and Management was established to ensure there is a structure for implementing mental health policies developed by the VHA. The OMHO reports directly to the deputy undersecretary for operations and management who is also the direct supervisor of all the VISN directors (see Figure 4-4). That makes one administrative entity responsible for ensuring that organizational priorities related to mental health care are met. In the reorganization, the OMHO will be responsible for monitoring compliance and providing technical assistance to networks to support implementation of national policies. Priorities related to mental health treatment, services, and policies will continue to be guided by the Office of Mental Health Services, which will work closely with OMHO to support common efforts. The realignment is expected to reduce variation in the delivery of mental health services throughout the system. The Office of Mental Health Services will also take the lead in the VHA's joint participation with the DoD in the development and dissemination of evidence-based practice guidelines for the screening and diagnosis of and treatment for PTSD.

PTSD Services and Programs

After the Vietnam War, a small number of medical centers developed local specialized treatment programs for PTSD. In the mid 1980s, congressional funding spurred the expansion of the number of such programs throughout the VA health care system. The programs were locally developed and were largely distinct from one another in organizational structure and treatment approach. They were predominantly residential or inpatient programs that drew patients from large geographic areas. During the 1990s, centralized seed money and local initiatives led to an expansion of outpatient PTSD programs. PTSD outpatient clinical teams that had uniform staffing patterns and expectations were established. However, the deployment of specialized PTSD programs in the VHA health care system was uneven and varied among the VISNs; some VISNs had established specialized programs, but others had done little specialized programming. Box 4-2 provides a selected list of programs and services offered by the VA. Many of the programs and services—especially those that are not specialized treatment programs—are not PTSD specific, but provide benefits and services that may be applicable to persons who have PTSD or other mental disorders.

BOX 4-2
Selected Examples of VA Programs and Services for PTSD[a]

Prevention:
LifeGuard
Families OverComing Under Stress (FOCUS)
FOCUS (couples version)
Moving Forward: A Problem-Solving Approach to Achieving Life's Goals
Psychological First Aid Manual for Direct Care Staff

Specialized Outpatient Treatment:
PTSD Clinical Teams
Substance Use PTSD Program
Women's Stress Disorder Treatment Team

Specialized Intensive Treatment:
Evaluation and Brief Treatment PTSD Unit
PTSD Day Hospital
PTSD Domiciliary
PTSD Residential Rehabilitation Program
Specialized Inpatient PTSD Unit
Women's Trauma Recovery Program

Rehabilitation, Readjustment, and Disability[b]:
Vocational Rehabilitation and Employment Program
Compensated Work Therapy
Individual Placement and Support
Specialized Homelessness Services
Strength at Home
Stand Down
Supportive Housing Services
Community-Supported Homeless Prevention Programs
Vet Centers

---

[a] This is not a comprehensive list of programs offered by the VA, and not all those listed are exclusively for persons who have PTSD.
[b] These programs are discussed in more detail in Chapter 8.

During FY 2010, the VA provided medical care to 5,232,182 veterans, of whom 438,091 (8.4%) received care for a diagnosis of PTSD (NEPEC, 2011a). Spurred by the return of large numbers of veterans from OIF and OEF, the VA has substantially increased the number of services for veterans who have PTSD and worked to improve the consistency of access to such services. Every medical center and at least the largest community-based outpatient clinics are expected to have specialized PTSD services available on site. Mental health staff members devoted to the treatment of OIF and OEF veterans have also been deployed throughout the system (Zeiss, 2011).

The National Center for PTSD is a VA-funded center of excellence for PTSD (VA, 2012h). Created in response to a congressional mandate in 1989, the center is made up of seven divisions around the United States—the Executive Division, the Behavioral Science Division, the Clinical Neurosciences Division, the Dissemination and Training Division, the Pacific Islands Division, and the Women's Health Sciences Division (VA, 2012i)—which "provide a unique infrastructure within which to implement multidisciplinary initiatives regarding the etiology, pathophysiology, diagnosis, and treatment of PTSD" (VA, 2012j). The center is at the forefront of research and education on PTSD.

Resilience Services

Resilience services provided by the VHA are designed to improve the readjustment of veterans to civilian life, to reduce the number and intensity of stress reactions to levels below those required for a diagnosis of PTSD, and to prevent comorbidities. Several joint VA and DoD initiatives are being developed and piloted. For example, the goal of the Integrated Mental Health Strategy is to focus on broad psychological prevention and resilience activities. Although not related specifically to PTSD, the goal of Action 24 of the Integrated Mental Health Strategy is to "ensure that emerging resilience and prevention programs being developed and implemented in VA are informed by lessons learned from DoD's resilience and prevention programs." In addition, the VA and the DoD have been developing national inventories of their resilience and prevention programs for mental health to identify and share best practices throughout the two departments (Schiffner, 2011).

As previously discussed, a robust resilience program is an integral part of the Vet Center program. Services targeted to improving readjustment include individual, group, and family counseling; employment counseling; counseling related to military sexual trauma (MST), a term used in the VA for "sexual harassment that is threatening in character or physical assault of a sexual nature that occurred while the victim was in the military, regardless of geographic location of the trauma, gender of the victim, or the relationship to the perpetrator" (VA, 2012k); outreach; substance abuse assessment and referral; bereavement counseling; referral for other mental health, substance abuse, and medical problems; and guidance on VA benefits (VA, 2009).

Several other VA programs and services are specific to resilience, including LifeGuard, which aims to promote psychological resilience on the basis of acceptance and commitment; FOCUS, a family-centered preventive intervention program; and Moving Forward, a group-based program focused on early intervention and prevention of mental health problems. The VA has also implemented programs and services that are not specific to prevention of PTSD, but instead aim to prevent comorbidities that tend to co-occur with PTSD (see Chapter 8 for a more complete discussion of comorbidities).

Screening and Diagnosis

It is VA policy to screen every patient seen in primary care in VA medical settings for PTSD, MST, depression, and problem drinking. It takes place during a patient's first appointment. Screenings for depression and problem drinking are repeated annually for as long as the veteran uses services. PTSD screening is repeated annually for the first 5 years and every 5 years thereafter (Schoenhard, 2011; VA, 2008). To screen for PTSD, the VA generally uses the four-item PC-PTSD screen. In 2005, the definition of a positive screen changed from at least two affirmative responses to at least three affirmative responses to the four questions (VA, 2005). A positive screen for PTSD or depression (using the two-item Patient Health Questionnaire) results in an additional screening for suicide. MST is screened for only once, generally at the first appointment, unless new data entered into the record indicate the need for additional screenings. Every veteran who receives services at a Vet Center is screened for PTSD and MST. Screening for PTSD is also available for all veterans through the VA's My Health*e*Vet website (VA, 2012l). It is VA policy that all veterans who are given mental health referrals are contacted within 24 hours to evaluate any immediate medical needs they may have. If the situation is not an emergency, veterans are required to receive follow-up care within 14 days after the referral (GAO, 2011a). Of the 5,372,354 veterans who used VA services in FY 2011, 12% of those screened for PTSD had a positive screen (a screen is considered positive if a score of three or more is obtained on the PC-PTSD assessment instrument) (Schiffner, 2012). The numbers of referrals to diagnosis and referrals to treatment could not be determined because such referrals are not coded in a consistent way in the administrative medical record.

Treatment

Every VA medical facility provides a full array of treatment services for PTSD, including pharmacotherapy, face-to-face mental health screening and assessment, group and individual therapy, and psychotherapy. The VA tracks where the treatment is given by assigning a code to every inpatient or residential bed setting and every outpatient clinic; this permits uniform definitions for the nature of the beds or clinics throughout the system. Services vary in frequency and intensity among treatment venues. The VA encourages the use of evidence-based treatments such as CPT and PE, although CAM treatment approaches are also common in the VA specialized treatment programs. A recent VA survey found that 96% of 125 PTSD programs surveyed used some type of CAM (Schiffner, 2011). Of those programs, about 77% offered mindfulness, 72% offered stress management or relaxation, 66% offered progressive muscle relaxation, and 59% offered guided imagery; almost one-third of the PTSD programs offered yoga and one-third offered art therapy. The VA is piloting and researching expanded use of CAM approaches that are the most promising (Schiffner, 2011). The committee will consider this topic in more detail during phase 2 of its study.

Table 4-2 provides data for FY 2010 on PTSD treatment venues in the VHA for 350,629 veterans who were given a primary diagnosis of PTSD. They constitute a substantial subset of the total of 438,091 veterans who received care for PTSD during that year. Some veterans received care in more than one venue, so the total in the table is greater than 350,629. The most common outpatient treatment venue for PTSD is in general mental health outpatient clinics. Treatment in those settings is usually provided by mental health practitioners who also provide services for other mental disorders. Each VA medical center has at least one "PTSD specialist" (VA, 2012a) who is expected to have expertise in treatment for PTSD. The mental health

TABLE 4-2 Care Setting in the VA for Veterans with a Primary Diagnosis of PTSD, FY 2010[a]

Venue	Veterans Treated
General mental health clinics	275,838
PTSD specialists	31,023
Nonmental health clinics	67,871
PTSD clinical teams	117,313

[a] The data do not include patients seen in Vet Centers.
SOURCE: NEPEC, 2011b.

providers enter their PTSD treatment data into the electronic medical record by using a specialized PTSD encounter code; however, because PTSD specialists are not part of designated specialized PTSD treatment programs, their actions and qualifications are not monitored.

Much outpatient PTSD treatment for veterans occurs in clinics that are not specifically designated as mental health clinics, such as primary care. Treatment includes medication prescribed by non-psychiatrists for PTSD and care given by some mental health professionals who work outside mental health clinics. A substantial portion of the workload would be assigned to staff in the new OIF and OEF outreach teams. Because there is no centralized monitoring of the PTSD treatment workload provided outside of specialized PTSD programs, no additional data on the patients treated outside the programs or on the nature or intensity of their care are available, although it appears that such data could be developed.

Readjustment counseling is offered through community-based Vet Centers. Any veteran or family member of a veteran who served in a combat zone is eligible for this service, which includes individual and group counseling, family counseling for military-related issues, MST counseling and referral, and substance abuse assessment and referral (VA, 2012m). If a veteran needs medications or immediate care, then staff can make a referral to a VA medical center (VA, 2009). If a veteran receives treatment through a Vet Center, then no information about that treatment will be released to any person or agency (including the VA) without the veteran's consent (VA, 2012n).

Primary Care in the Department of Veterans Affairs

The Primary Care Program Office is housed within the VHA and, similar to the DoD, is implementing a patient-centered medical home model at all VHA primary care sites. The Patient Aligned Care Teams are managed by primary care providers with support from other clinical and nonclinical staff to provide accessible, coordinated, comprehensive, patient-centered care to veterans. This model of health care has been associated with increased quality improvement, patient satisfaction, and fewer hospital visits and readmissions. To support the Patient Aligned Care Teams, the Primary Care Program Office has developed a variety of tools to assist primary care staff with implementing the patient-centered medical home model (VA, 2011c).

Like the DoD, the VA in recent years has substantially expanded the embedding of mental health providers (primarily psychologists) in primary care clinics. That facilitates the immediate assessment and treatment of patients who are identified by primary care providers as being in need of mental health services, including patients who screen positive for PTSD or are otherwise identified as having PTSD or other stress-related disorders. Beginning in 2008, the VA has been employing mental health professionals to work as an integral part of primary care teams (GAO, 2011a). In FY 2010, at least 155,554 veterans were seen by mental health staff deployed in primary care clinics (Schoenhard, 2011). VA policy requires mental health staff to be available for consultation to VA emergency departments and urgent care centers during all hours of operation (GAO, 2011a).

Primary Care for Veterans Outside the Department of Veterans Affairs

About 60% of veterans do not receive care in the VA system (VA, 2011a). Thus, primary care clinicians in the non-DoD, non-VA sector are likely to see a considerable portion of the OEF and OIF veterans who are living with PTSD. As these engagements wind down, the number of veterans who have PTSD is likely to increase. Many of the clinicians probably have little knowledge of PTSD, little understanding of the DoD and VA medical resources that might be available for a veteran or military family, and limited familiarity of military culture (Boscarino et al., 2010).

Non-VA, non-DoD primary care providers constitute a heterogeneous group, and this results in variation in the types of care they provide to veterans who have PTSD—variation in the types of practice and the geographic locations; in the psychiatric, psychologic, social services, and financial resources that are available; in the providers' training and expertise related to PTSD care; and in the providers' level of involvement in the care of the spouses and children of veterans. These primary care providers include physicians, nurse practitioners, and physician assistants who are employed in large health systems, public clinics, rural health centers, and solo private practices. The resources and financial support they can access for their PTSD patients vary commensurately from extensive resources in some health systems and communities to very few in others. The presentation of veterans who have PTSD will also vary. In the VA, the established screening programs may bring patients of concern to the attention of clinicians who are generally attentive to the possibility of PTSD and other underlying clinical presentations. In contrast, nonmilitary primary care practices do not typically screen for such conditions as PTSD, given the small proportion of the U.S. population that has served in the military.

The evolution of primary practices in recent years has included, and over the next several years will probably include, a transition that embraces patient-centered medical home concepts, electronic medical records, advances in information technology, and the active use of registry and case management systems to promote adequate follow-up and treatment adjustment for those with mental health and chronic medical conditions.

Specialized Programs

The VA provides almost 200 specialized PTSD treatment programs (VA, 2012n), mainly through specialized outpatient and intensive PTSD programs. There are three types of specialized outpatient PTSD programs in the total of 127 throughout the VA system: 119 PTSD clinical teams, 4 substance-use PTSD teams, and 4 women's stress-disorder treatment teams. The teams are interdisciplinary and are structured according to centralized staffing protocols. There is no uniform, national policy on admission criteria for specialized PTSD treatment programs. Individual programs may have specific inclusion or exclusion criteria, such as substance use disorder status or legal status (for example, not awaiting trial or sentencing), or in the case of specialized women's programs, gender. In general, referral processes to specialized programs are very liberal; programs generally accept self-referrals and referrals from other health care providers and community resources. Services provided by PTSD clinical teams may include assessment and diagnosis; individual, group, and family therapy; psychoeducation; pharmacotherapy and medication management; supportive therapy; CBT, PE, and CPT; and referrals to other services or clinics. It is important to note that the provision of treatment by the staff on the specialized outpatient PTSD program teams is not standardized and may not be consistent among programs. Substance use PTSD teams provide assessment, symptom management (for example, in the form of pharmacotherapy, anger management, and counseling), and group and individual psychotherapy to treat co-occurring substance abuse and PTSD symptoms. Women's stress disorder treatment teams are similar in structure to the PTSD clinical teams and provide face-to-face and group treatment to female veterans who have PTSD. Treatment options—such as psychologic assessment and consultation, psychiatric and medication services, and psychotherapy—do not vary markedly from those of VA-wide programs, but the teams target only female veterans, and their goal is for patients to feel more comfortable and thus improve treatment outcomes.

The 117,313 veterans treated in the specialized outpatient PTSD programs during FY 2010 were tracked in a centralized program evaluation system in the VHA, so more is known about the characteristics of this population than about characteristics of patients who are treated outside the specialized programs (NEPEC, 2011b). On the average, patients seen in the specialized outpatient PTSD programs made 7.8 visits during FY 2010 at a direct cost of $1,066 per person (this includes only the cost of the salaries of the program staff, not such indirect costs as facility and administrative overhead and supplies) (NEPEC, 2012a,b). According to intake forms filled out by the 21,104 new veterans who entered the programs during FY 2010, most had served in the Persian Gulf (includes the 1990–1991 Gulf

War, OIF, and OEF; 51%), were male (91%), were adjudicated as having their PTSD related to their time in service and were receiving compensation (62%), had been exposed to enemy or friendly fire (85%), and were prescribed psychotropic medications (63%) (NEPEC, 2011c).

Among veterans in outpatient services, comorbidities were high; 33% had a concurrent diagnosis of substance use disorder, 54% had a non-psychotic axis I diagnosis,[1] 4% had a psychotic axis I diagnosis, and 68% had a current chronic medical problem (NEPEC, 2011c). Most (64%) were not currently working, including 25% who were looking for but were unable to find work (NEPEC, 2011c). Only 2% were currently on active duty, but 13% were still active in the reserves or National Guard (NEPEC, 2011c). MST during time in service was reported by 9%, and an equal percentage reported sexual trauma either before or after their time in service (NEPEC, 2011c).

In addition to outpatient programs, the VA maintains 41 specialized intensive PTSD programs of six types: evaluation and brief treatment PTSD units, PTSD residential rehabilitation programs, PTSD domiciliary programs, PTSD day hospitals, specialized PTSD inpatient programs, and female trauma recovery programs. In FY 2010, specialized intensive PTSD programs had 3,967 admissions.

The specialized inpatient and outpatient settings seek to create a "therapeutic community" as a part of the treatment program and include counseling and social, recreation, and vocational training (VA, 2012n). The programs were locally developed, and therefore are different from each other in structure (for example, residential vs. day hospital), length of stay (average 43.9 days), and treatment approach. Most programs are comprehensive, offering a variety of interventions and treatment options. The VA monitors patients in the programs through a more robust national evaluation effort. Consequently, much is known because patient characteristics and outcome data are collected.

PTSD day hospitals provide intensive outpatient care for 3–6 weeks in individual or group settings (VA, 2010c). Evaluation and brief treatment PTSD units provide 14–28 days of care for acute cases of PTSD in inpatient psychiatric units with mandatory follow-up care after a stay. Specialized inpatient PTSD units provide trauma-focused care for 28–90 days for veterans who require more intense and monitored care. PTSD residential rehabilitation programs and PTSD domiciliary programs also

---

[1] The American Psychiatric Association *Diagnostic and Statistical Manual of Mental Disorders* uses a five-axis system to diagnose mental health disorders (APA, 2000): axis I includes clinical disorders, axis II includes personality disorders and mental retardation, axis III includes general medical conditions, axis IV includes psychosocial and environmental problems, and axis V includes global assessment of functioning.

provide longer-term care, generally 28–90 days, in a residential therapeutic environment to prepare veterans to re-enter the civilian community with better "self care and self control capabilities" (VA, 2010c). Some specialized services for women are met through women's trauma recovery programs, 60-day live-in rehabilitation programs that include PTSD treatment and coping skills for re-entering the community. There are only two of these programs in the VA, and they served fewer than 60 patients during FY 2009. Overall, about 5% of participants in all VA specialized intensive PTSD programs and 8% of all patients in specialized outpatient PTSD programs are female (NEPEC, 2011c,d).

Most patients treated in specialized intensive PTSD programs (75%) had PTSD that was connected to their service and were receiving compensation, almost all (91%) of these patients were prescribed psychotropic medication, 49% had served in the Persian Gulf (including the 1990–1991 Persian Gulf War, OEF, and OIF), 47% had a concurrent substance abuse diagnosis, and 45% had another axis I disorder. Almost all (96%) patients had some type of prior treatment for PTSD. At admission, 83% were not working, including 18% who reported that they were looking for and not able to find work (NEPEC, 2011d). A robust program evaluation effort tracked the progress of these patients through treatment.

An attempt was made to follow up with patients 4 months after discharge from the specialized intensive PTSD programs. Two-thirds were contacted and completed follow-up evaluations. The VA provided the committee with only overall combined data from all the programs. There was a modest improvement on measures of PTSD symptoms and substance abuse and a stronger improvement for PTSD symptoms and violence. It must be noted that there was no control group, and the programs that were combined to yield overall results are very different from one another (NEPEC, 2011b).

Provider Training

The VA has implemented a national initiative to train providers in evidence-based psychotherapies for PTSD (Schiffner, 2011). National experts have been employed to train a cadre of VA staff in both CPT and PE. The training includes an initial intensive experientially based workshop (3–5 days long) and weekly telephone-based consultations with an expert in the therapy for about 6 months. At of the end of FY 2011, about 3,300 VA clinicians had been trained in CPT, 1,500 in PE, and 800 in both (Schiffner, 2011). Recently, the VA announced that it plans to hire about 1,600 nurses, psychiatrists, psychologists, social workers, and other mental health staff and about 300 administrative support staff. This is in addition to the VA's current mental health staff of about 20,590 employees (VA, 2012g).

The emphasis has been on training clinicians who have large caseloads of patients who have PTSD. About one-third of those who are trained work in specialized PTSD programs, and about one-third work in general outpatient mental health settings, in which PTSD patients are also seen. There are plans to train an additional 400 clinicians in FY 2012 (Schiffner, 2011). Rates of participation in the consultation process after training workshops are very high (88%) for PE (Karlin et al., 2010). Master trainers are to be trained for each of the VISNs and for the Vet Centers to expand the training of clinicians closer to their work sites. The VA also continues to develop tools to enhance the delivery of the therapies, such as motivational educational videos for patients and supplemental training materials. The VA has reported good results from initial evaluations of the acceptance and impact of the program (Karlin et al., 2010). The VHA has also reported that the system has adequate staffing capacity to provide CPT or PE for PTSD to all OEF and OIF veterans in the VHA and is close to having full capacity to provide these therapies to VHA users of all combat eras (Schiffner, 2011).

The VHA has reported that barriers to the full implementation of treatment regimes remain (Schiffner, 2011). Most notable is the amount of time that clinicians have to provide a particular intervention in the time frame that is desirable for each patient. There are also problems with giving clinicians time to participate in post-workshop consultations and accessing the supplies and resources required to implement the evidence-based care. The VHA reports that it is attempting to address those barriers by implementing policies that make the requirements for the full implementation of evidence-based care at the local-facility level explicit. It also reports that it has developed a national performance measure that requires OEF and OIF veterans with a primary diagnosis of PTSD to receive at least eight sessions of psychotherapy within a 14-week period. And it has developed metrics for tracking psychotherapy delivery for all veterans who have PTSD that will be part of a comprehensive national dashboard of performance metrics. It has developed an initiative to expand the delivery of evidence-based therapies through telemental health modalities (Schiffner, 2011).

There is no mechanism for tracking the delivery of evidence-based therapies in the VA centralized databases. The VHA is developing progress note templates for CPT and PE that will allow documentation of the care in the computerized record in a manner that will facilitate the collection of centralized aggregate data (Desai, 2011).

VA clinicians also participate in seminars, courses, workshops, and other continuing education efforts that are not part of the new centralized VA initiative in evidence-based care for PTSD. These offerings may be sponsored by professional groups, educational institutions, local VA facilities, or a national VA educational center. Internet-based educational programs in PTSD are offered by the VA National PTSD Center and professional organizations such as the International Society for Traumatic Stress Studies. No centralized tracking is conducted on how many PTSD-related educational efforts are attended by local VA clinical staff. The currently untracked training encounters would include attendance at seminars and workshops on pharmacotherapy for PTSD attended by VHA prescribers of medication. Specific training in screening of veterans for mental health conditions and in discussing treatment options is in place for primary care physicians (GAO, 2011a).

All VA-independent professional mental health staff (including psychiatrists, psychologists, social workers, and advanced practice nurses) are credentialed and privileged at the local-facility level. There are broad guidelines for the process, but local professional standards boards and credentialing bodies are given latitude to delineate special competences and to grant privileges to engage in a particular therapeutic activity or treatment for specific disorders.

Among providers at 27 randomly selected Vet Centers, 98% of those who had been employed at a Vet Center for at least a year had attended mandatory training for PTSD assessment and counseling through the Readjustment Counseling Service. Nearly half had also attended VHA-sponsored training for PTSD; 37% reported receiving supplemental training in cognitive behavioral therapy, and 12% and 5% reported receiving supplemental training in cognitive exposure therapy and PE, respectively (VA, 2011a).

COLLABORATIVE EFFORTS BETWEEN THE DEPARTMENT OF DEFENSE AND THE DEPARTMENT OF VETERANS AFFAIRS

The committee was asked in its charge to identify collaborative activities between the DoD and the VA with respect to the prevention, screening, diagnosis, and treatment of PTSD. Some of these efforts, such as the original development of the joint *VA/DoD Clinical Practice Guideline for Management of Post-Traumatic Stress* in 2004 and updated in 2010 (VA and DoD, 2010), are required to be used by VA and DoD mental health providers. The VA and the DoD have also issued joint guidelines for other medical conditions that are frequently comorbid with PTSD, such as post-deployment health, concussion and mild traumatic brain injury, substance use disorder, major depressive disorder, and several types of pain.

Other collaborative efforts between the DoD and the VA include multiple joint executive councils, coordinating offices, working groups, and direct sharing agreements between VA medical centers and DoD medical facilities (VA and DoD, 2011). There have also been a number of conferences on military health issues sponsored and attended by staff from both departments. For example, the 2009 *Report of (VA) Consensus Conference: Practice Recommendations for Treatment of Veterans with Comorbid TBI,*

Pain, and PTSD was produced by participants from both the VA and the DCoE (VA and DCoE, 2009). In 2009, the National Institutes of Health (NIH), the DCoE, the VA, and other federal agencies held the Second Annual Trauma Spectrum Disorders Conference: A Scientific Conference on the Impact of Military Service on Families and Caregivers; it focused on the impact of trauma spectrum disorders on military and veteran families and caregivers across deployment, homecoming, and reintegration. Trauma spectrum disorder encompasses injury or illness that occurs as a result of combat or an unexpected traumatic event, and covers a broad range of psychological health and traumatic brain injury issues.

The VA and the DoD have recently released the *VA/DoD Collaboration Guidebook to Healthcare Research* (2011) as part of the VA/DoD Joint Strategic Plan for 2009–2011. Although this research guide is not PTSD-specific, both departments allocate millions of research dollars for PTSD research, and this guide is intended to help facilitate collaborations in human subject health care research between the two departments.

The DoD and the VA also collaborate to transition service members from active duty to the VA, as discussed in detail in the earlier section on transitioning in this chapter. VA facilities near military bases may assign VA staff at an MTF to facilitate the transfer of injured service members to VA care as they are discharged. VA personnel coordinate with DoD personnel to receive dates and locations of PDHRA administration and are present during the administration of the PDHRA to National Guard and reserve service members to inform them of eligibility for VA benefits and services.

There appear to be several other VA and DoD collaborative efforts, but these seem to focus on working groups, such as those that issue clinical practice guidelines, and hosting joint conferences. The committee asked the DoD and the VA to provide information on PTSD-related programs and services for screening, diagnosis, prevention, treatment, or rehabilitation, including information on eligibility, setting, treatments used, costs per participant, and outcomes to identify areas where there may be overlap or duplication. However, such a list was not provided by the DoD, and the RAND Corporation report on DoD psychological health programs (Weinick et al., 2011) does not include this level of detail. The committee hopes to have this information for phase 2. Given the lack of information on program specifics from the DoD for this Phase 1 report, the committee is unable to comment on issues such as collaboration or duplication of programs between the VA and the DoD. However, the committee is able to note that there is one program that is used by both the DoD, specifically the Navy and Marine Corps, and the VA. This program, FOCUS, is a family-centered program discussed earlier. Because the VA and the DoD service different populations, some duplication of programs is expected and appropriate as it may help with continuity as service members, including National Guard and reservists, move from active duty to veteran status.

RESEARCH IN THE DEPARTMENT OF DEFENSE AND THE DEPARTMENT OF VETERANS AFFAIRS

Numerous research efforts are under way in the DoD and the VA to develop a better understanding of all aspects of PTSD, including causes, treatments, prevention, barriers to care, and comorbidities. For example, since FY 1992, the DoD has funded numerous extramural and intramural health-related studies through the Office of the Congressionally Directed Medical Research Programs and through the service branches. (For a listing of PTSD research projects up through 2009 see the DoD Biomedical Research Database at http://brd.dtic.mil/). The studies cover various topics, including PTSD, and are of various types, such as experimental animal models, epidemiologic studies, studies of behavioral and cognitive therapies, and studies of resilience interventions. For example, the Air Force Research Laboratory is conducting a study to determine the role of genetic susceptibility in the development of PTSD.

Funding for congressionally directed PTSD-related studies has increased substantially in recent years. One research effort that has benefited the understanding of PTSD barriers is that of the MHATs (U.S. Army, 2012c). As previously discussed, these teams have been assembled and sent to Iraq since 2003 and to Afghanistan since 2007 to obtain information on symptoms of anxiety and depression, barriers to care (including stigma), symptoms of anxiety and depression, PTSD, and other mental health care issues (see Chapter 9 for more information on barriers identified through MHAT survey collections).

Several other PTSD research efforts are going on in the DoD. For example, the Center for the Study of Traumatic Stress, which was established in 1987, is part of the USUHS Department of Psychiatry and is partnering with DCoE. Its work was started to investigate the physical and psychologic effects of traumatic events. The work has since grown beyond service members to research on the impact of war, deployments, and injuries on children and families (Center for the Study of Traumatic Stress, 2012). The Army and the DoD have supported the work of the Walter Reed Army Institute of Research for over 100 years (U.S. Army, 2012d). The institute aims to be at the forefront of biomedical research, including deployment psychology and the psychologic impacts of the recent conflicts in Iraq and Afghanistan (Hoge et al., 2011). The Army has partnered with the National Institute of Mental Health (NIMH) to investigate risk and protective factors associated with service members' mental health symptoms and illness (NIMH, 2011). Mental health research is also carried out in the U.S. Army

Medical Research and Material Command, which is headquartered at Fort Detrick, Maryland. Psychologic health research managed by the Medical Research and Material Command totaled $524 million in FY 2006–2011 (255 projects); 57% of that research ($297 million, 162 projects) pertained to PTSD, 21% ($110 million, 24 projects) pertained to suicide, and 10% ($53 million, 25 projects) pertained to resilience (Hoover, 2011).

The VA has a separate line-item appropriation for research and development. During FY 2010, the VA research and development budget was $581 million (OMB, 2010), which supported more than 2,000 studies at VA facilities (U.S. Congress, 2011). The research portfolio is broad—from preclinical studies that use animal models or human biologic specimens, to health services and translational research—and includes large cooperative studies. VA researchers collaborate closely with academic affiliates and also receive funding from sources outside VA, including the NIH, nonprofit associations, and industry. Many VA medical centers have established VA-affiliated nonprofit research foundations that facilitate collaboration and that leverage VA research funding.

A recent GAO report noted that during FY 2009, VA research funding for PTSD totaled $24.5 million (4.8% of the VA research budget, an increase from 2.5% in FY 2005) (GAO, 2011e). The funding supported 96 intramural research studies in PTSD. VA research funding ($6.6 million) for one of the largest randomized controlled trials of PE in female veterans has recently concluded. The study provided a foundation for the VA's initiative to expand evidence-based treatment for PTSD throughout the system.

The VHA Office of Research and Development has focused its efforts on prevention and diagnosis of, and treatment for, PTSD using many approaches. Research related to psychotherapy has included virtual reality simulations and guided imagery, and on the basis of strong positive research findings, the VA has systematically adopted PE. Other research has focused on pharmacotherapy, determining the biologic basis of PTSD (by eliciting the role of stress-related hormones and examining functional brain images), and examining clinical and lifestyle factors that may increase or decrease a person's risk of PTSD. Additional research initiatives include collaborating with the DoD to create a PTSD registry and developing and improving telehealth models to improve PTSD care, especially for veterans in rural areas (VA, 2010b).

With clinical-care appropriations, the VA funds 10 mental illness research, education, and clinical centers that are located throughout the system. The centers were established to research the causes and treatments of mental disorders and to apply new knowledge to the VA's routine clinical practice. Four of the centers have at least a partial emphasis on PTSD and postdeployment issues, and all may conduct studies relevant to PTSD and its comorbidities. Two new VA PTSD centers of excellence focus on

TABLE 4-3 Current Clinical Trials on PTSD Funded by the DoD, the VA, and the NIH by Topic Area[a]

Topic Area	DoD	VA	NIH
Epidemiologic	1	13	1
Neurobiologic	3	4	8
Resilience/Prevention	2	6	
Assessment	1		
Treatment			
CAM	7	16	
Comorbidities	3	31	5
Delivery	8	17	
Pharmacotherapy	8	29	5
Psychosocial	10	32	5
Rehabilitation/Disability	1	4	
Other[b]	2	8	4
Total[c]	33	131	21

[a] This list reflects the number of studies that were found on Clinicaltrials.gov on April 4, 2012.
[b] Primary focus of study is not PTSD.
[c] This sum denotes the total number of studies identified on the website. Studies were classified under multiple categories, so the sum of studies for each organization may exceed the total.

coordinated care for veterans returning from OIF and OEF, including coordination of care for those who have PTSD. The VA's strategic plans for PTSD research include increased cooperation with DoD, the NIMH, the Centers for Disease Control and Prevention, and the Substance Abuse and Mental Health Services Administration.

Clinical trials on PTSD that are sponsored by the DoD, the VA, and the NIH are shown in Table 4-3. The committee categorized these studies by topic area. The number of studies on the Clinicaltrials.gov website changes frequently as studies are funded, completed, or discontinued. As can be seen from the table, the VA funds about four times as many studies on PTSD as does the DoD. Most of the studies funded by the NIH might be considered basic research on PTSD.

COST CONSIDERATIONS

It is difficult to estimate the costs of screening and treating for PTSD in DoD and VA settings. Screening for PTSD in civilian primary care settings is likely to be similar in cost to screening for depression, which cost $23 per patient in 2004 (National Business Group on Health, 2011). However, that is unlikely to reflect the costs of screening in VA or DoD settings because of differences in how care is organized and delivered. In addition to the cost of resources directly involved in screening (which primarily involve caregiver time), false positive results increase the cost of screening by leading to further testing and inconvenience. For people who screen positive, adequate resources need to be in place to cover the costs of treatment. Finally, in addition to the direct benefits of treatment to people, screening and early intervention may lead to economic benefits in averting productivity loss associated with PTSD. Not factored into the cost projections are substantial administrative expenditures associated with managing and overseeing the screening and general and specialized mental health treatment programs.

To the committee's knowledge, there have been only two studies of the costs associated with PTSD. The first, originally published in a RAND report (Eibner, 2008) and later updated by Kilmer et al. (2011), used a microsimulation model to estimate the burden of PTSD from a societal perspective. The second was a naval postgraduate school master of science thesis (Kwan and Tan, 2008) that used administrative data from MTFs and TRICARE to estimate costs of PTSD treatment.

In the RAND microsimulation model (Eibner, 2008; Kilmer et al., 2011), future costs of PTSD in a hypothetical group of simulated people were computed. The group was based on the 261,827 soldiers who were deployed as part of OEF or OIF on June 30, 2008, and their health care trajectories and costs were modeled over a 2-year period. As part of the simulation, the hypothetical people were allowed to experience comorbid conditions, health care treatments, and secondary outcomes, such as unemployment. An advantage of that approach is that PTSD could be treated as a chronic condition with episodes of remission and relapse. Probabilities associated with the course of disease (for example, receipt of evidence-based treatment, remission, and relapse) were based on published studies. Costs of health care services were based on published TRICARE and Medicare reimbursement rates, and pharmaceutical costs were based on average wholesale prices. Costs of secondary outcomes, such as unemployment and suicide, were gathered from published studies. The studies estimated that costs associated with PTSD for service members returning from Iraq and Afghanistan ranged from $708 million to $1.2 billion, which translated into a cost per patient of $5,904–$10,298 in the 2 years after discharge from the military. The majority of the costs were due to productivity loss, which accounted for 55.3–94.5% of total costs (Eibner, 2008). Only 4% of the cost was attributable to treatment (Kilmer et al., 2011).

The Kwan and Tan study (2008) took a different approach, using administrative data from FY 2001–2006 to estimate costs from the perspective of the military health care system of treatment for PTSD. The analyses examined officers and enlisted personnel separately and estimated costs by branch of service. Overall, the authors found that costs varied considerably by location of care (MTF versus TRICARE) and branch of service. Among officers, inpatient costs per patient ranged from $7,027 to $12,954 for PTSD treatment among the four military services, outpatient costs from $1,812 to $3,514, and pharmacy costs from $125 to $238. TRICARE inpatient costs ranged from $2,917 to $28,986, and outpatient costs from $976 to $1,106; no pharmacy costs under TRICARE were reported. Costs among enlisted personnel were similar, ranging from $10,723 to $12,954 for inpatient care in an MTF and from $684 to $1,130 for outpatient care received from TRICARE providers. It was not clear whether these were annual costs or costs over the entire study period (FY 2001–2006). Another limitation was the small sample sizes for some types of care in some of the services and outliers, which can have a considerable effect on the mean. For example, only two people who served in the Marine Corps received inpatient services from a TRICARE provider.

In addition to those published studies, there are some data from the VA on the costs of specialized PTSD programs, which treat about 25% of veterans who have PTSD. In FY 2010, the VA spent $112,460,032 on specialized outpatient PTSD programs that served 105,531 veterans, for an average cost of $1,066 per veteran. Veterans averaged 10.2 visits per year in those programs, for a cost of $105 per visit (NEPEC, 2012b). The VA also spent $42,716,581 on specialized intensive PTSD programs in FY 2010 (NEPEC, 2012c); the 5,128 admissions during the year cost an average of $8,330. Cost data on PTSD services delivered outside the specialized programs have not been reported (NEPEC, 2012c).

Thus, it is difficult to monetize the costs of PTSD treatment. Although the microsimulation model estimated societal costs associated with PTSD, few details were given about the costs of treatment. The Kwan and Tan study also lacked the detail needed for a thorough assessment of PTSD treatment costs. Although some data are available from the VA, they are limited to specialized programs, which treat a minority of PTSD patients. Finally, no data on costs of PTSD services have been reported by the DoD.

SUMMARY

The DoD and the VA have played an active and pivotal role in the prevention of, screening for, diagnosis of, and treatment for PTSD. This chapter has sought to describe what is known about mental health care, specifically care for PTSD, in the DoD and the VA. Both organizations have contributed much time, funding, and effort to PTSD health care and research. The foundational information provided in this chapter has set the stage for further discussion of PTSD prevention and prophylaxis, screening, diagnosis, treatment, co-occurring medical conditions and psychosocial complexities, and barriers to, facilitators of, and access to care.

In phase 2 of this study, the committee will gather data from the DoD and the VA and from visits to bases and medical centers to gain a better understanding of the success of different PTSD services and programs. The committee will also take a deeper look at costs associated with treatment and rehabilitation for PTSD.

REFERENCES

APA (American Psychiatric Association). 2000. *Diagnostic and statistical manual of mental disorders, fourth edition, text revision (DSM-IV-TR)*. Washington, DC: American Psychiatric Association.

Batres, A. R. 2011. Readjustment counseling service. Presentation to the Committee on the Assessment of Ongoing Efforts in the Treatment of PTSD.Washington, DC, April 21.

Boscarino, J. A., S. Larson, I. Ladd, E. Hill, and S. J. Paolucci. 2010. Mental health experiences and needs among primary care providers treating OEF/OIF veterans: Preliminary findings from the Geisinger Veterans Initiative. *International Journal of Emergency Mental Health* 12(3):161-170.

Brunwasser, S. M., J. E. Gillham, and E. S. Kim. 2009. A meta-analytic review of the Penn Resiliency Program's effect on depressive symptoms. *Journal of Consulting and Clinical Psychology* 77(6):1042-1054.

Carnes, R. 2011. Yoga and yoga nidra meditation at the Deployment Health Clinical Center's specialized care program. Presented at the Defense Centers of Excellence monthly Webinar, Bethesda, MD. 28 July.

Center for the Study of Traumatic Stress. 2012. *About us*. http://www.cstsonline.org/about-us/ (accessed January 30, 2012).

Cigrang, J. A., S. A. M. Rauch, L. L. Avila, C. J. Bryan, J. L. Goodie, A. Hryshko-Mullen, A. L. Peterson, and the STRONG STAR Consortium. 2011. Treatment of active-duty military with PTSD in primary care: Early findings. *Psychological Services* 8(2):104-113.

Conway, T. L., P. S. Hammer, M. R. Galarneau, G. E. Larson, N. K. Edwards, E. A. Schmied, H. L. Ly, K. J. Schmitz, J. A. Webb-Murphy, W. C. Boucher, D. C. Johnson, and S. G. Ghaed. 2011. Theater mental health encounter data (TMHED): Overview of study design and methods. *Military Medicine* 176(11):1243-1252.

DCoE (Defense Centers of Excellence for Psychological Health and Traumatic Brain Injury). 2012a. *DCoE—what we do*. http://www.dcoe.health.mil/DCoEv2/WhatWeDo.aspx (accessed January 30, 2012).

DCoE. 2012b. *PTSD: Treatment options*. http://www.dcoe.health.mil/ForHealthPros/PTSD TreatmentOptions.aspx (accessed January 30, 2012).

DCoE. 2012c. *PTSD and TBI training events*. http://www.dcoe.health.mil/TrainingCalendar.aspx (accessed January 30, 2012).

Desai, R. 2011. NEPEC and PTSD program evaluation. Presentation to the Committee on the Assessment of Ongoing Efforts in the Treatment of PTSD. February 28, 2011. Washington, DC.

Dinneen, M. 2011. Military health systems overview. Presentation to the Committee on the Assessment of Ongoing Efforts in the Treatment of PTSD. February 28, 2011. Washington, DC.

DoD (Department of Defense). 2004. *Subject: Force health protection (FHP)*. 6200.04. http://www.dtic.mil/whs/directives/corres/pdf/620004p.pdf (accessed April 27, 2012).

DoD. 2006. *Subject: Periodic health assessment policy for active duty and selected reserve members*. HA Policy: 06-006. http://www-nehc.med.navy.mil/downloads/ PHA/PHA_Policy_Signed.pdf (accessed April 27, 2012).

DoD. 2007. *An achievable vision: Report of the Department of Defense Task Force on Mental Health.* Falls Church, VA: Defense Health Board.

DoD. 2010. *Guidance for mental health provider training for the treatment of post-traumatic stress disorder and acute stress disorder.* Memorandum. Washington, DC: Department of Defense, Office of the Assistant Secretary of Defense. December 13.

DoD. 2011a. *Maintenance of psychological health in military operation.* Instruction 6490.05.

DoD. 2011b. Welcome to the RESPECT-MIL program. *RESPECT-Mil Newsletter* Fall. http://www.pdhealth.mil/respect-mil/index1.asp (accessed January 30, 2012).

DoD. 2012. *About the Department of Defense (DoD).* http://www.defense.gov/about/ (accessed January 30, 2012).

Eibner, C. 2008. *Invisible wounds of war: Quantifying the societal costs of psychological and cognitive injuries.* Arlington, VA: RAND Corporation.

Eidelson, R. 2011. The dark side of "comprehensive soldier fitness." *Psychology Today* 66(7):643-644.

FHP&R (Force Health Protection & Readiness). 2012. *What is force health protection and readiness?* http://home.fhpr.osd.mil/about/what-is-fhpr.aspx (accessed January 30, 2012).

GAO (U.S. Government Accountability Office). 2006. *Post-traumatic stress disorder: DoD needs to identify the factors its providers use to make mental health evaluation referrals for service members.* Washington, DC: GAO.

GAO. 2008a. *DoD health care: Mental health and traumatic brain injury screening efforts implemented, but consistent pre-deployment medical records review needed.* Washington, DC: GAO.

GAO. 2008b. *VA and DoD health care: Administration of DoD's post-deployment health reassessment to National Guard and reserve servicemembers and VA's interaction with DoD.* Washington, DC: GAO.

GAO. 2011a. *VA mental health: Number of veterans receiving care, barriers faced, and efforts to increase access.* GAO 12-12. Washington, DC: GAO.

GAO. 2011b. *DOD and VA health care—Action needed to strengthen integration across care coordination and case management programs.* Washington, DC: GAO.

GAO. 2011c. *Federal Recovery Coordination Program: Enrollment, staffing, and care coordination pose significant challenges.* GAO-11-572T. Washington, DC: GAO.

GAO. 2011d. *DOD and VA health care: Federal recovery coordination program continues to expand but faces significant challenges.* GAO-11-250. Washington, DC: GAO.

GAO. 2011e. *VA health care:VA spends millions on post-traumatic stress disorder research and incorporates research outcomes into guidelines and policy for post-traumatic stress disorder services.* GAO 11-32. Washington, DC: GAO.

Glover, W., C. Kamin, J. Wang, J. Srinivasan, C. R. Kenley, and D. Nightingale. 2011. Continuum of care for post-traumatic stress in the US military enterprise. *Proceedings of the 2011 Society of Health Systems Conference*, Orlando, FL, February 17–19.

Hoge, C. W., J. L. Auchterlonie, and C. S. Milliken. 2006. Mental health problems, use of mental health services, and attrition from military service after returning from deployment to Iraq or Afghanistan. *Journal of the American Medical Association* 295(9): 1023-1032.

Hoge, W. G., A. B. Adler, K. M. Wright, P. D. Bliese, A. Cox, D. McGurk, C. Milliken, and C. A. Castro. 2011. Chapter 5: Walter Reed Army Institute of Research Contributions During Operations Iraqi Freedom and Enduring Freedom: From Research to Public Health Policy. In *Combat and Operational Behavioral Health.* Textbooks of Military Medicine. Office of the Surgeon General and U.S. Army Medical Department Center and School.

Hoover, R. 2011. PTSD therapies with ongoing research: Updates. Paper read at Trauma Spectrum Conference, December 9, Bethesda, MD.

IOM (Institute of Medicine). 2006. *Improving the quality of health care for mental and substance-use conditions.* Washington, DC: The National Academies Press.

IOM. 2010a. *Returning home from Iraq and Afghanistan: Preliminary assessment of readjustment needs of veterans, service members, and their families.* Washington, DC: The National Academies Press.

IOM. 2010b. *Provision of mental health counseling services under TRICARE.* Washington, DC: The National Academies Press.

Karlin, B. E., J. I. Ruzek, K. M. Chard, A. Eftekhari, C. M. Monson, E. A. Hembree, P. A. Resick, and E. B. Foa. 2010. Dissemination of evidence-based psychological treatments for posttraumatic stress disorder in the Veterans Health Administration. *Journal of Traumatic Stress* 23(6):663-673.

Kilmer, B., C. Eibner, J. S. Ringel, and R. L. Pacula. 2011. Invisible wounds, visible savings? Using microsimulation to estimate the costs and savings associated with providing evidence-based treatment for PTSD and depression to veterans of Operation Enduring Freedom and Operation Iraqi Freedom. *Psychological Trauma-Theory Research Practice and Policy* 3(2):201-211.

Kizer, K. W. 2012. Veterans and the Affordable Care Act. *Journal of the American Medical Association* 307(8):789-790.

Kizer, K. W., and R. A. Dudley. 2009. Extreme makeover: Transformation of the veterans health care system. *Annual Review of Public Health* 30:313-339.

Koffman, R. L. Navy Combat/Operational Stress Control (COSC) Update. 2007. Cited in *Invisible Wounds of War. Psychological and Cognitive Injuries, Their Consequences, and Services to Assist Recovery.* RAND. 2008.

Kwan, B. W., and L. Y. I. Tan. 2008. Economic analysis of post-traumatic stress disorder (PTSD) in the Global War on Terror (GWOT), Management, Naval Postgraduate School.

Larson, G. E., P. S. Hammer, T. L. Conway, E. A. Schmied, M. R. Galarneau, P. Konoske, J. A. Webb-Murphy, K. J. Schmitz, N. Edwards, and D. C. Johnson. 2011. Predeployment and in-theater diagnoses of American military personnel serving in Iraq. *Psychiatric Services* 62(1):15-21.

McPherson, F., and M. A. Schwenka. 2004. Use of complementary and alternative therapies among active duty soldiers, military retirees, and family members at a military hospital. *Military Medicine* 169(5):354-357.

Meredith, L. S., C. D. Sherbourne, S. Gaillot, L. Hansell, H. V. Ritschard, A. Parker, and G. Wrenn. 2011. *Promoting psychological resilience in the U.S. Military.* Santa Monica, CA: RAND Corporation.

MHAT VII (Mental Health Advisory Team VII). 2011. *Joint mental health advisory team 7 (J-MHAT 7) Operation Enduring Freedom 2010.* Washington, DC: Office of the Surgeon General U.S. Army Medical Command.

MHS (Military Health System). 2012. *MHS organization.* http://www.health.mil/About_MHS/Organizations/Index.aspx (accessed January 30, 2012).

Miller, G. 2011. Healing the brain, healing the mind. *Science* 333(6042):514-517.

National Business Group on Health. 2011. *Evidence statement. Clinical preventive service recommendations.* http://www.businessgrouphealth.org/preventive/topics/depression.cfm (accessed April 17, 2012).

NEPEC (VA Northeast Program Evaluation Center). 2011a. *Number of specialized PTSD programs for FY2010, by program type.* Response to data request by the Committee on the Assessment of Ongoing Efforts in the Treatment of PTSD, August 26, 2011.

NEPEC. 2011b. Long Journey Home, Table 5-24. *VA PTSD outpatient treatment by specialized PTSD programs, PTSD specialists, mental health and non-mental health stops for FY2010 by VISN.* Response to data request by the Committee on the Assessment of Ongoing Efforts in the Treatment of PTSD, October 19, 2011.

NEPEC. 2011c. Part 2. *Treatment of veterans by specialized outpatient PTSD teams FY2010.* Response to data request by the Committee on the Assessment of Ongoing Efforts in the Treatment of PTSD, August 15, 2011.

NEPEC. 2011d. Part 3. *Treatment of veterans by specialized intensive PTSD teams FY2010.* Response to data request by the Committee on the Assessment of Ongoing Efforts in the Treatment of PTSD, August 15, 2011.

NEPEC. 2012a. Table 1-9. *The number of visits, number of veterans seen, and the number of visits per veterans seen in specialized outpatient PTSD programs for FY2004, FY2010, and the FY2004-FY2010 Difference (%) by VISN.* Response to data request by the Committee on the Assessment of Ongoing Efforts in the Treatment of PTSD, January 23, 2012. Washington, DC.

NEPEC. 2012b. Table 1-19. *Workload and direct cost for specialized outpatient PTSD programs for FY2004, FY2010, and the FY2004-2010 difference by VISN.* Response to data request by the Committee on the Assessment of Ongoing Efforts in the Treatment of PTSD, January 23, 2012.

NEPEC. 2012c. Table 1-21. *Workload and direct cost for specialized intensive PTSD programs for FY2010 and the FY2004-FY2010 difference by VISN.* Response to data request by the Committee on the Assessment of Ongoing Efforts in the Treatment of PTSD, January 23, 2012.

NIMH (National Institute of Mental Health). 2011. *The making of Army STARRS: An overview.* http://www.nimh.nih.gov/health/topics/suicide-prevention/suicide-prevention-studies/the-making-of-army-starrs-an-overview.shtml (accessed January 30, 2012).

OMB (U.S. Office of Management and Budget). 2010. *Budget of the U.S. government fiscal year 2011.* Washington, DC: U.S. Government Printing Office.

Oxman, T., A. Dietrich, J. W. Williams, C. C. Engel, M. Friedman, P. Schnurr, S. Rosenberg, and S. Barry. 2008. *Primary care clinician's manual.* RESPECT-Mil. http://sud.editme.com/files/Seeds/Respect-mil%20suicide.pdf (accessed April 27, 2012).

Patient-Centered Primary Care Collaborative. 2007. *Joint principles of the patient-centered medical home.* http://www.pcpcc.net/content/joint-principles-patient-centered-medical-home (accessed January 30, 2012).

Quick, J. C. 2011. Missing: Critical and skeptical perspectives on comprehensive soldier fitness. *American Psychologist* 66(7):645.

Saito, C. 2011. Warrior transition brigade helps wounded soldiers determine next step in life. *YNN Austin/Round Rock/San Marcos.* http://austin.ynn.com/content/top_stories/281019/warrior-transition-brigade-helps-wounded-soldiers-determine-next-step-in-life (accessed January 30, 2012).

Schiffner, S. 2011. *Data request on mental health providers in the VA, provider training, and the use of complementary and alternative medicine and treatments.* Response to data request by the Committee on the Assessment of Ongoing Efforts in the Treatment of PTSD. October 18, 2011. Washington, DC.

Schiffner, S. 2012. *Data request on the number of veterans screened for PTSD, the number of positive screens for PTSD, and the number of veterans diagnosed with PTSD.* Response to data request by the Committee on the Assessment of Ongoing Efforts in the Treatment of PTSD. January 18, 2012. Washington, DC.

Schoenhard, W. 2011. *Statement to the Senate Committee on Veterans' Affairs.* July 14, 2011. http://veterans.senate.gov/hearings.cfm?action=release.display&release_id=796c41ee-3006-4647-b461-920653c6425e (accessed April 27, 2012).

Seligman, M. E. P. 2011. Helping American soldiers in time of war: Reply to comments on the comprehensive soldier fitness special issue. *American Psychologist* 66(7):646-647.

Smith, T. C., M. A. Ryan, B. Smith, R. J. Reed, J. R. Riddle, F. R. Gumbs, and G. C. Gray. 2007. Complementary and alternative medicine use among US Navy and Marine Corps personnel. *BMC Complementary and Alternative Medicine* 7:16.

STRONG STAR (South Texas Research Organization Network Guiding Studies on Trauma and Resilience). 2012a. *STRONG STAR*. https://delta.uthscsa.edu/strongstar/ (accessed January 30, 2012).

STRONG STAR. 2012b. *STRONG STAR research projects: Finding the best ways to prevent and treat combat-related PTSD*. https://delta.uthscsa.edu/strongstar/research.asp (accessed January 30, 2012).

Tanielian, T. L., and L. Jaycox. 2008. *Invisible wounds of war: Psychological and cognitive injuries, their consequences, and services to assist recovery*. Arlington, VA: RAND Corporation.

TRICARE (TRICARE Management Activity). 2008. *The Fort Bliss Restoration & Resilience Center*. http://www.tricare.mil/twr/downloads/RRCENTER.pdf (accessed January 30, 2012).

TRICARE. 2011. *Evaluation of the TRICARE program: Fiscal year 2011 report to Congress*. Washington, DC: Department of Defense.

TRICARE. 2012. *TRICARE—media center*. http://www.tricare.mil/mediacenter/press_resources.aspx (accessed January 30, 2012).

Tyson, M., and VA. 2009. Mobile Vet Centers: Reaching out in rural areas. http://www.va.gov/health/newsfeatures/20091116a.asp (accessed January 30, 2012).

U.S. Air Force. 2006. *Traumatic stress response*. Washington, DC: Department of the Air Force.

U.S. Air Force. 2011. *Primary behavioral health care services: Practice manual*. Lackland AFB, TX: Airforce Medical Operations Agency (AFMOA), Mental Health Division/SGHW.

U.S. Army. 2012a. *Comprehensive solder fitness*. http://csf.army.mil/ (accessed January 30, 2012).

U.S. Army. 2012b. *Carl R. Darnall Army Medical Center—Ft. Hood, Texas*. http://www.crdamc.amedd.army.mil/default.asp (accessed January 30, 2012).

U.S. Army. 2012c. *Army behavioral health*. http://www.behavioralhealth.army.mil/research/index.html (accessed January 30, 2012).

U.S. Army. 2012d. *Walter Reed Army Institute of Research*. http://wrair-www.army.mil/ (accessed January 30, 2012).

U.S. Congress. 2011. *Military construction, veterans affairs, and related agencies appropriations bill, 2012*. 112-94. Washington, DC: Government Printing Office.

U.S. Marine Corps. 2012. *About COSC*. http://www.usmc-mccs.org/cosc/cosc.cfm?sid=ml&smid=2 (accessed January 30, 2012).

USUHS (Uniformed Services University of the Health Sciences). 2012. *About Uniformed Services University*. http://www.usuhs.mil/usuhs/ (accessed January 30, 2012).

VA (Department of Veterans Affairs). 2002a. *Content of Vet Center files and counseling notation*. Memorandum No. 3-9. Washington, DC: VA.

VA. 2002b. *Review of clinical records*. Memorandum No. 3-10. Washington, DC: VA.

VA. 2005. *Implementation of the national clinical reminder for Afghan and Iraq post-deployment screening*. Washington, DC: VA. http://www1.va.gov/vhapublications/ViewPublication.asp?pub_ID=1346 (accessed April 27, 2012).

VA. 2008. *Uniform mental health services in VA medical centers and clinics*. VHA Handbook 1160.01. Washingon, DC: Veterans Health Administration. http://www1.va.gov/vhapublications/ViewPublication.asp?pub_ID=1762 (accessed April 27, 2012).

VA. 2009. *Healthcare inspection. Readjustment counseling service—Vet Center report*. Washington, DC: VA Office of the Inspector General. http://www.va.gov/oig/54/reports/VAOIG-08-02589-171.pdf (accessed April 27, 2012).

VA. 2010a. *2010 Organizational briefing book.* Washington, DC: VA. http://www.va.gov/ofcadmin/docs/vaorgbb.pdf (accessed April 27, 2012).

VA. 2010b. Posttraumatic stress disorder. In *VA brochure series*, edited by Veterans Health Affairs Research and Development. VA ORD Office of Communications. http://www.research.va.gov/resources/pubs/docs/ptsd-brochure.pdf (accessed April 27, 2012).

VA. 2010c. Programs for Veterans with Post-traumatic Stress Disorder (PTSD). VHA Handbook 1160.03. March 12, 2010. http://www1.va.gov/vhapublications/ViewPublication.asp? pub_ID=2174 (accessed April 26, 2012).

VA. 2011a. *Department of Veterans Affairs: Statistics at a glance.* http://www.va.gov/vetdata/docs/quickfacts/Homepage-slideshow.pdf (accessed April 27, 2012).

VA. 2011b. *Healthcare Inspection. Post traumatic stress disorder counseling services at Vet Centers.* Washington, DC: VA Office of the Inspector General. http://www.va.gov/oig/54/reports/VAOIG-10-00628-170.pdf (accessed April 27, 2012).

VA. 2011c. *Patient aligned care team.* http://www.va.gov/PRIMARYCARE/PACT/index.asp (accessed April 4, 2012).

VA. 2012a. *Treatment of PTSD.* http://www.PTSD.va.gov/public/pages/treatment-PTSD.asp (accessed January 30, 2012).

VA. 2012b. *Course modules.* http://www.PTSD.va.gov/professional/PTSD101/course-modules/course-modules.asp (accessed January 30, 2012).

VA. 2012c. *About us.* http://www.va.gov/health/about VHA.asp (accessed March 20, 2012).

VA. 2012d. *Where do I get the care I need?* http://www.va.gov/health/findcare.asp (accessed January 30, 2012).

VA. 2012e. *Vet Center home.* http://www.vetcenter.va.gov/ (accessed January 30, 2012).

VA. 2012f. *VA deploying 20 new mobile Vet Centers.* http://www.va.gov/opa/pressrel/press release.cfm?id=2241 (accessed January 30, 2012).

VA. 2012g. *VA to increase mental health staff by 1,900.* http://www.va.gov/opa/pressrel/pressrelease.cfm?id=2302 (accessed April 12, 2012).

VA. 2012h. *What is the National Center for PTSD.* http://www.PTSD.va.gov/about/index.asp (accessed January 30, 2012).

VA. 2012i. *History of the National Center for PTSD.* http://www.PTSD.va.gov/about/mission/history_of_the_national_center_for_PTSD.asp (accessed January 30, 2012).

VA. 2012j. *Mission and overview.* http://www.PTSD.va.gov/about/mission/mission-and-overview.asp (accessed January 30, 2012).

VA. 2012k. *Military sexual trauma.* http://www.ptsd.va.gov/public/pages/military-sexual-trauma-general.asp (accessed January 30, 2012).

VA. 2012l. *My HealtheVet—the gateway to veteran health and wellness.* https://www.myhealth.va.gov/index.html (accessed January 30, 2012).

VA. 2012m. *Services.* http://www.vetcenter.va.gov/Vet_Center_Services.asp (accessed January 30, 2012).

VA. 2012n. *PTSD treatment programs in the U.S. Department of Veterans Affairs.* http://www.PTSD.va.gov/public/pages/va-PTSD-treatment-programs.asp (accessed January 30, 2012).

VA and DCoE. 2009. *Report of (VA) consensus conference: Practice recommendations for treatment of veterans with comorbid TBI, pain, and PTSD.* http://www.ptsd.va.gov/professional/pages/handouts-pdf/ TBI_PTSD_Pain_ Practice_ Recommend.pdf (accessed April 4, 2012).

VA and DoD. 2010. *VA/DOD clinical practice guideline for management of post-traumatic stress.* Washington, DC: VA and DoD.

VA and DoD. 2011. *VA/DoD collaboration guidebook to healthcare research.* Washington, DC: VA and DoD.

Warner, C. H., G. N. Appenzeller, J. E. Breitbach, J. T. Lange, A. Mobbs, and E. C. Ritchie. 2011. Psychiatric consultation to command. In *Combat and Operational Behavioral Health*, edited by E. C. Ritchie. Fort Detrick, MD: Borden Institute. Pp. 171-188.

Weinick, R. M., E. B. Beckjord, C. M. Farmer, K. T. Martin, E. M. Gillen, J. D. Acosta, M. P. Fisher, J. Garnett, G. C. Gonzalez, T. C. Helmus, K. H. Jaycox, K. A. Reynolds, N. Salcedo, and D. M. Scharf. 2011. Programs addressing psychological health and traumatic brain injury among U.S. military servicemembers and their families. Arlington, VA: RAND Corporation.

White, M. R., I. G. Jacobson, B. Smith, T. S. Wells, G. D. Gackstetter, E. J. Boyko, and T. C. Smith. 2011. Health care utilization among complementary and alternative medicine users in a large military cohort. *BioMed Central Complementary and Alternative Medicine* 11:27-37.

Zeiss, A. 2011. Veterans Affairs efforts in identification and treatment of PTSD. Presentation to the Committee on on the Assessment of Ongoing Efforts in the Treatment of PTSD. February 28, 2011. Washington, DC.

5

Prevention

Prevention of posttraumatic stress disorder (PTSD) in active-duty and veteran populations is important to support their overall health and well-being, to preserve personnel resources, and to maximize force readiness. This chapter examines prevention of and prophylaxis for PTSD in active-duty and veteran populations. It begins by defining primary, secondary, and tertiary prevention and then summarizes the state of the science with regard to prevention programs and current research. That is followed by a discussion of what the Department of Defense (DoD) and the Department of Veterans Affairs (VA) are doing with regard to prevention at each level and a discussion of the VA/DoD guideline and other guidelines and programs, including evidence of the efficacy of prevention programs.

OVERVIEW OF PTSD PREVENTION

Prevention is broadly defined as measures taken to avoid the occurrence of disease or "interventions that are applied before the onset of a clinically diagnosable disorder with the aim of reducing the number of new cases of that disorder" (Munoz et al., 1996, as cited by Boyce et al., 2007). The term can also be applied to an intervention aimed at limiting the disorder's progression, relapse, or associated disability. Prevention of PTSD in active-duty personnel is provided via programs aimed at preparing service members for combat and other deployment-related stressors. Some programs focus on reducing the risk of exposure to traumatic events (such as interventions aimed at reducing the risk of military sexual trauma) and on training service members to respond effectively to such events if they occur.

Other prevention efforts seek to detect and treat disorder in its early stages (for example, treat those who meet the criteria for acute stress disorder [ASD]) often before it presents clinically as chronic PTSD. Several studies (for example, Bryant et al., 1999, 2003; Shalev et al., 2011) have demonstrated that early interventions for ASD result in significant reductions of ASD symptoms and the prevention of the onset of PTSD in the majority of individuals treated. Prophylactic interventions can be implemented immediately after a trauma (within 48 hours) or during the acute period (within weeks) to prevent full onset of PTSD symptoms (Litz, 2008), although the efficacy of this approach is unknown. And prevention may refer to measures taken to mitigate the consequences of existing symptoms by improving functioning and reducing complications. The latter type of PTSD prevention includes interventions in patients who have subthreshold PTSD symptoms, ASD, and ancillary problems; it provides treatment for clinical PTSD and recurrence prevention through rehabilitation programs. Treatment and rehabilitation programs for PTSD are covered in depth in Chapter 7 and 8, respectively; the present chapter discusses interventions to limit the development of clinical PTSD (that is, beyond subclinical symptoms) and to prevent recurrence.

Prevention is considered here in three phases:

1. Interventions that are applied to an entire population before a traumatic event and regardless of the potential for exposure. These are often called primary or universal interventions.
2. Interventions that are applied to individuals who are known to have been exposed to a traumatic event and thus to be at risk for PTSD and who may or may not be showing symptoms of stress. These are called secondary or selective interventions.
3. Interventions aimed at individuals who are displaying symptoms of or have received a diagnosis of PTSD with the goals of preventing worsening of the symptoms and improving functioning. These are called tertiary or indicated interventions.

As noted by Lau and Rapee (2011), universal interventions do not require screening, and they reduce the possibility that specific persons will be labeled unfavorably by others for having a mental illness. Selective and indicated interventions are targeted at persons viewed to be vulnerable, and therefore, pose a risk that such persons will be labeled as mentally disordered and viewed unfavorably.

PRETRAUMA PREVENTION EFFORTS

Much research related to the prevention of trauma has focused on the prevention of unwanted sexual contact in civilian and military populations (Casey and Lindhorst, 2009; Exner and Cummings, 2011; Langhinrichsen-Rohling et al., 2011; McMahon and Banyard, 2012; Moor, 2011; Moynihan and Banyard, 2008; Rau et al., 2011; Vladutiu et al., 2011). Research has identified modifiable and nonmodifiable risk factors for unwanted sexual contact in these populations. Those data have been used to inform the development of preventive interventions in both civilian and military personnel. Modifiable factors include unit culture, whereby reporting sexual assault by a fellow service member may considered to be "breaking a code" and may result in ostracization; leadership behavior that may implicitly or explicitly condone, tolerate, or ignore sexual assault and harassment; and facilitating situations such as excessive use of alcohol by any of the involved parties (Allard et al., 2011; Sadler et al., 2001; Street et al., 2009; Suris and Lind, 2008). Nonmodifiable risk factors among service members include female sex, young age, low rank, and prior sexual abuse history.

Several prevention programs in civilian populations and in the U.S. military have focused on decreasing the likelihood that individuals exposed to trauma will develop PTSD. Many of the programs emphasize the development of mental or emotional resilience. In this context, mental resilience refers to a person's capacity to adapt or change successfully in the face of adversity (Pietrzak et al., 2010b). Most importantly, resilience and PTSD appear to be inversely correlated (Nishi et al., 2010). Those who perceive a trauma as a crisis but are able to confront distressing memories and emotions and integrate them into a coherent meaning may be resilient, whereas those who cope by avoiding distressing emotions appear to be at risk for PTSD (Larner and Blow, 2011). In a RAND report on resilience factors in military personnel, Meredith et al. (2011) found 20 evidence-informed factors associated with resilience. Individual-level factors were positive coping, positive affect, positive thinking, realism, behavioral control, physical fitness, and altruism. Family-level factors were emotional ties, communication, support, closeness, nurturing, and adaptability. Military unit-level factors were positive command climate, teamwork, and cohesion. And community-level factors were belongingness, cohesion, connectedness, and collective efficacy.

Other factors thought to protect against the development of PTSD are social support and confidence in the military mission and training. Pietrzak et al. (2010b) found that resilience, unit support, and postdeployment social support are psychosocial buffers of PTSD even at 2 years after deployment in veterans of Operation Enduring Freedom (OEF) and Operation Iraqi Freedom (OIF). In a study of U.S. Air Force medical personnel deployed to Iraq or Afghanistan, unit cohesion, positive attitudes about the military mission and the military in general, and confidence in their military training were all protective factors for PTSD when service members were experiencing increased combat-related or health-care–related stressors (Dickstein et al., 2010).

Some early work suggested that characteristics of deployment conditions and support are risk factors or protective factors for PTSD. The Mental Health Advisory Team surveyed marines and soldiers deployed to OEF and OIF in 2006 and found the level of combat experienced was the most important determinant of their mental health (MHAT, 2006). Similar to deployment stressors reported by 1990–1991 Gulf War veterans, OEF and OIF deployment stressors include being in the vicinity of explosions, direct combat duty, witnessing death of a person, being exposed to dead and dismembered bodies, and having a combat-related injury (IOM, 2008). In a sample of active-duty, National Guard, and reserve soldiers deployed in the 1990–1991 Gulf War, the stressors most highly associated with PTSD were all combat related and included having a buddy killed or wounded in action, exposure to dead or dying people, and being fired on by the enemy (Stretch et al., 1996). In a 2003 survey of combat infantry service members (2,856 soldiers and 815 marines) deployed to either Iraq or Afghanistan, Hoge et al. (2004) found the majority had been attacked or ambushed; shot at; saw dead bodies or human remains; received incoming artillery, rocket, or mortar fire; or knew someone who was seriously injured or killed. Fewer combat experiences were reported for soldiers deployed to Afghanistan than those deployed to Iraq; however, rates of PTSD increased with more exposure to firefights and for service members who were wounded or injured. See Table 5-1 for the combat experiences reported by the soldiers and marines surveyed.

A recent study found that soldiers who reported higher preparedness appraised the threat involved in different levels of combat exposure more realistically, whereas less prepared soldiers perceived even low-level combat as highly threatening (Renshaw, 2011). Perceived threat is thought to be an important link between combat experience and PTSD (the greater the perceived threat, the greater the likelihood of developing PTSD after the experience) (Green et al., 1990; King et al., 1995, 2008; Vogt and Tanner, 2007). Preparedness, therefore, may play a role in the development of PTSD through its relation with perceived threat. If service members are better prepared, they may perceive specific situations as less threatening (Renshaw, 2011). Other studies suggest a positive influence of high levels of unit support and cohesion on mental health in UK and U.S. soldiers in OEF and OIF who experienced combat (Brailey et al., 2007; Dickstein et al., 2010; Du Preez et al., 2012; Rona et al., 2009). Receiving support from one's unit during deployment may promote soldiers' resilience to PTSD by increasing

TABLE 5-1 Combat Experiences Reported by Members of the U.S. Army and Marine Corps Following Deployment to Iraq or Afghanistan

	Army Groups		Marine Group
Experience	% in Afghanistan (n = 1,962)	% in Iraq (n = 894)	% in Iraq (n = 815)
Being attacked or ambushed	58	89	95
Receiving incoming artillery, rocket, or mortar fire	84	86	92
Being shot at or receiving small-arms fire	66	93	97
Shooting or directing fire at the enemy	27	77	87
Being responsible for the death of an enemy combatant	12	48	65
Being responsible for the death of a noncombatant	1	14	28
Seeing dead bodies or human remains	39	95	94
Handling or uncovering human remains	12	50	57
Seeing dead or seriously injured Americans	30	65	75
Knowing someone who was seriously injured or killed	43	86	87
Participating in demining operations	16	38	34
Seeing ill or injured women or children and being unable to help them	46	69	83
Being wounded or injured	5	14	9
Having a close call, being shot or hit, but being saved by protective gear	Not asked	8	10
Having a buddy shot or hit nearby	Not asked	22	26
Clearing or searching homes or buildings	57	80	86
Engaging in hand-to-hand combat	3	22	9
Saving the life of a soldier or civilian	6	21	19

SOURCE: Adapted with permission from Hoge et al., 2004.

self-efficacy (belief in one's ability to handle situations or perform well) or mitigating the psychologic consequences of war zone stressors through strengthened coping abilities.

Studies of OEF, OIF, and Vietnam veterans have also documented post-event social support as a strong predictor of PTSD and other psychopathologic conditions (Brewin et al., 2000; Fikretoglu et al., 2006; Fontana et al., 1997; King et al., 1998; Pietrzak et al., 2009; Taylor and Seeman, 1999). Receiving support from others after a traumatic event may enhance a person's coping abilities or influence how he or she evaluates the stressful situation and later reacts to it emotionally and behaviorally and may buffer the psychologic consequences of traumatic events. Psychologic resilience and social support are hypothesized to protect against the development of both PTSD and depression and may preserve or improve functioning in those with PTSD. In a study of 284 OEF and OIF veterans with and without PTSD, Pietrzak et al. (2009) found that veterans without PTSD had a higher resilience score than those with PTSD; the greatest difference was in personal control, and this suggests lower coping self-efficacy in those with PTSD. Longer dwell time, at least twice the length of the deployment, has also been shown to reduce the odds of PTSD and other mental health disorders (MacGregor et al., 2012). See Chapter 2 for a longer discussion on the effect of dwell time and PTSD.

A relatively new concept associated with PTSD is that of posttraumatic growth—positive personal changes resulting from coping with a traumatic event. This concept is being explored, as is enhancement of resilience and hardiness, as a method for protecting against adverse sequelae, such as PTSD and depression, in military personnel who experience extreme stress and trauma (Gallaway et al., 2011; Larner and Blow, 2011; MacDermott, 2010; Nelson, 2011; Pietrzak et al., 2010a; Prati and Pietrantoni, 2009; Tedeschi, 2011). The effectiveness of programs to encourage posttraumatic growth has yet to be determined.

INTERVENTIONS FOR TRAUMA-EXPOSED PEOPLE

Interventions to prevent PTSD in trauma-exposed persons are aimed at interfering with overconsolidation of the fear memory and accelerating extinction of the fear memory. The interventions may be pharmacologic or behavioral and may be given to all exposed persons or targeted to people who show high levels of acute distress. This section reviews research on early psychosocial interventions for the prevention of PTSD. First, psychologic debriefing that is usually conducted immediately or within few days after a traumatic event is reviewed and then the literature on cognitive behavioral therapy (CBT) and non-CBT interventions used for severe PTSD symptoms or ASD within the first month after the trauma is discussed.

Immediate psychoeducation and advice for acute distress management and such interventions as psychologic support, nonspecific stress management, family interventions, and family-centered decision making have all been proposed to prevent PTSD, but no randomized controlled trials (RCTs) have been conducted to demonstrate their efficacy. Psychoeducation can be used to encourage resiliency and adaptation and, ultimately, help-seeking, but its content and dissemination need to be appropriate for the audience and time after trauma exposure (Wessely et al., 2008). The use of CBT in the weeks or days after exposure for people who display symptoms of posttraumatic stress have proved to be effective in RCTs and meta-analytic reviews, but there are no studies of the use of CBT immediately after trauma exposure. These effective trauma-focused therapies include psychoeducation, relaxation and stress management, affective expression and modulation, cognitive coping, prolonged imaginal exposure, in vivo exposure, and cognitive reprocessing. The use of multisession psychologic interventions delivered up to 72 hours after trauma does not appear to be effective in preventing PTSD (Agorastos et al., 2011). Evidence on the use of collaborative care interventions (discussed in more detail later in the chapter) and virtual-reality–based interventions (Agorastos et al., 2011) is still lacking.

Psychologic Debriefing

Psychologic debriefing includes a variety of single-session individual and group interventions that involve survivors' or other affected persons' revisiting of the trauma for the purpose of encouraging them to talk about their experiences during the trauma; to recognize and express their thoughts, emotions, and physical reactions during and since the event; and to learn coping methods. Specially trained debriefers lead the sessions, which usually focus on normalization of symptoms, group support, and provision of psychoeducation and information about resources. Two main psychologic debriefing protocols have been examined empirically. Critical incident stress debriefing (CISD) is a group-based formalized structured review that was first developed to assist first responders, such as fire and police personnel, and has expanded to include disaster victims and their relatives. Critical incident stress management includes precrisis intervention, disaster or large-scale incident demobilization and informational briefings, "town meetings," staff advisement, defusing, CISD, one-on-one crisis counseling or support, family crisis intervention, organizational consultation, and follow-up and referral mechanisms for assessment and treatment.

Most RCTs that have examined psychologic debriefing for the prevention of PTSD have used individually administered, one-time debriefings of victims of motor vehicle incidents or crimes, such as rape. Numerous reviews and meta-analyses of these studies have determined that this treatment is ineffective and sometimes even harmful (McNally et al., 2003; Rose et al., 2002). In particular, two RCTs that included long-term follow-up indicated that psychologic debriefing may be related to a poorer outcome than that in controls (Bisson et al., 1997; Mayou et al., 2000). However, the two studies suffered from methodologic flaws so it cannot be presumed that early interventions can interfere with recovery. Bisson et al. (2009) reviewed 10 studies that compared psychologic debriefing with wait list (WL) and found that two studies showed that psychological debriefing decreased PTSD symptoms compared with results of WL, five showed no difference between the two methods, and three showed that people who received the intervention experienced worsened PTSD symptoms compared with results of WL. Overall, Bisson et al. found no evidence to support the preventive value of individual debriefing delivered in a single session. Cuijpers et al. (2005) reviewed studies examining psychologic debriefing and found the risk of PTSD was somewhat, but not statistically significantly, increased after debriefing. Similarly, a meta-analysis of individual, single-session interventions immediately after a trauma found that non-CISD interventions (which typically included 30 minutes of individual counseling, education, and group debriefing focusing on the objective facts pertaining to the disaster or trauma) and an absence of intervention improved symptoms of PTSD but that CISD did not (van Emmerik et al., 2002).

Deahl et al. (2000) found no difference in PTSD symptoms between patients who received group-based debriefing and those who received assessment. Campfield and Hills (2001) randomly assigned robbery victims to immediate CISD (sooner than 10 hours) or delayed CISD (later than 48 hours) and found that immediate CISD produced more pronounced reduction in PTSD symptoms. However, the findings are limited by the lack of a control group, and it is unclear how many people would have recovered without the need for an intervention. No conclusions regarding treatment efficacy can be drawn from other studies (e.g., Eid et al., 2001; Richards, 2001) because they used small samples and nonrandom assignment.

Two RCTs conducted by Adler et al. examined group psychologic debriefing in military samples. Adler et al. (2008) randomized 1,050 soldiers who served in Kosovo as peacekeepers into 62 groups that were subjected to three conditions—CISD (23 groups), stress education (20 groups), and WL (19 groups)—and focused on the entire deployment period. No differences were found between groups with respect to all mental health outcomes, although it should be noted that soldiers in this study experienced relatively few traumas. In a second RCT, Adler et al. (2009) studied U.S. soldiers returning from Iraq who had been exposed to direct combat throughout their deployment. Soldiers received either stress education or Battlemind debriefing (*Battlemind* is an Army program to foster resilience;

see the "Prevention Efforts in the Army" section for more information on Battlemind). The authors (2009) found that Battlemind debriefing did not result in a reduction in PTSD symptoms compared with stress education.

In a review of RCTs of psychologic debriefing immediately after trauma exposure, Agorastos et al. (2011) found no evidence of its efficacy in reducing PTSD symptoms. In summary, there is no evidence of efficacy of psychologic debriefing in preventing PTSD in trauma-exposed people. And there is insufficient evidence of the efficacy of group psychologic debriefing in PTSD prevention.

Brief Early Interventions

Treatment of early symptoms of PTSD usually begins with CBT in an effort to prevent the development of chronic PTSD (Feldner et al., 2007). Brief specialized interventions (for example, four or five sessions) delivered within weeks of a traumatic event may effectively prevent PTSD in survivors of sexual and nonsexual assault (Foa et al., 1995), motor vehicle incidents, industrial accidents, and traumatic brain injuries (Bryant et al., 1998, 1999, 2003). Trauma-focused CBT has also been found to be effective in both reducing and preventing PTSD symptoms in people who experienced PTSD symptoms soon after a traumatic event and those who met the criteria for ASD (Roberts et al., 2009a; Stapleton, 2006). This particular intervention focused on the traumatic experience through memories and trauma reminders, sometimes combined with cognitive therapy or other behavioral interventions. Another study showed that combined imaginal and in vivo exposure is significantly more effective than cognitive restructuring only in reducing PTSD in people diagnosed with ASD (Bryant et al., 2008). Ehlers et al. (2003) found that CBT was more effective in reducing symptoms than a self-help booklet or repeated assessment.

In a pilot RCT, Kazak et al. (2005) studied stress in caregivers of children who had new diagnoses of cancer. A three-session integrated CBT and family-therapy intervention, surviving cancer competently intervention program—newly diagnosed (SCCIP-ND), was compared with the usual treatment. Results indicated that families who received SCCIP-ND had lower anxiety and parental posttraumatic stress symptoms than families that did not.

Zatzick et al. (2004) found that in acutely injured trauma survivors, a stepped-care approach of CBT, pharmacotherapy, or a combination of the two for 6–12 months after injury did not reduce PTSD, but fewer patients developed PTSD than in the usual-care group when pharmacotherapy or CBT was initiated 3 months after injury. Roberts et al. (2009b) conducted a meta-analysis of early interventions (within 3 months of trauma) for the prevention of PTSD. If patients received an intervention regardless of their symptoms, there was no statistically significant difference between those who received and those who did not receive an intervention. If patients who manifested traumatic-stress symptoms received an intervention within 3 months of a traumatic event, significant differences were found in those who received trauma-focused CBT and supportive counseling (but not structured writing) compared with controls. In those who were given a diagnosis of ASD or acute PTSD within 3 months of a trauma, only trauma-focused CBT resulted in significant improvement compared with the WL control or supportive counseling. The authors concluded that multiple-session interventions aimed at everyone exposed to trauma were ineffective and that people who were symptomatic but did not have a diagnosis of PTSD showed a variable response. Those who had diagnosed ASD or PTSD showed the greatest response to intervention within 3 months of the trauma.

A few other non-CBT interventions have been examined as potential preventive treatments for PTSD, but none have been found to be effective in reducing or preventing PTSD symptoms. For example, brief structured writing has been found ineffective in preventing PTSD in two studies (Bugg et al., 2009; van Emmerik et al., 2008) and a memory-restructuring intervention was no more effective than a control condition (Gidron et al., 2007). Providing self-help information as a preventive psychoeducation strategy has not been found efficacious (Scholes et al., 2007; Turpin et al., 2005).

Two caveats should be noted. First, it has yet to be determined how much time should pass before CBT interventions are used in traumatized people (Litz and Bryant, 2009). If prophylactic treatment is provided too early, people who may not need therapy will consume valuable resources; it is for this reason that trials do not usually begin before 2 weeks after the trauma (Bryant et al., 1998, 1999, 2003). Second, studies that have targeted all trauma survivors, regardless of the levels of stress reactions, have not been effective in preventing PTSD (Roberts et al., 2009a).

Pharmacotherapy

It is standard practice to manage acute PTSD symptoms by using pharmaceuticals to inhibit sleep disturbance, pain, or hyperarousal. However, it is unknown whether that helps to prevent the development of PTSD. The VA/DoD guideline states that "due to the limited support of evidence, the use of medications in the early posttrauma period to prevent PTSD cannot be recommended" (VA and DoD, 2010). Drugs that are mentioned in the 2010 VA/DoD guideline as having the potential to prevent PTSD are opioids, benzodiazepines, and propranolol. Research has been conducted on the use of pain medicines, especially the opioid morphine, and the prevention of PTSD. The work of Bryant et al. (2009) and Holbrook et al. (2010)

showed lower rates of PTSD in patients who received pain medication after traumatic injury. The guideline states that pharmacotherapy aids in treating some PTSD symptoms like pain, but it does not recommend the use of morphine to prevent PTSD.

Although benzodiazepines have historically been used as effective treatments for anxiety and insomnia, the guidelines do not recommend their use as preventive measures "due to lack of evidence for effectiveness and risks that may outweigh potential benefits" (VA and DoD, 2010). Studies using propranolol have had mixed results, and overall the VA/DoD guideline concludes that despite some positive results "the size and weak study designs of the investigations do not allow for definitive conclusions regarding the value of these medications in preventing the development of PTSD symptoms after traumatic events."

The use of hydrocortisone has also been studied in small trials. Two controlled trials in high-risk patients who had septic shock or who underwent cardiac surgery found that stress (high) doses of hydrocortisone administered over a few days were associated with lower rates of PTSD at long-term follow-up (Schelling et al., 2001, 2004). In a third study by the same group, hydrocortisone given at stress doses over a 4-day taper resulted in better post-operative adjustment after cardiac surgery, on the basis of measures of quality of life, stress, and PTSD (Weis et al., 2006). A prospective, randomized, placebo-controlled, double-blind trial in civilians found the best results at 1-month and 3-month follow-up with a single high intravenous dose (100–400 mg) of hydrocortisone given within hours of trauma (Zohar et al., 2011).

In an RCT of early interventions with psychopharmaceuticals (Shalev et al., 2011), Israeli trauma survivors who met the criteria for PTSD received one of the following treatments for 12 weeks: weekly prolonged exposure (PE) therapy, CBT, the selective serotonin reuptake inhibitor (SSRI) escitalopram, placebo pills, or WL. At 5 months, the prevalence of PTSD was significantly lower in the PE group (21.6%) and CBT group (20.0%) compared with the two WL groups (57.1% and 58.7%) (odds ratio [OR] 0.21, 95% confidence interval [CI] 0.09–0.46, and OR 0.18, 95% CI 0.06–0.48, respectively), the SSRI group (55.6%), and the placebo group (61.9%). There was no difference in PTSD outcome between those receiving PE versus CBT (OR 0.87, 95% CI 0.29–2.62). At 9 months, the prevalence of PTSD in the PE (21.2%), CBT (22.9%), and WL (22.8%) groups was about half that in the SSRI (42.1%) and placebo (47.1%) groups. About 40% of those on the WL who initially met the criteria for PTSD no longer did so at 5 months, and only 23% met the criteria at 9 months. Trauma survivors who had symptoms of PTSD but did not meet the full criteria for PTSD at the first assessment did not benefit from CBT.

Fletcher et al. (2010) reviewed the evidence on the use of pharmaceutical agents to prevent PTSD after a traumatic event. Alcohol is the most frequently used prophylactic, and it has been shown that intoxicated people have less PTSD after trauma than those who are not intoxicated, but the harmful effects of alcohol outweigh the beneficial effects.

Many psychopharmacologic agents have been proposed to prevent the development of PTSD if administered in the acute aftermath of a traumatic event, but the current evidence of the effectiveness of these agents, such as glucocorticoids and benzodiazepines, is disappointing (see Chapter 3 for a description of the agents). Chapter 7 discusses the use of psychopharmacologic agents in combination with psychotherapies for PTSD treatment.

PREVENTION IN THE DEPARTMENT OF DEFENSE

In this section the committee considers service-wide PTSD prevention efforts that have been mandated by the DoD, including directives and instructions for establishing plans, procedures, and responsibilities for managing stress before it causes PTSD, and treating symptoms of PTSD after they develop. The committee then looks at examples of PTSD prevention programs in each service. The examples are not exhaustive but are used to indicate the wide variety of approaches that are used to acclimate service members to the rigors of deployment and combat, to help them mitigate the effects of traumatic exposure after they occur, and to assist service members who have symptoms of PTSD to regain function.

Service-wide Prevention Efforts

The DoD has issued directives and instructions on stress control programs for many years; however, the instructions and programs deal with general combat stress and are not always PTSD-specific (Brusher, 2011; Stokes et al., 2003). For example, DoD Instruction 6490.05 (DoD, 2011) "Maintenance of Psychological Health in Military Operations" (which replaced Directive 6490.05 "Combat Stress Control [CSC] Programs" [DoD, 1999]) is applicable to all service branches and established requirements for the "early detection and management of combat and operational stress reactions in order to preserve mission effectiveness and war fighting capabilities and mitigate the adverse physical and psychological consequences of exposure to severe stress." The goal of CSC programs is to manage combat stress reactions as close to unit level as possible. Furthermore, "psychological interventions for combat and operational stress reactions shall be implemented by first-responders on the same parity with physical injuries in order to mitigate the risk of potential longer-term physical and psychological consequences of combat and other military operations." The instruction also requires the mental health providers "be trained in command consultation, coaching techniques, resilience skills, motivational interviewing, psychological first aid, management of COSRs [combat and operational stress reactions], cognitive-behavioral techniques for managing post-traumatic stress disorder and acute stress disorder, and all related regulations pertinent to the COSC [combat and operational stress continuum] mission" and that other health care providers be familiar with the general principles of COSR management. It should be noted that Instruction 6490.05 deals with all types of combat stress and is not PTSD-specific.

CSC primary prevention "involves the effort to monitor, identify, modify, avoid, or reduce stressors before they cause dysfunction—and build stress-coping skills within individuals" (Stokes et al., 2003). CSC personnel talk with service members at the squad and crew levels to provide advice on stress control techniques and other preventive measures. CSC personnel work at the individual level to teach and build "confidence, competence, communication and coordination" and at the organizational level to foster "community, cooperation, comfort and concern" (Stokes et al., 2003). Those principles need to be incorporated into the functioning of a military unit, and the unit's force-health protection team, which comprises personnel in mental health and preventive medicine, must demonstrate its own usefulness to its unit by understanding the unit, developing a sense of membership and identification with the unit, and doing actual force-health protection work.

Prevention efforts in the DoD are directed to all service personnel who face the risk of exposure to traumatic events during deployment. Preparing service members for the stressful environment they may encounter in the theater of war before an encounter occurs may make it possible to limit the development or severity of PTSD. Primary prevention within the DoD is intended to promote the skills in at-risk populations necessary to cope with the traumatic experiences associated with combat. A large number of PTSD prevention programs have been developed by each service and are discussed in the RAND report *Programs Addressing Psychological Health and Traumatic Brain Injury Among U.S. Military Servicemembers and Their Families* (Weinick et al., 2011).

The DoD Defense Centers of Excellence for Psychological Health and Traumatic Brain Injury (DCoE) have a Resilience and Prevention Directorate that assists the services and the DoD in optimizing resilience, psychologic health, and readiness for service members and their families (Meredith et al., 2011). Navy and Marine Corps COSC is color-coded to indicate a service member's ability to function (see Chapter 4 for more details on the Marine Corps Operational Stress Control and Readiness [OSCAR] program). DCoE has a Resiliency Continuum that is similar and emphasizes a leader's responsibility to mitigate service members' risk of psychologic damage.

The focus on *stress resilience* training before deployment reflects a quantum shift in military culture and can now be seen to emanate from the highest levels of command in the military. For example, in a recent article in *American Psychologist,* Army General George Casey (Casey, 2011) makes the case that "soldiers can 'be' better *before* deploying to combat so they will not have to 'get' better *after* they return," and he then calls for a shift in the military "to a culture in which psychological fitness is recognized as every bit as important as physical fitness." That level of endorsement can be seen in practice in the substantial funding and resources applied to stress-resilience training in the Comprehensive Soldier Fitness program (Cornum et al., 2011). The core aims of such approaches are to promote psychologic fitness to better prepare service members for the psychologic stressors they may experience during combat deployment, and ultimately to reduce the incidence of stress reactions and PTSD on their return home.

The DoD has a number of programs to promote psychologic resilience in service members and their families, but most have not been evaluated. Of the ones that have, few have been subject to RCTs, and therefore, do not appear to have used evidence-based practices (Meredith et al., 2011). Furthermore, there were numerous barriers to the use of the programs in the military, but the barriers were not peculiar to these types of programs; that is, the barriers existed for other DoD programs as well. RAND recommended that the DoD define resilience, integrate the concept of resilience into policy decisions for each service, strengthen existing resilience programs by evaluating and publishing the evaluations, base the evaluations on such standardized resilience measures as the Global Assessment Tool being developed for the Army's Comprehensive Soldier Fitness program, provide a resource guide to service members and their families, have new programs incorporate factors supported by the most evidence, engage senior military leaders in building resilience, and promote a flexible program curriculum, such as the Marine Corps OSCAR program, to coordinate with existing training and community-based programs (Weinick et al., 2011).

In a review of DoD approaches to primary care, Hourani et al. (2011) note that educational briefings and stress control techniques are two types of primary prevention that have been used in civilian populations to reduce stress reactions and are being used by the U.S. military. Prevention efforts in the DoD are built on the recognition that stressors and traumatic exposures can vary among the services. The cultures of the services are different, and these differences can affect service members' training, exposures, and perceptions of possible traumatic events. The committee considers service-specific prevention efforts next.

Prevention Efforts in the Army

U.S. Army activities to prevent or mitigate mental health symptoms after exposure to combat and deployment stress have included the use of Army CSC teams (Reger and Moore, 2006). The mission of the teams is to provide prevention and treatment as close to a soldier's unit as possible to keep the soldier with his or her unit in the theater of war. Guidelines for treating COSRs focus on proximity, immediacy, expectancy, and simplicity. Proximity is based on the premises that soldiers will seek refuge from stress but want to remain loyal to their unit and that if they are removed from their unit they will have more incentive not to return, which may increase the potential for long-term psychiatric issues. A CSC team consists of a psychologist or psychiatrist, a social worker, and two mental health specialists. Prevention consists of presentations at command meetings or informally on how to recognize initial signs of COSRs and assess unit climate surveys. Teams also work directly with soldiers via briefings on suicide, stress and anger management, home-front issues, and reintegration tips for returning home. Walkouts to talk informally with soldiers are conducted to mitigate soldiers' fear of stigmatization. CSC members can also provide crisis debriefings after a traumatic event to help normalize feelings and challenge distressing beliefs in a safe environment.

Resilience training (formerly called Battlemind) is an Army program designed to foster resilience to combat stress by teaching self-confidence and mental toughness in the context of deployment and transitioning home. It is a psychologic-educational intervention given to all U.S. Army soldiers and uses a cognitive and skills-based approach to normalize reactions to operational stress, build resilience, and promote self-recognition of psychologic problems, help seeking, and identification of difficulties in others (Brusher, 2011). Resilience training is also used at intervals during deployment to reduce mental health symptoms in a deployed unit overall (Hourani et al., 2011). Some randomized trials of the earlier Battlemind training have been conducted (Adler et al., 2009). Although the benefits of Battlemind training were modest, it did appear to reduce binge drinking after deployment. The program is being implemented and evaluated in service members, but there is no empirical evidence of the effectiveness of the current resilience training in preventing or reducing mental health problems, including PTSD.

Attitudes regarding mental health screening, stigma, and barriers to mental health care were examined in 2,678 soldiers returning from OEF and OIF (Warner et al., 2008). Participants reported fewer barriers and diminished stigma relative to the Hoge et al. (2004) study. Approximately 41% of respondents reported receiving Battlemind psychological resiliency training, and those that did reported that they were more likely to seek treatment for mental health problems. These findings suggest that preventive interventions may help reduce mental health stigma and enhance access to care in active-duty populations. However, RCTs are needed to determine whether Battlemind psychological resiliency training itself or nonspecific factors such as receiving any type of psychologic training are responsible for stigma reduction.

Morgan and Bibb (2011) describe several programs used by the services to promote postdeployment resilience to the development of PTSD. One prevention program that has received wide attention is the Army's Comprehensive Soldier Fitness (CSF) program. The CSF program is based, in part, on the Penn Resiliency Program, which was developed by Martin Seligman (Seligman and Fowler, 2011). The Penn Resiliency Program is based on cognitive-behavioral theories of depression and includes training in assertiveness, negotiation, social skills, creative problem-solving, and decision making. The CSF program is designed to prevent adverse mental health consequences of trauma exposure by increasing resilience in service members before deployment.

The CSF resilience-building program encompasses four components that enhance the service member's mental, spiritual, physical, and social capabilities: master resilience training, a 10-day, hands-on, face-to-face training course that includes the principles of positive psychology (Reivich et al., 2011); comprehensive resilience modules (formerly known as Battlemind) are online training modules that focus on specific resilience skills using precepts of positive psychology, cognitive restructuring, mindfulness, and research on posttraumatic stress, unit cohesion, occupational health models, organizational leadership, and deployment to prepare service members for military life, combat, and transitioning home; the global assessment tool (GAT), a confidential online 105-question survey that must be taken annually; and institutional resilience training that is expected to occur at every level of the Noncommissioned Officer Education System and the Officer Education System (U.S. Army, 2012). Master resilience training for noncommissioned officers and midlevel supervisors is a "train the trainer" component of CSF for sergeants to use with their troops. Versions of the CSF program are also available for military families and Army civilians. Anecdotal feedback from those attending the course has been favorable, but there is no evidence on the short-term or long-term effectiveness of the program in increasing resilience among either the sergeants or the troops they train. The CSF GAT measures psychosocial well-being in four domains: emotional fitness, social fitness, family fitness, and spiritual fitness. Results of the GAT are used to refer soldiers to programs to enhance their strengths and improve in elements of weakness, for example, training in flexible thinking if scores are lower than the norm. A similar instrument, the Family GAT, is being developed for soldiers' spouses and partners to provide advice about possible resources for building assets.

Prevention Efforts in the Navy and Marine Corps

The Marine Corps developed the OSCAR program in the 1990s to prevent and manage stress reactions as early as possible. It is not PTSD-specific, but attempts to provide support to marines in dealing with deployment and nondeployment stressors. It uses embedded personnel who have been trained to combat stigma and to connect marines with mental health professionals when necessary. This peer support can also help marines to handle daily stress. OSCAR is being expanded throughout the corps and is in the process of being evaluated by the RAND Corporation (Meredith et al., 2011).

The Navy and Marine Corps COSC program, based on the stress injury model, assesses service members' resilience. A color-coded continuum for indicating stress ranges from red, representing illness, to green, representing readiness (Nash, 2011). The COSC program distinguishes between combat stress and operational stress, with the understanding that the latter can be experienced with or without deployment. The program focuses on positive emotions to foster resilience (Morgan and Garmon Bibb, 2011).

The Navy provides boot camp survival training for new recruits (Boot Strap) in which it uses a series of COSC modules to target specific issues and phases before, during, and after deployment, including modules for spouses and significant others. The Navy also has training for caregiver occupational stress control (Morgan and Garmon Bibb, 2011).

Families OverComing Under Stress (FOCUS) is a Navy and Marine Corps family-centered stress preventive-intervention strategy for military families, particularly those affected by multiple deployments. FOCUS incorporates COSC and the Stress Continuum Model and was piloted at Camp Pendleton, California, by the Navy Bureau of Medicine and Surgery. The eight-module program focuses on individual family-resilience training for parents and children (separately and combined) by offering a variety of services aimed at prevention of family dysfunction. Other services include training or briefing base commanders and workshops and consultations for groups of families, individual families, and family members. The resilience training was modified to address the needs of young children and children of service members who are wounded or ill. FOCUS staff work with mental health providers, and families may be referred to the program from a variety of sources, including self-referral, school, military social service, and mental health providers. The program is based on evidence-based interventions, and although no RCTs have been conducted, some program evaluation has occurred (Beardslee et al., 2011; Lester et al., 2011).

Prevention Efforts in the Air Force

The Air Force has also been studying risk factors for PTSD and resilience in its OEF- and OIF-deployed members. Service members deployed to the Air Force Theater Hospital at Joint Base Balad, Iraq, were surveyed before, during, and at 1, 6, and 12 months after deployment to identify factors related to psychologic risk and resiliency (Peterson et al., 2011). Although no PTSD prevention interventions were used, results of the survey indicated that increased preparedness and training of high-risk groups, such as those who are not normally exposed to combat or medical-exposure incidents, would be beneficial in reducing war zone stress.

The Air Force also has several tiers of resilience training in the Total Force Resiliency Program, including airman resilience training for new recruits; and the Comprehensive Airman Fitness program, on whose effectiveness information is lacking (Morgan and Garmon Bibb, 2011). The authors note that virtually all these new programs lack empirical evidence of effectiveness.

The Air Force is helping to develop the Deployment Anxiety Reduction Training (DART) program to prevent PTSD in service members exposed to combat stress. DART is being launched as a small pilot program in Afghanistan; medical personnel are training service members to recognize their own stress responses and teaching them exercises to monitor and control them. DART includes muscle relaxation and grounding; the latter focuses on deflecting attention from a traumatizing event. Service members can complete the training within hours of experiencing a traumatic battlefield event (UCSF News Release, 2010). There is no information on the efficacy of the program or expanding its use.

Prevention of Sexual Trauma in the Military

The DoD has made substantial efforts to reduce service members' exposure to sexual trauma, which is a known risk factor for PTSD (Allard et al., 2011). Suris and Lind (2008) in a review of the literature on sexual trauma in the military reported that the overall prevalence rates of sexual trauma in military personnel and veterans ranges from 20% to 43%. They also found that female respondents who were using VA services reported "significantly higher rates of sexual assault while on active duty compared with current active-duty [respondents]"; this suggested that such trauma "results in mental and physical health conditions that require further medical attention … or that those with [military sexual trauma] MST receive medical services from VA for service-connected injuries." Female veterans who had a history of sexual assault were five times more likely to meet the criteria for PTSD than female veterans who had no such history; in those with a history of MST specifically, the risk of PTSD was ninefold higher (Suris and Lind, 2008).

The DoD Defense Manpower Data Center tracks the incidence of unwanted sexual contact, which includes unwanted sexual touching, with the Workplace and Gender Relations Survey of Active Duty Members. In 2010, 4.4% of women and 0.9% of men indicated experiencing unwanted sexual contact (DMDC, 2011). The survey also showed that the vast majority of respondents in all service branches had had sexual-assault prevention training in the prior 12 months; of those, 85% of women and 88% of men indicated that their training was moderately or very effective in reducing or preventing sexual assault or behaviors related to sexual assault.

The DoD has instituted the myduty.mil website to encourage service members to participate in active-bystander intervention to prevent sexual assault (DoD, 2012b). That program seeks to engage service members to be responsible for their own behavior, to help those who may be targets of sexual assault, and to prevent other service members from perpetrating sexual assault. The site provides practical suggestions for ensuring everyone's safety, gauging whether a situation requires intervention, and preventing situations in which sexual assault may occur. The site also provides a confidential 24/7 hotline, "Safe Helpline," for sexual-assault victims (www.SafeHelpline.org; DoD, 2012a). The DoD also provides a sexual assault response coordinator and a victim advocate at each installation or ship and Sexual Assault Awareness Month programs at each installation or ship (DMDC, 2011).

VA/DoD Clinical Practice Guideline for Management of Post-Traumatic Stress

In an attempt to ameliorate the adverse stress response that some service members may experience during and after deployment, the 2010 VA/DoD guideline recommends a dual system of education and resilience training to prepare them for possible deployment experiences and to maintain their psychologic health. The 2007 DoD Task Force on Mental Health encourages the use of crisis intervention and management to prevent the progression of subclinical to clinically significant PTSD.

To that end, the DoD programs to enhance the psychologic resilience and promote the concept of hardiness as protective against the development of PTSD rely on the following precepts (VA and DoD, 2010):

- Provide realistic training—Repeated exposure to stimuli consistent with combat in a controlled environment in an effort to condition a response of reduced anxiety or reduced emotional arousal.

- Strengthen perceived ability to cope—Practice in responding to traumatic stimuli and positive encouragement from peers and superiors to reinforce appropriate coping techniques.
- Create supportive interpersonal work environments—Social support through team building, families, peer stress-management consultants, and leadership to protect against adverse psychologic reactions.
- Develop and maintain adaptive beliefs—Realistic expectations about the experience of combat and ensuing stress reactions bolstered by confidence in coping ability, leadership management, and the value of military service.
- Develop workplace-specific comprehensive traumatic-stress management programs—Encouragement of the use and promotion of the benefits of programs tailored to support service members after trauma.

Other Prevention Activities

Decompression at a "third location" is used by Canada and the UK to provide a transition back into the home environment. Although no formal definition exists, decompression in this situation refers to a stopover at a location that is neither home or in the theater of war, where service members may begin to unwind after leaving the theater of war (Hacker Hughes et al., 2008). A literature review by Fertout et al. (2011) states that decompression programs have common elements, including permitting units to unwind together in a structured but informal manner and having the environment of the decompression location be superior to the deployment location. The length of the decompression program is variable: the UK uses 36 hours, and Canada 5 days. Questions surrounding the use of decompression programs focus on the optimal length of the program, who should participate (all troops versus only those exposed to combat or trauma), and whether the program should be carried out at a location that is neither home nor the deployment position (Cyprus is used by the UK and Canada) but rather conducted on the troops' home base but with adjustments (the third location). Fertout notes that the use of decompression programs has not been subjected to formal trials of efficacy, but one survey of troops just returned from decompression (Jones et al., 2011) found that although the majority initially resisted the use of the decompression program, the overwhelming majority found it to be useful after they completed the decompression period. Officers found that the time was not helpful in that they were still in charge of their troops and could not decompress.

The committee will consider the emerging evidence on these and other PTSD prevention activities in phase 2 of this study.

PREVENTION IN THE DEPARTMENT OF VETERANS AFFAIRS

The VA is not involved in the early military life of active-duty personnel and thus does not have a role in preventing service members' exposure to traumatic events. As discussed in Chapter 4, the VA/DoD integrated mental health strategy focuses on broad psychologic health and resilience activities and builds on the resilience programs in the DoD.

Vet Centers also provide prevention services to veterans who may have been exposed to trauma or who are suffering from PTSD symptoms. The services are available to any veteran and have the advantage of being available for the veterans' families as well as veterans themselves. They include individual, group, and family counseling; employment counseling; sexual counseling; and referrals to other mental health and medical health programs.

There are other considerations for veterans who receive treatment at VA medical facilities. Many veterans are members of the National Guard or reserve and never expected to be deployed to a war zone. Unlike active-duty service members, National Guard and reservists may cycle between civilian and military life over several deployments with little or no support from colleagues who are familiar with the stresses of deployment, and they can face stressors such as job loss that do not affect active-duty personnel (Riviere et al., 2011). Furthermore, these service members may not receive the same level of predeployment training as active-duty personnel, and this increases the risk of PTSD after exposure to a traumatic event during deployment.

VA programs and services specific to prevention and resilience include

- Life Guard—This program promotes psychologic resilience based on acceptance and commitment therapy. It has been implemented at one local site and is designed to facilitate reintegration of returning OEF and OIF veterans (Blevins et al., 2011; Schiffner, 2011).
- FOCUS—This is a family-centered preventive intervention program. It was designed on the basis of a skills-building pyschoeducational model that integrates traumatic-stress research, theories of child development, and the COSC model. FOCUS has been piloted and expanded to encompass more issues surrounding couples and issues surrounding wounded veterans (Schiffner, 2011); see the discussion of the Navy FOCUS program in this chapter and in Chapter 4.
- Moving Forward—A Problem-Solving Approach to Achieving Life's Goals—This is a multisite (12 sites) pilot training program that includes a four-session group-based curriculum focused on early intervention and prevention of mental health problems (not

specifically PTSD) by teaching "specific skills that veterans can use to constructively address a wide range of problems that may arise in their lives" (Schiffner, 2011).

The VA has also developed a program on MST. The VA has a different definition of sexual trauma than the DoD. MST is a VA-specific term, and thus the prevalence of MST pertains only to the VA. The prevalence of MST in VA users is tracked by the Veterans Health Administration and includes experiences of sexual assault or repeated, threatening acts of sexual harassment (VA, 2012). The VA mandated that each facility identify a MST coordinator to oversee the universal screening and treatment referral process for MST. Each Vet Center also has one staff member to address issues of MST.

The VA provides a guide for returning service members on what to expect after deployment and return to civilian life, including how to deal with children, spouses, family and friends, finances, and emotions. Advice is given on coping with common reactions to trauma and how to resume routine activities of work, family, and life.

SUMMARY

The DoD supports a number of programs that are aimed at preventing the development of PTSD by building resilience and helping service members to anticipate some of the traumatic events they may experience in a combat zone. In particular, the Army has had a variety of prevention programs including Battlemind and, most recently, the CSF program that will be used for all Army personnel before deployment. The Navy and Marine Corps and the Air Force have similar training. All four services also have programs to help service members who have symptoms of PTSD avoid chronic PTSD by using a variety of treatments.

The VA does not have the responsibility for predeployment programs but, like the DoD, it does attempt to prevent chronic PTSD by working with veterans who have symptoms. Furthermore, the VA has programs that help veterans with PTSD to regain functioning in civilian life and to prevent further PTSD-related disability. The VA and the DoD have collaborated in the development of PTSD management guidelines to minimize the impact of PTSD on service members, veterans, and their families.

While there are a variety of DoD and VA programs that target PTSD prevention, it is important to note that, at present, none of them has evidence for their effectiveness in preventing or reducing PTSD or stress in service members or their families. Evaluation of some of these programs is ongoing, and the committee hopes that such information will be available for phase 2 of this study.

REFERENCES

Adler, A. B., B. T. Litz, C. A. Castro, M. Suvak, J. L. Thomas, L. Burrell, D. McGurk, K. M. Wright, and P. D. Bliese. 2008. A group randomized trial of critical incident stress debriefing provided to U.S. Peacekeepers. *Journal of Traumatic Stress* 21(3):253-263.

Adler, A. B., P. D. Bliese, D. McGurk, C. W. Hoge, and C. A. Castro. 2009. Battlemind debriefing and battlemind training as early interventions with soldiers returning from Iraq: Randomization by platoon. *Journal of Consulting & Clinical Psychology* 77(5):928-940.

Agorastos, A., C. R. Marmar, and C. Otte. 2011. Immediate and early behavioral interventions for the prevention of acute and posttraumatic stress disorder. *Current Opinion in Psychiatry* 24(6):526-532.

Allard, C. B., S. Nunnink, A. M. Gregory, B. Klest, and M. Platt. 2011. Military sexual trauma research: A proposed agenda. *Journal of Trauma & Dissociation* 12(3):324-345.

Beardslee, W., P. Lester, L. Klosinski, W. Saltzman, K. Woodward, W. Nash, C. Mogil, R. Koffman, and G. Leskin. 2011. Family-centered preventive intervention for military families: Implications for implementation science. *Prevention Science* 12(4):339-348.

Bisson, J. I., P. L. Jenkins, J. Alexander, and C. Bannister. 1997. Randomised controlled trial of psychological debriefing for victims of acute burn trauma. *British Journal of Psychiatry* 171:78-81.

Bisson, J. I., A. C. McFarlane, S. R. Rose, J. I. Ruzek, and P. J. Watson. 2009. Psychological debriefing for adults. Chapter 4. In *Effective treatments for PTSD: Practice guidelines from the International Society for Traumatic Stress Studies*, edited by E. B. Foa, 2nd. ed. New York: Guilford Press.

Blevins, D., J. V. Roca, and T. Spencer. 2011. Life guard: Evaluation of an ACT-based workshop to facilitate reintegration of OIF/OEF veterans. *Professional Psychology-Research and Practice* 42(1):32-39.

Boyce, C. A., R. Heinssen, C. B. Ferrell, R. K. Nakamura. 2007. Prospects for the prevention of mental illness: Integrating neuroscience and behavior. In *Recognition and prevention of major mental and substance use disorders*, edited by W. S. Stone and M. J. Lyons. Washington, DC: American Psychiatric Publishing.

Brailey, K., J. J. Vasterling, S. P. Proctor, J. I. Constans, and M. J. Friedman. 2007. PTSD symptoms, life events, and unit cohesion in U.S. soldiers: Baseline findings from the neurocognition deployment health study. *Journal of Traumatic Stress* 20(4):495-503.

Brewin, C. R., B. Andrews, and J. D. Valentine. 2000. Meta-analysis of risk factors for posttraumatic stress disorder in trauma-exposed adults. *Journal of Consulting and Clinical Psychology* 68(5):748-766.

Brusher, E. A. 2011. Combat and operational stress control. Chapter 4. In *Textboooks of military medicine: Combat and operational behavioral health*, edited by E. C. Ritchie. Fort Detrick, MD: Office of the Surgeon General, Borden Institute.

Bryant, R. A., A. G. Harvey, S. T. Dang, T. Sackville, and C. Basten. 1998. Treatment of acute stress disorder: A comparison of cognitive-behavioral therapy and supportive counseling. *Journal of Consulting and Clinical Psychology* 66(5):862-866.

Bryant, R. A., T. Sackville, S. T. Dang, M. Moulds, and R. Guthrie. 1999. Treating acute stress disorder: An evaluation of cognitive behavior therapy and supportive counseling techniques. *American Journal of Psychiatry* 156(11):1780-1786.

Bryant, R. A., M. L. Moulds, and R. V. D. Nixon. 2003. Cognitive behaviour therapy of acute stress disorder: A four-year follow-up. *Behaviour Research and Therapy* 41(4):489-494.

Bryant, R. A., M. L. Moulds, R. M. Guthrie, S. T. Dang, J. Mastrodomenico, R. D. V. Nixon, K. L. Felmingham, S. Hopwood, and M. Creamer. 2008. A randomized controlled trial of exposure therapy and cognitive restructuring for posttraumatic stress disorder. *Journal of Consulting and Clinical Psychology* 76(4):695-703.

Bryant, R. A., M. Creamer, M. O'Donnell, D. Silove, and A. C. McFarlane. 2009. A study of the protective function of acute morphine administration on subsequent posttraumatic stress disorder. *Biological Psychiatry* 65(5):438-440.

Bugg, A., G. Turpin, S. Mason, and C. Scholes. 2009. A randomised controlled trial of the effectiveness of writing as a self-help intervention for traumatic injury patients at risk of developing post-traumatic stress disorder. *Behaviour Research and Therapy* 47(1):6-12.

Campfield, K. M., and A. M. Hills. 2001. Effect of timing of critical incident stress debriefing (CISD) on posttraumatic symptoms. *Journal of Traumatic Stress* 14(2):327-340.

Casey, E. A., and T. P. Lindhorst. 2009. Toward a multi-level, ecological approach to the primary prevention of sexual assault: Prevention in peer and community contexts. *Trauma Violence Abuse* 10(2):91-114.

Casey, G. W. 2011. Comprehensive soldier fitness a vision for psychological resilience in the U.S. Army. *American Psychologist* 66(1):1-3.

Cornum, R., M. D. Matthews, and M. E. P. Seligman. 2011. Comprehensive soldier fitness building resilience in a challenging institutional context. *American Psychologist* 66(1):4-9.

Cuijpers, P., A. Van Straten, and F. Smit. 2005. Preventing the incidence of new cases of mental disorders—a meta-analytic review. *Journal of Nervous and Mental Disease* 193(2): 119-125.

Deahl, M., M. Srinivasan, N. Jones, J. Thomas, C. Neblett, and A. Jolly. 2000. Preventing psychological trauma in soldiers: The role of operational stress training and psychological debriefing. *British Journal of Medical Psychology* 73(Pt 1):77-85.

Dickstein, B. D., C. P. McLean, J. Mintz, L. M. Conoscenti, M. M. Steenkamp, T. A. Benson, W. C. Isler, A. L. Peterson, and B. T. Litz. 2010. Unit cohesion and PTSD symptom severity in Air Force medical personnel. *Military Medicine* 175(7):482-486.

DMDC (Defense Manpower Data Center), L. Rock, R. Lipari, P. Cook, and A. Hale. 2011. *2010 workplace and gender relations survey of active duty members: Overview report on sexual assault.* Ft. Belvoir, VA: DMDC.

DoD (Department of Defense). 1999. *Combat stress control (CSC) programs.* DoD Directive 6490.5 [cancelled]. February 23. http://biotech.law.lsu.edu/blaw/dodd/corres/html2/d64905x.htm.

DoD. 2011. *Maintenance of psychological health in military operation.* DoD Instruction 6490.05. November 22. http://www.dtic.mil/whs/directives/corres/pdf/649005p.pdf.

DoD. 2012a. *Army, Navy, Marine, Air Force and Coast Guard rape, sexual assault and harassment help.* https://safehelpline.org/ (accessed January 30, 2012).

DoD. 2012b. *Myduty.Mil.* http://myduty.mil/ (accessed January 30, 2012).

Du Preez, J., J. Sundin, S. Wessely, and N. T. Fear. 2012. Unit cohesion and mental health in the UK armed forces. *Occupational Medicine (London)* 62(1):47-53.

Ehlers, A., D. M. Clark, A. Hackmann, F. McManus, M. Fennell, C. Herbert, and R. Mayou. 2003. A randomized controlled trial of cognitive therapy, a self-help booklet, and repeated assessments as early interventions for posttraumatic stress disorder. *Archives of General Psychiatry* 60(10):1024-1032.

Eid, J., B. H. Johnsen, and L. Weisaeth. 2001. The effects of group psychological debriefing on acute stress reactions following a traffic accident: A quasi-experimental approach. *International Journal of Emergency Mental Health* 3(3):145-154.

Exner, D., and N. Cummings. 2011. Implications for sexual assault prevention: College students as prosocial bystanders. *Journal of American College Health* 59(7):655-657.

Feldner, M. T., C. M. Monson, and M. J. Friedman. 2007. A critical analysis of approaches to targeted PTSD prevention: Current status and theoretically derived future directions. *Behavior Modification* 31(1):80-116.

Fertout, M., N. Jones, N. Greenberg, K. Mulligan, T. Knight, and S. Wessely. 2011. A review of United Kingdom armed forces' approaches to prevent post-deployment mental health problems. *International Review of Psychiatry* 23(2):135-143.

Fikretoglu, D., A. Brunet, J. Poundja, S. Guay, and D. Pedlar. 2006. Validation of the deployment risk and resilience inventory in French-Canadian veterans: Findings on the relation between deployment experiences and postdeployment health. *Canadian Journal of Psychiatry—Revue Canadienne de Psychiatrie* 51(12):755-763.

Fletcher, S., M. Creamer, and D. Forbes. 2010. Preventing post traumatic stress disorder: Are drugs the answer? *Australian & New Zealand Journal of Psychiatry* 44(12):1064-1071.

Foa, E. B., D. Hearstikeda, and K. J. Perry. 1995. Evaluation of a brief cognitive-behavioral program for the prevention of chronic PTSD in recent assault victims. *Journal of Consulting and Clinical Psychology* 63(6):948-955.

Fontana, A., R. Rosenheck, and T. Horvath. 1997. Social support and psychopathology in the war zone. *Journal of Nervous and Mental Disease* 185(11):675-681.

Gallaway, M. S., A. M. Millikan, and M. R. Bell. 2011. The association between deployment-related posttraumatic growth among U.S. Army soldiers and negative behavioral health conditions. *Journal of Clinical Psychology* 67(12):1151-1160.

Gidron, Y., R. Gal, G. Givati, A. Lauden, Y. Shir, and J. Benjamin. 2007. Interactive effects of memory structuring and gender in preventing posttraumatic stress symptoms. *Journal of Nervous and Mental Disease* 195(2):179-182.

Green, B. L., M. C. Grace, J. D. Lindy, G. C. Gleser, and A. Leonard. 1990. Risk factors for PTSD and other diagnoses in a general sample of Vietnam veterans. *American Journal of Psychiatry*147(6):729-733.

Hacker Hughes, J., M. Earnshaw, N. Greenberg, R. Eldridge, N. T. Fear, C. French, M. Deahl, and S. Wessely. 2008.The use of psychological decompression in military operational environments. *Military Medicine* 173:534-538.

Hoge, C. W., C. A. Castro, S. C. Messer, D. McGurk, D. I. Cotting, and R. L. Koffman. 2004. Combat duty in Iraq and Afghanistan, mental health problems, and barriers to care. *New England Journal of Medicine* 351(1):13-22.

Holbrook, T. L., M. R. Galarneau, J. L. Dye, K. Quinn, and A. L. Dougherty. 2010. Morphine use after combat injury in Iraq and post-traumatic stress disorder. *New England Journal of Medicine* 362(2):110-117.

Hourani, L. L., C. L. Council, R. C. Hubal, and L. B. Strange. 2011. Approaches to the primary prevention of posttraumatic stress disorder in the military: A review of the stress control literature. *Military Medicine* 176(7):721-730.

IOM (Institute of Medicine). 2008. *Gulf War and health. Volume 6. Physiologic, psychologic, and psychosocial effects of deployment-related stress.* Washington, DC: The National Academies Press.

Jones, N., H. Burdett, S. Wessely, and N. Greenberg. 2011. The subjective utility of early psychosocial interventions following combat deployment. *Occupational Medicine (London)* 61(2):102-107.

Kazak, A. E., S. Simms, M. A. Alderfer, M. T. Rourke, T. Crump, K. McClure, P. Jones, A. Rodriguez, A. Boeving, W. T. Hwang, and A. Reilly. 2005. Feasibility and preliminary outcomes from a pilot study of a brief psychological intervention for families of children newly diagnosed with cancer. *Journal of Pediatric Psychology* 30(8):644-655.

King, D., L. King, G. Leskin, and D. W. Foy. 1995. The Los Angeles symptom checklist: A self-report measure of posttraumatic stress disorder. *Assessment* 2:1-17.

King, L. A., D. W. King, J. A. Fairbank, T. M. Keane, and G. A. Adams. 1998. Resilience-recovery factors in post-traumatic stress disorder among female and male Vietnam veterans: Hardiness, postwar social support, and additional stressful life events. *Journal of Personality and Social Psychology* 74(2):420-434.

King, L. A., D. W. King, E. E. Bolton, J. A. Knight, and D. S. Vogt. 2008. Risk factors for mental, physical, and functional health in Gulf War veterans. *Journal of Rehabilitation Research and Development* 45(3):395-407.

Langhinrichsen-Rohling, J., J. D. Foubert, H. M. Brasfield, B. Hill, and S. Shelley-Tremblay. 2011. The men's program: Does it impact college men's self-reported bystander efficacy and willingness to intervene? *Violence Against Women* 17(6):743-759.

Larner, B., and A. Blow. 2011. A model of meaning-making coping and growth in combat veterans. *Review of General Psychology* 15(3):187-197.

Lau, E. X., and R. M. Rapee. 2011. Prevention of anxiety disorders. *Current Psychiatry Reports* 13(4):258-266.

Lester, P., W. R. Saltzman, K. Woodward, D. Glover, G. A. Leskin, B. Bursch, R. Pynoos, and W. Beardslee. 2011. Evaluation of a family centered prevention intervention for military children and families facing wartime deployments. *American Journal of Public Health* 102(Suppl 1):S48-S54.

Litz, B. T. 2008. Early intervention for trauma: Where are we and where do we need to go? A commentary. *Journal of Traumatic Stress* 21(6):503-506.

Litz, B. T., and R.A. Bryant. 2009. Early cognitive-behavioral interventions for adults. In *Effective treatments for PTSD: Practice guidelines from the International Society For Traumatic Stress Studies*, edited by E. B. Foa, 2nd ed. New York: Guilford Press.

MacDermott, D. 2010. Psychological hardiness and meaning making as protection against sequelae in veterans of the wars in Iraq and Afghanistan. *International Journal of Emergency Mental Health* 12(3):199-206.

MacGregor, A. J., P. P. Han, A. L. Dougherty, and M. R. Galarneau. 2012. Effect of dwell time on the mental health of US military personnel with multiple combat tours. *American Journal of Public Health* 102(Suppl 1):S55-S59.

Mayou, R. A., A. Ehlers, and M. Hobbs. 2000. Psychological debriefing for road traffic accident victims—three-year follow-up of a randomised controlled trial. *British Journal of Psychiatry* 176:589-593.

McMahon, S., and V. L. Banyard. 2012. When can I help? A conceptual framework for the prevention of sexual violence through bystander intervention. *Trauma Violence Abuse* 13(1):3-14.

McNally, R. J., R. Bryant, and A. Ehlers. 2003. Does early psychological intervention promote recovery from posttraumatic stress? *Psychological Science in the Public Interest* 4(2).

Meredith, L. S., C. D. Sherbourne, S. Gaillot, L. Hansell, H. V. Ritschard, A. Parker, and G. Wrenn. 2011. *Promoting psychological resilience in the U.S. military*. Santa Monica, CA: RAND Corporation.

MHAT (Mental Health Advisory Team IV). 2006. *Mental health advisory team (MHAT) IV Operation Iraqi Freedom 05-07 final report.* Office of the Surgeon Multinational Force-Iraq, Office of the Surgeon General United States Army Medical Command.

Moor, A. 2011. The efficacy of a high school rape prevention program in Israel. *Violence & Victims* 26(3):283-295.

Morgan, B. J., and S. C. Garmon Bibb. 2011. Assessment of military population-based pyschological resilience programs. *Military Medicine* 176(9):10.

Moynihan, M. M., and V. L. Banyard. 2008. Community responsibility for preventing sexual violence: A pilot study with campus greeks and intercollegiate athletes. *Journal of Prevention and Intervention in the Community* 36(1-2):23-38.

Munoz, R. F., P. J. Mrazek, and R. J. Haggerty. 1996. Institute of Medicine report on prevention of mental disorders. Summary and commentary. *American Psychologist* 51(11): 1116-1122.

Nash, W. P. 2011. US Marine Corps and Navy combat and operational stress continuum model: A tool for leaders. Chapter 7. In *Textboooks of military medicine: Combat and operational behavioral health,* edited by E. C. Ritchie. Fort Detrick, MD: Office of the Surgeon General, Borden Institute.

Nelson, S. D. 2011. The posttraumatic growth path: An emerging model for prevention and treatment of trauma-related behavioral health conditions. *Journal of Psychotherapy Integration* 21(1):1-42.

Nishi, D., Y. Matsuoka, N. Yonemoto, H. Noguchi, Y. Kim, and S. Kanba. 2010. Peritraumatic distress inventory as a predictor of post-traumatic stress disorder after a severe motor vehicle accident. *Psychiatry and Clinical Neurosciences* 64(2):149-156.

Peterson, A. L., B. Litz, R. J. McNally, W. C. Isler, M. Baker, J. Mintz, and J. P. Hatch. 2011. *Risk and resilience in deployed Air Force medical personnel study.* San Antonio, TX: UT Health Science Center San Antonio.

Pietrzak, R. H., D. C. Johnson, M. B. Goldstein, J. C. Malley, and S. M. Southwick. 2009. Psychological resilience and postdeployment social support protect against traumatic stress and depressive symptoms in soldiers returning from Operations Enduring Freedom and Iraqi Freedom. *Depression and Anxiety* 26(8):745-751.

Pietrzak, R. H., M. B. Goldstein, J. C. Malley, A. J. Rivers, D. C. Johnson, C. A. Morgan, and S. M. Southwick. 2010a. Posttraumatic growth in veterans of Operations Enduring Freedom and Iraqi Freedom. *Journal of Affective Disorders* 126(1-2):230-235.

Pietrzak, R. H., D. C. Johnson, M. B. Goldstein, J. C. Malley, A. J. Rivers, C. A. Morgan, and S. M. Southwick. 2010b. Psychosocial buffers of traumatic stress, depressive symptoms, and psychosocial difficulties in veterans of Operations Enduring Freedom And Iraqi Freedom: The role of resilience, unit support, and postdeployment social support. *Journal of Affective Disorders* 120(1-3):188-192.

Prati, G., and L. Pietrantoni. 2009. Optimism, social support, and coping strategies as factors contributing to posttraumatic growth: A meta-analysis. *Journal of Loss & Trauma* 14(5):364-388.

Rau, T. J., L. L. Merrill, S. K. McWhorter, V. A. Stander, C. J. Thomsen, C. W. Dyslin, J. L. Crouch, M. M. Rabenhorst, and J. S. Milner. 2011. Evaluation of a sexual assault education/prevention program for female U.S. Navy personnel. *Military Medicine* 176(10):1178 1183.

Reger, G. M., and B. A. Moore. 2006. Combat operational stress control in Iraq: Lessons learned during operation Iraqi freedom. *Military Psychology* 18(4):297-307.

Reivich, K. J., M. E. P. Seligman, and S. McBride. 2011. Master resilience training in the US Army. *American Psychologist* 66(1):25-34.

Renshaw, K. D. 2011. An integrated model of risk and protective factors for post-deployment PTSD symptoms in OEF/OIF era combat veterans. *Journal of Affective Disorders* 128(3): 321-326.

Richards, D. 2001. A field study of critical incident stress debriefing versus critical incident stress management. *Journal of Mental Health* 10(3):351-362.

Riviere, L. A., A. Kendall-Robbins, D. McGurk, C. A. Castro, and C. W. Hoge. 2011. Coming home may hurt: Risk factors for mental ill health in US reservists after deployment in Iraq. *British Journal of Psychiatry* 198(2):136-142.

Roberts, N. P., N. J. Kitchiner, J. Kenardy, and J. Bisson. 2009a. Multiple session early psychological interventions for the prevention of post-traumatic stress disorder. *Cochrane Database of Systematic Reviews* (3):CD006869.

Roberts, N. P., N. J. Kitchiner, J. Kenardy, J. I. Bisson, and F. R. C. Psych. 2009b. Systematic review and meta-analysis of multiple-session early interventions following traumatic events. *American Journal of Psychiatry* 166(3):293-301.

Rona, R. J., R. Hooper, M. Jones, A. C. Iversen, L. Hull, D. Murphy, M. Hotopf, and S. Wessely. 2009. The contribution of prior psychological symptoms and combat exposure to post Iraq deployment mental health in the UK military. *Journal of Traumatic Stress* 22(1):11-19.

Rose, S., J. Bisson, R. Churchill, and S. Wessely. 2002. Psychological debriefing for preventing post traumatic stress disorder (PTSD). *Cochrane Database of Systematic Reviews*(2): CD000560.

Sadler, A. G., B. M. Booth, B. L. Cook, J. C. Torner, and B. N. Doebbeling. 2001. The military environment: Risk factors for women's non-fatal assaults. *Journal of Occupational & Environmental Medicine* 43(4):325-334.

Schelling, G., J. Briegel, B. Roozendaal, C. Stoll, H. B. Rothenhausler, and H. P. Kapfhammer. 2001. The effect of stress doses of hydrocortisone during septic shock on posttraumatic stress disorder in survivors. *Biological Psychiatry* 50(12):978-985.

Schelling, G., B. Roozendaal, and D. J. F. De Quervain. 2004. Can posttraumatic stress disorder be prevented with glucocorticoids? In *Biobehavioral stress response: Protective and damaging effects*, edited by R. Yehuda and B. McEwen. *Annals of the New York Academy of Sciences* 1032:158-166.

Schiffner, S. 2011. *Data request on mental health providers in the VA, provider training, and the use of complementary and alternative medicine and treatments.* Response to data request by the Committee on the Assessment of Ongoing Efforts in the Treatment of PTSD. October 18, 2011. Washington, DC.

Scholes, C., G. Turpin, and S. Mason. 2007. A randomised controlled trial to assess the effectiveness of providing self-help information to people with symptoms of acute stress disorder following a traumatic injury. *Behaviour Research and Therapy* 45(11):2527-2536.

Seligman, M. E. P., and R. D. Fowler. 2011. Comprehensive soldier fitness and the future of psychology. *American Psychologist* 66(1):82-86.

Shalev, A. Y., Y. Ankri, Y. Israeli-Shalev, T. Peleg, R. Adessky, and S. Freedman. 2011. Prevention of posttraumatic stress disorder by early treatment: Results from the Jerusalem trauma outreach and prevention study. *Archives of General Psychiatry* 69(2):166-176.

Stapleton, J. A., S. Taylor, and G. J. G. Asmundson. 2006. Effects of three PTSD treatments on anger and guilt: Exposure therapy, eye movement desensitization and reprocessing, and relaxation training. *Journal of Traumatic Stress* 19(1):19-28.

Stokes, J. W., H. Green, and P. S. Hammer. 2003. Combat stress control and force health protection. Chapter 16. In *Military preventive medicine: Mobilitzation and deployment*, edited by P. W. Kelley. Vol. 1. http://www.bordeninstitute.army.mil/published_volumes/mpmVol1/mpmvol1.html.

Street, A. E., D. Vogt, and L. Dutra. 2009. A new generation of women veterans: Stressors faced by women deployed to Iraq and Afghanistan. *Clinical Psychology Review* 29(8):685-694.

Stretch, R. H., P. D. Bliese, D. H. Marlowe, K. M. Wright, K. H. Knudson, and C. H. Hoover. 1996. Psychological health of gulf war-era military personnel. *Military Medicine* 161(5):257-261.

Suris, A., and L. Lind. 2008. Military sexual trauma—a review of prevalence and associated health consequences in veterans. *Trauma Violence & Abuse* 9(4):250-269.

Taylor, S. E., and T. E. Seeman. 1999. Psychosocial resources and the SES-health relationship. *Annals of the New York Academy of Science* 896:210-225.

Tedeschi, R. G. 2011. Posttraumatic growth in combat veterans. *Journal of Clinical Psychology in Medical Settings* 18(2):137-144.

Turpin, G., M. Downs, and S. Mason. 2005. Effectiveness of providing self-help information following acute traumatic injury: Randomised controlled trial. *British Journalof Psychiatry* 187:76-82.

UCSF News Release. 2010. *Can post-traumatic stress disorder be stopped before it begins?* http://www.ucsf.edu/news/2010/08/6001/post-traumatic-stress-disorder-PTSD-prevention-military (accessed January 30, 2012).

U.S. Army. 2012. *Comprehensive soldier fitness.* http://csf.army.mil/ (accessed January 30, 2012).

VA (Department of Veterans Affairs). 2012. *Military sexual trauma.* http://www.PTSD.va.gov/public/pages/military-sexual-trauma-general.asp (accessed January 30, 2012).

VA and DoD. 2010. *VA/DoD clinical practice guideline for management of post-traumatic stress.* Washington, DC: VA/DoD.

van Emmerik, A. A. P., J. H. Kamphuis, A. M. Hulsbosch, and P. M. G. Emmelkamp. 2002. Single session debriefing after psychological trauma: A meta-analysis. *Lancet* 360(9335):766-771.

van Emmerik, A. A. P., J. H. Kamphuis, and P. M. G. Emmelkamp. 2008. Treating acute stress disorder and posttraumatic stress disorder with cognitive behavioral therapy or structured writing therapy: A randomized controlled trial. *Psychotherapy and Psychosomatics* 77(2):93-100.

Vladutiu, C. J., S. L. Martin, and R. J. Macy. 2011. College- or university-based sexual assault prevention programs: A review of program outcomes, characteristics, and recommendations. *Trauma Violence Abuse* 12(2):67-86.

Vogt, D. S., and L. R. Tanner. 2007. Risk and resilience factors for posttraumatic stress symptomatology in Gulf War I veterans. *Journal of Traumatic Stress* 20(1):27-38.

Warner, C. H., G. N. Appenzeller, K. Mullen, C. M. Warner, and T. A. Grieger. 2008. Soldier attitudes toward mental health screening and seeking care upon return from combat. *Military Medicine* 173(6):563-569.

Weinick, R. M., E. B. Beckjord, C. M. Farmer, L. T. Martin, E. M. Gillen, J. D. Acosta, M. P. Fisher, J. Garnett, G. C. Gonzalez, T. C. Helmus, L. Jaycox, K. A. Reynolds, N. Salcedo, and D. M. Scharf. 2011. *Programs addressing psychological health and traumatic brain injury among U.S. military servicemembers and their families.* Santa Monica, CA: RAND Corporation.

Weis, F., E. Kilger, B. Roozendaal, D. J. de Quervain, P. Lamm, M. Schmidt, M. Schmolz, J. Briegel, and G. Schelling. 2006. Stress doses of hydrocortisone reduce chronic stress symptoms and improve health-related quality of life in high-risk patients after cardiac surgery: A randomized study. *Journal of Thoracic Cardiovascular Surgery* 131(2):277-282.

Wessely, S., R. A. Bryant, N. Greenberg, M. Earnshaw, J. Sharpley, and J. H. Hughes. 2008. Does psychoeducation help prevent post traumatic psychological distress? *Psychiatry-Interpersonal and Biological Processes* 71(4):287-302.

Zatzick, D. F., P. Roy-Byrne, J. Russo, F. P. Rivara, R. Droesch, A. Wagner, C. Dunn, G. J. Jurkovich, E. Uehara, and W. Katon. 2004. A randomized effectiveness trial of stepped collaborative care for acutely injured trauma survivors. *Archives of General Psychiatry* 61(May):498-506.

Zohar, J., H. Yahalom, N. Kozlovsky, S. Cwikel-Hamzany, M. A. Matar, Z. Kaplan, R. Yehuda, and H. Cohen. 2011. High dose hydrocortisone immediately after trauma may alter the trajectory of PTSD: Interplay between clinical and animal studies. *European Neuropsychopharmacology* 21(11):796-809.

6

Screening and Diagnosis

This chapter begins with the rationale for screening in general and then looks at screening for posttraumatic stress disorder (PTSD) specifically. After a discussion of the goals of screening for PTSD, especially in the military and veteran populations, key considerations in screening for PTSD are examined, such as when, how, and by whom screening should be conducted and the potential effect of stigma on screening. That is followed by descriptions of screening and barriers to screening in the Department of Defense (DoD), the Department of Veterans Affairs (VA), and nonmilitary settings and the different types of screening instruments that are used or are being developed. The screening section ends with a consideration of what should be done with screening results. The second part of the chapter discusses clinical assessment for and diagnosis of PTSD, including the current guidelines for diagnostic interviews and the use of various scales for diagnosing PTSD in military and veteran populations.

SCREENING

Screening has been defined as the examination of a generally healthy population to identify people as likely or unlikely to have a particular condition (Morrison, 1992). In light of the fact that screening is not without cost or potential damage, six criteria have been proposed for determining the acceptability of any given screening procedure (Rona et al., 2005):

- The identified condition should be an important health problem.
- The test should be clinically, socially, and ethically acceptable.

- The test should be simple, precise, and valid.
- The test should lead to reduced morbidity.
- Staffing and facilities for all aspects of the screening program must be adequate.
- Benefits of screening should outweigh potential harms.

It is inherent in those criteria that the test used should detect the condition at an early stage and that treatment at an early stage is of more benefit than treatment at a later stage (Wilson and Jungner, 1968). It is generally accepted that screening for PTSD, depression, and other mental health problems is ineffective unless it is integrated into a total management program with adequate follow-up to confirm or refute a positive screening result and adequate capability to provide appropriate treatment. An illustrative example is depression, in which screening alone without follow-up care and treatment is unlikely to improve management and is believed to be associated with an unacceptable ratio of cost to benefit (Gilbody et al., 2006; Lang and Stein, 2005; U.S. Preventive Services Task Force, 2002). Similar considerations are likely to apply to PTSD screening.

Screening is not meant to replace assessment or diagnosis, but it can serve as a decision support tool. A person who has a positive screening result should undergo a clinical assessment that can be used by a trained clinician to make appropriate diagnoses—including diagnoses of comorbid conditions, such as depression or traumatic brain injury (TBI)—and to acquire additional information that is required to plan treatment. Such an assessment should take into account the symptoms that the person is experiencing and the severity of and functional impairment associated with the symptoms. Although it is widely believed that screening for PTSD among current and former service members is important for identifying affected people and directing them to treatment as early as possible to prevent chronic suffering and maladjustment, there is no strong evidence to support this belief.

Traumas associated with military service, such as combat and sexual assault, have been associated with a high prevalence of PTSD in this population, and several factors should be considered in implementing broad screening directives in this group (Kessler et al., 1995; Skinner et al., 2000). For a screening program to be effective, adequate resources need to be in place to support it, such as appropriate personnel and time (VA and DoD, 2010). The choice of instrument, method of delivery (such as self-report vs. clinician-administered), place of delivery (such as in the theater of war vs. on the home front), and intended use of the results of the screen are all important in designing a screening program.

Many PTSD screening instruments are available. The VA/DoD guideline notes there is insufficient evidence to recommend one PTSD screening tool over another, but several screening tools have been validated and should be considered for use: the Primary Care PTSD screen (PC-PTSD) (Prins et al., 2003), the PTSD Brief Screen (Leskin and Westrup, 1999), the Short Screening Scale for the *Diagnostic and Statistical Manual-IV* PTSD (Breslau et al., 1999), and the PTSD Checklist (PCL) (Blanchard et al., 1996, civilian version; Weathers et al., 1991, military version). The four-item PC-PTSD is the most widely used of those (see Box 6-1). In the DoD, the PC-PTSD screening questions are incorporated into longer surveys—the post-deployment health assessment (PDHA) and the post-deployment health reassessment (PDHRA). In DoD clinic settings, the PCL is commonly used. Before deployment, in addition to screening for PTSD itself, determination of the presence of factors that might increase a service member's risk of PTSD may be an associated undertaking.

For those who screen positive for PTSD or when evidence suggests the presence of other disorders or comorbidities, the screening program should ensure rapid diagnostic evaluation by a trained provider that includes the assessment of other possible causes of the symptoms and issues that are important for treatment planning. The use of a structured interview may improve the validity and reliability of such an evaluation. Evaluation should address comorbidities—such as TBI, depression, other anxiety disorders,

BOX 6-1
Primary Care PTSD Screen

In your life, have you ever had any experience that was so frightening, horrible, or upsetting that, in the past month, you:

1. Have had nightmares about it or thought about it when you did not want to?
   YES / NO

2. Tried hard not to think about it or went out of your way to avoid situations that reminded you of it?
   YES / NO

3. Were constantly on guard, watchful, or easily startled?
   YES / NO

4. Felt numb or detached from others, activities, or your surroundings?
   YES / NO

SOURCE: VA (2012a).

alcohol or substance abuse—and the presence of risky behaviors (discussed in more detail in Chapter 8). In addition, determining the severity of symptoms, the degree and nature of functional impairments, and suicide risk are important in selecting treatment. During the evaluation, the people being evaluated should be educated regarding PTSD and other relevant diagnoses, have their treatment options explained, and participate and be in agreement with treatment decisions. The latter is key to later engagement with and adherence to treatment.

Identifying those who have established PTSD and offering them treatment is a DoD and VA priority (VA, 2002; VA and DoD, 2010). In planning a program involving screening of active-duty service members or veterans, it is important to be clear about the goals of the activity. As will be discussed below, screening in this environment is not benign. It carries financial costs, and more important, it can lead to anxiety, further testing, and in some cases change in the course of a military career, which leads to pressure for underreporting. The costs and benefits of screening and assessment must be weighed. However, there are costs of *not* screening and assessing; allowing a physically or mentally impaired service member to continue to serve when not battle ready may jeopardize the service member's or the unit's safety. Allowing problems to go undetected may compound them and lead to comorbid disorders and increased disability; it then becomes even more complicated and expensive to treat than if the initial problem had been detected and treated earlier.

The major psychologic conditions currently screened for in populations of active-duty military personnel and veterans are PTSD, depression, alcohol use disorders, sexual trauma, suicidality, and mild TBI. All those are addressed in the DoD-administered PDHA and PDHRA, discussed in detail in Chapter 4. Here, the committee focuses on PTSD, acknowledging that partial or subthreshold PTSD should not be overlooked inasmuch as it is associated with substantial functional disability (Stein et al., 1997; Walker et al., 2002).

In active-duty service members, screening can identify those who have impaired operational readiness and ideally can lead to the care necessary to restore their previous levels of functioning. In veteran populations, screening and assessment can identify diagnosable disorders and functional impairments and thereby guide treatment and lead to fulfilling lives out of the military. As covered in Chapter 5, to implement an effective early intervention and potentially eradicate a developing problem or mitigate its effect, a candidate for intervention must first be identified. Therefore, wide-scale screening of all those at risk must be implemented. It is easier to define "at risk" for some other conditions than for PTSD. For example, all persons within 35 meters of a blast are considered "at risk" for TBI, but "at risk" is much harder to determine for PTSD. There are a few screening tools that capture PTSD and other health issues. Although the General Health Questionnaire (Goldberg, 1972) and the 10-item and 6-item Kessler scales (Kessler et al, 2002) have been used extensively worldwide for the detection of mental health disorders, those instruments do not target specific disorders.

In conducting assessments of the effects of trauma exposure in the theater of war, it is important to attempt to discriminate between a normative stress response and a pathologic condition that requires diagnosis and intervention. War by its nature is an extreme stressor and a life-threatening situation, and humans should be expected to react accordingly. A detailed discussion of adaptive and maladaptive responses to stress is presented in Chapter 3. The intention is not to treat a normal or adaptive stress response, which is imperative to survival, but instead to detect when it has become maladaptive and interferes with functioning. A primary purpose of the evaluation is to lead to maintaining individual service member and unit functioning and readiness.

CONSIDERATIONS REGARDING SCREENING IN THE DEPARTMENT OF DEFENSE AND THE DEPARTMENT OF VETERANS AFFAIRS

The *VA/DoD Clinical Practice Guideline for Management of Post-Traumatic Stress* (2010) considers that the evidence supporting screening with the PC-PTSD or three other scales is II-2—based on well-designed cohort or case–control studies rather than randomized controlled trials—and that the quality of the evidence is fair and the strength of recommendation is B, that is, the recommendation can be made on the basis of fair evidence that screening improves health outcomes and that the benefits outweigh the costs. In their review of seven PTSD guidelines, Forbes et al. (2010) note that there is a range of support for screening: the American Psychiatric Association concludes that level 1 evidence (defined as strong expert consensus) supports screening, and others, such as the British National Institute for Health and Clinical Excellence (NICE) and the Australian Guidelines, regard the evidence as weak, at the level of "good practice points" as distinct from good evidence. A key weakness in the literature is the paucity of evidence regarding the effect of screening on PTSD outcomes.

Delivery

In the DoD and the VA, screening for PTSD is usually not the sole focus of a clinical assessment but is combined with screening and assessment of other conditions. The VA/DoD clinical practice guideline (2010) supports assessment of patients for psychiatric and medical conditions, which includes "past and current psychiatric and substance use problems and treatment, prior trauma exposure, pre-injury psychological stressors, and existing social support." The number of deployments that a person has had should also be considered. PTSD screening can be divided into premilitary trauma, peritrauma, and posttrauma screening, each having specific considerations, which are addressed below.

The Role of the Screener

As previously discussed, the results of screening tests are usually integrated into a more comprehensive assessment, and positive or negative results require interpretation by qualified professionals. Service members must give informed consent before completing the pre-deployment health assessment, PDHA, or PDHRA, and this consent states that responses on the form "may result in a referral for additional healthcare that may include medical, dental or behavioral healthcare or diverse community support services" (10 U.S.C. 136, 1074f, 3013, 5013, 8013, and Executive Order 9397). A credentialed health care provider is required to review and discuss the service member's responses during the face-to-face part of the assessment. Physicians, physician's assistants, nurse practitioners, and others who are medically trained to administer the PDHA and PDHRA, such as independent corpsmen and technicians, are examples of such providers. A health care provider interviews the subject and completes the second part of the assessment, documents any concerns, and makes recommendations for further treatment or referral. The provider then signs off on the PDHA or PDHRA, documenting the nature of the service provided and of the referral given and whether the service member accepted the recommendations. PDHA and PDHRA assessments are filed in the service member's medical record and in the Defense Medical Surveillance System. A credentialed health care practitioner at the service member's home base is expected to review the findings and ensure that follow-up occurs and that necessary appointments are scheduled (GAO, 2008).

The Effect of Stigma

Regardless of the reliability and validity of a screening instrument in ideal testing environments, as long as there is the belief that being labeled with a given condition may affect one's future adversely, especially in the U.S. military, there will be an underreporting bias. It is only touched on here, but a more complete discussion of stigma can be found in Chapter 9. In one study that used a brigade of Army soldiers as the population of interest, service members first completed the PDHA, and then a subsample were invited to complete an anonymous survey that consisted of the same mental health questions found on the PDHA. A comparison of the PDHA and the anonymous survey (which would not be a part of the soldiers' records) found that the numbers of positive responses to the mental health questions overall and to the PTSD-specific questions more than doubled and in some cases quadrupled. On the PDHA, 3.3% of soldiers screened positive for PTSD, whereas on the anonymous survey, 7.7% screened positive. Of the service members that screened positive for either PTSD or depression on the anonymous survey (12.1%), 20.3% reported that they were not comfortable in reporting their answers honestly on the PDHA. The positive-screen group also indicated they were less likely to seek treatment for these issues (one-third indicated that they thought it would harm their careers) than the group that screened negative for PTSD or depression (Warner et al., 2011). Those results indicate a high level of underreporting of mental health symptoms, which may have adverse implications for the health and readiness of the armed forces. As discussed in the next section, additional specific stigma-related concerns are involved in screening before and after deployment.

Timing of Screening

One of the many considerations in screening for PTSD is when to screen. In the active-duty (and National Guard and reserve) force, screening can occur before deployment to a combat zone, during deployment in the theater of war, or after deployment. Because PTSD symptoms may not show for a number of months or years or may not be present when a service member transitions from active duty to the civilian population, screening for PTSD is also an important consideration in the VA.

Predeployment Screening

There are several approaches to predeployment screening of service members, including screening before accession, basic training and boot camp, and screening prior to the actual deployment. Service members undergo a rigorous selection process to ensure physical and mental fitness. Each of the different services has its own criteria for acceptance, including minimum scores on the Armed Forces Qualification Test, minimum level of education, and policies for waivers. Basic training also serves to test physical and mental strength and abilities, and this can lead to discharges of unqualified people. Because the resulting force consists of people who have high levels of physical and mental health, the value of additional screening for PTSD symptoms in this cohort before deployment is uncertain (Hyams, 2006).

Screening just before deployment has been proposed as an additional method of identifying persons who have disqualifying conditions and are not otherwise eliminated. However, the preponderance of evidence does not support that approach (Hyams, 2006). The pre-deployment health assessment has one mental health question: "During the past year, have you sought counseling or care for your mental health?" This question is of limited usefulness for the assessment of predeployment mental health concerns, particularly given the stigma associated with seeking mental health care or the assumption that a service member may not recognize that he or she has a mental health problem. An affirmative response to the question results in referral for an interview by a trained medical provider who may then sign a form indicating medical readiness for deployment.

One British study demonstrated that in a sample of soldiers deployed to Iraq, screening for common mental disorders, including PTSD, before deployment would not reduce morbidity or predicted PTSD (Rona et al., 2006). A prospective study of 22,630 service members enrolled in the Millennium Cohort Study found that those who reported one or more mental health disorders on a predeployment questionnaire were significantly more likely to screen positive for postdeployment PTSD symptoms (odds ratio 2.52, 95% confidence interval 2.01–3.16) (Sandweiss et al., 2011). However, this study did not assess morbidity and did not categorize service members' fitness for duty. Categorizing service members as unfit to deploy or unfit for military duty on the basis of such an unfounded approach may have unjustified adverse implications for their lives and careers.

A large nonrandomized controlled cohort study that compared screened and unscreened combat brigades deployed to Iraq showed that the combination of predeployment screening and subsequent contact with mental health services in the theater of war reduced the rate of combat stress reactions, behavioral health disorders, suicidal ideation, and occupational-duty restrictions (Warner et al., 2011). The purpose of the screening was not to keep service members from deploying but to link them to needed services in the theater of war. Predeployment screening opens the possibility of underreporting that is perhaps driven by service members' desire not to compromise their chance of deploying. Evidence supporting that argument comes in part from a retrospective cohort study of service members deployed in support of Operation Enduring Freedom (OEF) that found that fewer than half those who received a diagnosis of a mental health disorder during the predeployment period gave an affirmative response to the pre-deployment health assessment question "During the past year, have you sought counseling or care for your mental health?" That demonstrates the low validity of this instrument for identifying service members who have diagnosed mental health disorders before deployment (Nevin, 2009).

Postdeployment Screening

Evidence that screening for PTSD immediately after deployment may result in underreporting compared with screening later can be seen in results of a matched study of 509 soldiers returning from Iraq. Statistically significant increases in mental health symptoms of PTSD, depression, general psychologic distress, anger, and relationship problems were found 120 days after deployment compared with the immediate integration period (Bliese et al., 2007). Because the PDHA and the PDHRA are not anonymous, such underreporting may be due to fear of delaying family reunion and interference with an allocated extended period of leave after returning from deployment (Bliese et al., 2007; DoD, 2007; McClure, 2007). Another possible explanation for lower rates of symptom reporting in the immediate reintegration period is that some symptom clusters may not be present or may not have a recognized adverse effect on functioning during this time (Bliese et al., 2007). A third possibility may be that service members' relief at being home overshadows any mental health issues.

In a longitudinal follow-up of more than 88,000 soldiers returning from Iraq, Milliken et al. (2007) found that the rates of positive PTSD screening results were more than 50% higher in the PDHRA than in the initial PDHA. The increases were greatest in the National Guard and reserve components, in which the prevalence increased from 9% to 14%. In active-duty soldiers, the prevalence increased from 6% to 9%. However, the investigators observed a reduction in the rate of positive PTSD screening results in the PDHA sample on rescreening several months later. The implications are that PTSD symptoms in the early posttraumatic phase often resolve and that educational programs in the military promote recovery. One other important finding from the Milliken et al. study is that the rates of self-reported interpersonal problems increased substantially in the PDHRA. Inasmuch as those issues often involve spouses, there may be a case for greater involvement of spouses, partners, or close family members in some part of the screening process or for facilitating access of such people to the health care system (Milliken et al., 2007).

Screening, assessment, and diagnosis are different. Whereas screening instruments and tools are used to identify persons who are likely to have the condition of interest, in the case of PTSD, assessment and diagnosis are necessary to confirm diagnosis and plan treatment. A positive PTSD screening result on the PDHA and PDHRA is indicated by an affirmative response to two or more of the four PTSD-specific questions. From August 2010 through July 2011, a total of 231,822 active-duty service members in all services and 75,219 reserve-component members (National Guard and reserves) completed the PDHA. During the same period, 223,582 active-duty and 86,421 reserve-component members completed the PDHRA. In all the completed surveys, 8.3% of active-duty service members screened positive for PTSD on the PDHA and 9.5% on the PDHRA, and 9.2% of reserve members screened positive on the PDHA and 16.6% on the PDHRA. When stratified by service, both active-duty and reserve Army and Marine Corps personnel had the highest rates of positive PTSD screens on the PDHA and the PDHRA. Of all active-duty service members, 5.9% were referred for additional mental health assessment by a provider (for any mental health concern indicated, not specifically PTSD) after the PDHA, but 10.9% after the PDHRA. Of all reserve-component members, 4.9% were referred for additional mental health assessment after the PDHA and 16.2% after the PDHRA. Because the percentage of referrals for any mental health concern was reported, it is impossible to know how many service members who had affirmative responses to the PTSD questions were referred. Among both active-duty and reserve-component members, the percentage of mental health referrals increased between the PDHA and the PDHRA. Furthermore, 95.9% of all active-duty service members and 94.6% of reserve-component service members who were given referrals after the PDHA had a medical visit (according to records of outpatient or inpatient visits for either mental health or physical health concerns) within 6 months of the referrals (Armed Forces Health Surveillance Center, 2011).

Screening of Veterans

In the VA, positive screenings for PTSD, depression, suicidality, or military sexual trauma (sexual assault or extreme harassment that occurred during service in the military) result in referral of the veteran to a mental health professional for evaluation. Patients referred are to receive an initial evaluation within 24 hours and a full evaluation within 14 days after referral. However, no data are available to track what happens after referral—for example, what proportion engage and complete evaluations, enter and complete treatment, continue or return to active duty, or are discharged. A recent analysis of 125,729 Operation Iraqi Freedom (OIF) and OEF veterans screened for military sexual trauma in VA primary care and mental health clinics found that 15.1% of women and 0.7% of men reported military sexual trauma and that such trauma was associated with increased odds of PTSD, depression, and other mental health disorders (Kimerling et al., 2010).

SCREENING IN PRIMARY CARE

Given that an estimated 90% of patients who have received mental health diagnoses are seen in primary care (Gebhart and Neeley, 1996) and that persons who receive diagnoses of PTSD are more likely to seek medical care than mental health care (VA, 2002), screening for PTSD in primary care settings is paramount. A variety of primary care venues are available through the DoD, the VA, and private practices, each of which is discussed below. This section concludes with a brief overview of some of the challenges to implementing PTSD screening in primary care settings and how they might be overcome by using lessons learned from implementing screening for depression in primary care settings.

The Department of Defense

The DoD provides primary care through the individual services and through contracted TRICARE providers. Service members who received care in an integrated behavioral health and primary care setting had significantly reduced psychologic distress and significant improvement in clinical outcomes (Cigrang et al., 2006). One example of a successful implemented screening program that is Army-specific is the Re-Engineering Systems for Primary Care Treatment of Depression and PTSD in the Military (RESPECT-Mil) program, discussed in Chapter 4. Primary care providers are trained to screen and treat soldiers for PTSD and depression at every visit. It is an approach to establish collaboration between primary care and behavioral health professionals to overcome many of the barriers to effective management of PTSD in primary care settings in the DoD. Key elements of the program include universal primary care screening for PTSD and depression, including use of the single-item PTSD screener, developed for military primary care settings (Gore et al., 2008); brief standardized primary care diagnostic assessment for those who screen positive; and use of a nurse–care facilitator to ensure continuity of care for those who have unmet depression and PTSD treatment needs. The care facilitator assists primary care clinicians with follow-up, symptom monitoring, and treatment adjustment and enhances the primary care interface with specialty mental health services (Engel et al., 2008). Separate manuals that integrate care for PTSD with care for major depression guide the primary care clinician, behavioral health specialist, and care facilitator in their roles. As of Fall 2011, RESPECT-Mil had been implemented in 32 of 37 Army sites and in 84 primary care clinics. Since its inception, more than 1.1 million primary care visits have included screening for PTSD and depression, and approximately 13% of the screenings have been positive (DoD, 2011).

According to the official RESPECT-Mil website (DoD, 2011), "The US Army Medical Command has directed wide implementation of RESPECT-Mil in Army primary care facilities. Tri-service implementation is in the planning stages." During FY 2012–2016, as the DoD phases in its primary care model of the patient-centered medical home—that is, a health care setting model with goals of providing comprehensive primary care for all family members and facilitating partnerships between the patient, the physician, and members of the patient's family (if appropriate) (Patient-Centered Primary Care Collaborative, 2007)—it plans to use RESPECT-Mil as the basis of its delivery of behavioral health care.

The U.S. Air Force initiated the Behavioral Health Optimization Program (BHOP) to integrate behavioral health and primary care services administered by the Air Force Medical Service (U.S. Air Force, 2011). It has resulted in increased availability of behavioral health services for families, as well as service members, and reduced stigma by making behavioral health care a routine part of primary medical care. In surveys of BHOP patients, 97% indicated that they were satisfied or very satisfied with their care. Not only were there statistically significant reduced levels of psychologic distress, but fewer than 10% of patients had to be referred to more intensive, specialty care services, and this suggests that integrated providers are able to manage the needs of most mental health patients in the primary care setting (Air Force Medical Operations Agency, 2011).

The Navy has integrated behavioral health and primary care services through deployment health clinics. Staff include primary care providers, psychologists, psychiatrists, social workers, and certified medical assistants. The Navy has also piloted the Behavioral Health Integration Project, whose purpose is to ensure continuity of care by placing mental health providers in primary care facilities. Mental health providers serve as consultants to the primary care providers and "provide sailors with short, focused assessments, brief interventions, skill training, and behavioral change plans" (Weinick et al., 2011).

The Department of Veterans Affairs

The VA uses annual universal mental health screening for veterans who are seen in the VA as part of its primary care preventive-health assessment process (Kirchner, 2011; Zeiss and Karlin, 2008). The VA is increasingly using mental health professionals to work as an integral part of primary care teams. In FY 2010, 155,554 veterans were seen by mental health staff deployed in primary care clinics—an increase of 102% from FY 2008 (Schoenhard, 2011). The VA policy is to screen every patient who is seen in VA primary care settings for PTSD, military sexual trauma, depression, and problem drinking, usually during the first appointment. Screenings for depression and problem drinking are repeated annually for as long as the veteran uses VA services. Military sexual trauma is screened for only once unless new data are entered into the record that indicate the need for additional screenings. PTSD screening is repeated annually for the first 5 years and every 5 years thereafter (VA, 2010).

To screen for PTSD, the VA uses the four-item PC-PTSD screen. In

2005, the definition of a positive screen changed from two or more affirmative responses to any three or more affirmative responses to the four questions (VA, 2005). The purpose of the change was to maximize efficiency (0.85) while reducing the number of false positives (Calhoun et al., 2010; Prins et al., 2003, 2004). Positive screenings for PTSD or depression also result in an additional screening for suicidality.

In addition to screening in VA health facilities, veterans seen in any of the approximately 300 Vet Centers are screened for PTSD and sexual trauma. Counseling is provided on site for those conditions, and veterans can be referred to VA mental health services as needed. Of the 191,000 veterans seen at Vet Centers in 2011, 39% were not seen at a VA medical facility (Batres, 2011).

The Private Sector

In the private sector (non-DoD and non-VA settings), veterans may be seen in primary care settings either with funding provided by TRICARE or with no military-related connection or funding. Veterans who have private insurance may choose to be seen by providers in the private sector. It has been estimated that 90% of patient visits for a mental health disorder in the private sector are to primary care providers as opposed to mental health providers, so it is likely that clinicians, especially those who have veteran patients, will encounter patients who have mental health needs (VA, 2002). However, because there are no PTSD clinical practice guidelines for the private sector specific to people who have service-related PTSD, integration of screening for service-related PTSD into private-sector primary care faces several challenges.

Challenges to Screening in Primary Care

First, primary care clinicians may not be aware of the adverse effects of PTSD on physical health (Schnurr and Jankowski, 1999). Second, many primary care providers do not have much experience in dealing with PTSD and its consequences and may find it difficult to bring up to a patient whose chief concern is seemingly unrelated. Third, with increased patient loads and cost constraints, lack of clinician time can be serious; many providers do not have or take the time to discuss with patients issues that may not be directly visible or may not seem related to the primary presenting health complaints. Fourth, if a primary care provider wants to screen for PTSD or trauma, selection of the best screening tool can be confusing (VA, 2002). The 2010 VA/DoD guideline endorses screening, but, although it does not offer specific guidance on which of the more than 20 screens and assessment tools should be used, the VA preferentially uses the four-item PC-PTSD

Screen and the DoD also uses these questions in its regular screening practices (PDHA, PDHRA) and the PCL in clinical settings. Fifth, primary care clinicians may have knowledge gaps concerning both PTSD and VA resources for its care. A recent study of nonmilitary, rural primary care providers is illustrative. Over a 6-month period, the providers saw about 1,200 OEF and OIF veteran patients and 3,600 of their family members. Many of the patients had mental health problems. Substantial gaps in knowledge of mental health disorders are suggested by the fact that providers lacked knowledge of PTSD and were unaware of VA resources. Only 20% of the providers rated their mental health treatment skills as high, and only about 8% reported that they had adequate knowledge of current mental health treatment strategies (Boscarino et al., 2010).

Other obstacles to screening in primary care settings are persistent provider and patient attitudes regarding mental health and traumatic experiences. Concerns about upsetting, retraumatizing, or offending a patient and not knowing what to do with the results of screening contribute to a reluctance of primary care providers to screen for trauma and PTSD in their patients. Some patients may not want to be reminded of their experience because of the painful memories it evokes, shame about what happened, or a belief that the provider will not be able to help them even if they disclose, but others may not be aware of what PTSD is or that it is a maladaptive response. Some research has suggested that patients who have a history of trauma are willing to disclose such information in a primary care setting, but will not typically disclose their trauma history spontaneously (VA, 2002).

Lessons from Screening for Depression in Primary Care

Screening for major depressive disorder as an accepted and routine part of primary care practice has depended on a number of developments, which are illustrative for integrating screening for and management of PTSD in primary care practice. These are of particular concern in practices outside the DoD and the VA systems. The adoption of screening for PTSD in the private sector will require a number of barriers to be addressed, including those described below.

Brief Screening Measures Acceptable to Primary Care Clinicians

Evidence that screening leads to the identification of those who have previously undiagnosed PTSD and that this identification leads to improved outcomes in primary care settings is required before any PTSD screening program can be implemented. Validation is required both for initial (one-time) screening and for any recommendation for repeated screening, such as annually, as is the current policy in the VA. For private-sector (non-DoD and non-VA) practice, a two-step screening process—such as the use of the two-question Patient Health Questionnaire-2 (Kroenke et al., 2003) and the full Patient Health Questionnaire-9 (Kroenke et al., 2001) as the second step for major depressive disorder—has not been similarly defined for service-related PTSD. Given that current service members and veterans will usually make up a small portion of the total practice patient population and may not identify themselves as a veteran, a simple two-step process might involve, as the first step, questions like "Have you ever served in the U.S. military?", and then if the response is affirmative, a question from the PC-PTSD instrument like "Have you ever had any experience that was so frightening, horrible, or upsetting that, in the last month, you . . .?" Such an approach requires validation of effectiveness before it can be recommended.

Because national guidelines and quality metrics are not available for PTSD screening in the private sector, it is unlikely for clinicians in settings outside the DoD and the VA to perform this type of screening routinely. The committee could find no specific information or data on routine PTSD screening in the private sector. Perhaps a question that should be investigated in the private sector is whether the addition of screening for PTSD to screening for major depressive disorder in nonmilitary and non-VA primary care settings provides improved outcomes, possibly with only marginal increases in cost and effort compared with screening for major depression alone. This might occur through the addition of PTSD screening and management to established primary care depression programs or the de novo implementation of such combined PTSD and major depression screening and management programs.

Accessibility of Treatment to Primary Care Clinicians

Selective serotonin reuptake inhibitors provide primary care clinicians with a treatment option for depression that has been effective in some PTSD patients and in some communities. Telemedicine options may provide additional treatment strategies for primary care clinicians. However, guidelines for PTSD management are few and do not exist specifically for primary care physicians practicing outside the DoD and the VA. Measures and criteria specifically for evaluating and monitoring primary care practice performance regarding care for PTSD have not been developed.

SCREENING TOOLS

This section addresses the types of PTSD screening instruments that are most commonly used. The instruments can be used to assess exposure to trauma or to assess the presence of PTSD symptoms that are related to trauma. Some of the instruments listed in Tables 6-1 and 6-2 are more commonly used in research than in clinical care, and some of the longer instruments, such as the 201-item Deployment Risk and Resiliency Inventory, involve the use of only a subset of questions. Longer screening instruments have not been found to have any advantage over shorter ones (Brewin, 2005), and there is no evidence that one validated screening tool is superior to another (VA and DoD, 2010). The selection of a screening instrument depends ultimately on the goal of the screening (for example, clinical versus research settings or brief screening versus assessment of all symptoms). Although the screens have been validated to greater or smaller degrees, it is important to note that they cannot replace the knowledge of a trained clinician or leader (such as a first sergeant or chaplain) in detecting signs and symptoms of stress. Below, the section describes screening instruments used to screen for trauma exposure, symptom-based instruments, screens for stress reactions, novel technologies for screening, and biomarkers. The American Psychiatric Association is expected to release an update of the *Diagnostic and Statistical Manual of Mental Disorders (DSM)* in 2013. Changes to the diagnostic criteria will also affect screening instruments used (see Box 6-2).

TABLE 6-1 Instruments for Screening for Exposure to Trauma

Instrument	Reference
Abusive Violence Scale	Hendrix and Schumm, 1990
Childhood Trauma Questionnaire	Bernstein et al., 2003
Combat Exposure Index	Janes et al., 1991
Combat Exposure Scale	Keane et al., 1989
Comprehensive Trauma Inventory	Hollifield et al., 2005
Deployment Risk and Resilience Inventory	King et al., 2003
Graves Registration Duty Scale	Sutker et al., 1994
Harvard Trauma Questionnaire	Mollica et al., 1992
Life Events Checklist of the Clinician-Administered PTSD Scale	Blake et al., 1995
Military Stress Scale	Watson et al., 1988
Posttraumatic Diagnostic Scale	Foa et al.,1997
Sexual Experiences Questionnaire—DoD	Fitzgerald et al., 1999
Vietnam Era Stress Inventory—Specific Stressor Subscale	Wilson and Krause., 1980
War Events Scale	Unger et al., 1998
War Zone Stress Scale	King et al., 1995
Women's Wartime Stressor Scale	Wolfe et al., 1993

TABLE 6-2 Symptom-Based Screening Scales for PTSD

Scale	Reference
Beck Anxiety Inventory-Primary Care	Mori et al., 2003
Primary Care PTSD Screen	Prins et al., 2003
Short Screening Scale for PTSD	Breslau et al., 1999
SPAN	Davidson, 2002
Trauma Screening Questionnaire	Brewin et al., 2002
PTSD Brief Screen	Leskin and Westrup, 1999
PTSD Checklist (PCL)—Civilian and Military versions	Blanchard et al., 1996 (Civilian); Weathers et al., 1991 (Military)
Posttraumatic Adjustment Scale	O'Donnell et al., 2008
M-3 Checklist	Gaynes et al., 2010
Single item PTSD Screener	Gore et al., 2008
Five-item Primary Care Anxiety Screener	Means-Christensen et al., 2006
Anxiety and Depression Detector	Means-Christensen et al., 2006
Two-item and six-item PCL	Lang and Stein, 2005
Short Post-Traumatic Stress Disorder Rating Interview	Connor and Davidson, 2001
Post-Deployment Health Assessment	DoD, 1998; current DD form 2796, 2008
Post-Deployment Health Reassessment	DoD, 2005; current DD form 2900, 2008

Trauma Exposure

There are a number of self-reporting screens for exposure to trauma (Fitzgerald et al., 1999; Hendrix and Schumm, 1990; Janes et al., 1991; Keane et al., 1989; King et al., 1995, 2003; Sutker et al., 1994; Unger et al., 1998; Watson et al., 1988; Wilson and Krause, 1980; Wolfe et al., 1993). Trauma-exposure instruments may be limited to one type of event, such as military or combat-related trauma, or to a comprehensive list of events, including childhood trauma. Other trauma-exposure screening scales include the Childhood Trauma Questionnaire (Bernstein et al., 2003), which exists in long (70-item) and short (28-item) forms; the Comprehensive Trauma Inventory, a 104-item scale developed in refugee populations (Hollifield et al., 2005); and the Harvard Trauma Questionnaire (Mollica et al., 1992). Exposure to nonmilitary trauma can be assessed through interviews, such as those using the life events checklist of the Clinician-Administered PTSD Scale (CAPS) and the Posttraumatic Diagnostic Scale (Foa et al., 1997). A

BOX 6-2
Changes in Diagnostic Criteria for PTSD in the *Diagnostic and Statistical Manual-V* and Effect on Screening

Major revisions of the *Diagnostic and Statistical Manual* occur at variable intervals. Changes in the newest edition, *DSM-V*, are being piloted (see discussion in Chapter 2). Because some of the proposed changes, such as elimination of the A2 criterion (the person's response involved intense fear, helplessness, or horror), have direct effects on many of the questions in current screening instruments, these instruments will probably change to reflect the updates. For example, on the PDHA and PDHRA, the screening questions for PTSD begin with "Have you ever had any experience that was so frightening, horrible, or upsetting that in the past month you . . .?" Thus, it will be necessary to update guidelines around screening, especially with regard to preferred instruments. The proposed change from a three-pronged to a four-pronged model (see Chapter 2) may also affect current popular screening instruments, such as the four-item PC-PTSD screen (on which the PDHA and the PDHRA are based), in which each question seeks to elicit symptoms related to each of the main criteria. The proposed addition of four symptoms (anger and aggressive behavior, erroneous self- or other-blame regarding the cause or consequences of trauma, pervasive negative emotional states, and reckless and self-destructive behavior) to the current 17 may also require revision of current screening instruments. It may, therefore, become necessary to update guidelines around screening, especially with regard to preferred instruments, instrument items, and scoring.

representative list of questionnaires relevant to military service is shown in Table 6-1. Some of the questionnaires may have application only to particular groups, such as women, sexual trauma survivors, Vietnam-era veterans, or grave registration personnel.

Symptom-Based

Several short symptom-based screening scales are used to detect possible PTSD. The VA/DoD guideline (2010) notes that a symptom-driven scale that is cued to a particular event is more attractive to clinic staff, who may not be able to address a person's entire life history of trauma at the first visit. Those scales, which are listed in Table 6-2, are the seven-item Beck Anxiety Inventory-Primary Care (Mori et al., 2003), the four-item PC-PTSD (Prins et al., 2003), the seven-item Short Screening Scale for PTSD (Breslau et al., 1999), the four-item SPAN (Davidson, 2002), and the 10-item Trauma Screening Questionnaire (Brewin et al., 2002). All those assess symptoms that follow any type of trauma and can be completed in less than 4 minutes. The PC-PTSD is the most widely used screen in active-duty military (with PDHA and PDHRA screens) and veteran populations. Its introductory statement is as follows: "[In your life,] have you ever had any experience that was so frightening, horrible, or upsetting that, in the last month, you . . .?" The PDHA and PDHRA contain detailed questions about exposure to trauma in the course of military service and then frames the PC-PTSD symptom screen questions in the context of "any experience" (it could be related to either military or civilian life).

The 17-item PCL has separate formats for military and civilian situations (Blanchard et al., 1996; Weathers et al., 1991). Additional scales include the PTSD Brief Screen (Leskin and Westrup, 1999); the 17-item symptom subscale of the Posttraumatic Diagnostic Scale; the Posttraumatic Adjustment Scale, a 10-item self-rating based on pretraumatic, peritraumatic, and posttraumatic symptoms (O'Donnell et al., 2008); the M-3 Checklist, a 27-item screener for several disorders, including PTSD (Gaynes et al., 2010); the Single-Item PTSD Screener developed in the military primary care setting (Gore et al., 2008), which did not perform as well as the widely used four-item PC-PTSD; and the five-item primary care anxiety screener and Anxiety and Depression Detector (Means-Christensen et al., 2006). Lang and Stein have refined the PCL to shorter two-item and six-item screening options in primary care, and they have both performed adequately (Lang and Stein, 2005).

Stress Reactions: The Best Screen Is a Good First Sergeant

Related to screening for PTSD is screening for stress reactions. Identification of persons who are likely to have PTSD may be based on instruments or on personal knowledge and experience of a person. Instruments used to screen for stress reactions include the Perceived Stress Scale (Cohen et al., 1983), the Sheehan Perceived Stress Scale (Sheehan et al., 1990), the Posttraumatic Diagnostic Scale (Foa et al., 1997)—which are not used specifically in military or veteran populations—and the recently developed Response to Stressful Experiences Scale, which was developed by using active-duty and veteran populations (Johnson et al., 2011).

There has been an effort to identify service members who might be having reactions that decrease their combat readiness, but no scale has been developed for this purpose. It has been proposed that medics or embedded leaders who know their soldiers, airmen, sailors, or marines are in the best position to make such an informal assessment ("the best screen is a good first sergeant"). The idea is for the embedded leaders not to serve as counselors but to be trained to recognize and respond appropriately to signs that may be associated with stress reactions in service members for whom they are responsible. The emerging screens may elicit warning signs by asking questions like these:

- Has the service member exhibited or described a decline in operational readiness? Has he or she been forgetful, had problems falling or staying asleep during operational pauses, or displayed extreme emotional responses, such as excessive crying or excessive anger or violence?
- Has the service member been cut off or withdrawn from others? Does he or she appear depressed or overwhelmed? Has he or she withdrawn from friends, the squad, or the platoon? Does he or she appear numb or emotionally dazed?
- Is the service member a danger to himself or herself or to others?

If a service member is a danger to himself or herself or to others, he or she should be referred immediately to a credentialed provider. If he or she makes suicidal statement or comments or threatens others, he or she should be referred. And a service member should be referred to a credentialed provider if his or her condition worsens or does not improve after 4 days of psychologic first aid.

Event-triggered screening occurs at prescribed times and currently occurs before deployment, immediately after deployment (with the PDHA), and 3–6 months after deployment (with the PDHRA). Routine screening for disruptive emotional reactions after exposure to combat operational stressors has recently been adopted. It should be performed by the medic or embedded leader that knows the service members as described above. Target stress-exposed groups include

- All wounded personnel who require medical attention and all personnel who were in direct contact (defined as visual contact) with a seriously wounded or killed unit comrade;
- All personnel who were directly involved in actions that resulted in deaths or serious injuries of civilians, including women and children;
- All personnel who killed enemy combatants in close contact and had direct visual contact with the enemy before or after killing;
- All personnel who were involved in a combat or mob incident in which they believed or feared that they would die; and
- All personnel who meet screening criteria for TBI.

Novel Technologies

The use of computing and information technology tools for increasing availability, promoting access, and improving acceptance (reducing stigma) of screening and other clinically relevant services has evolved substantially during OEF and OIF, but research to document their efficiency and efficacy is still in its infancy. Computing and information technology applications include Internet-based mental health resources, social media, mobile applications, virtual worlds, and virtual reality. Some tools being used to screen for PTSD have been launched online (for example, afterdeployment.org, myhealth.va.gov, and braveheartveterans.org) or as mobile applications (for example, PTSD Coach and Mood Tracker). Such anonymous screening and education options may provide users with self-assessment results that can be used to instigate or encourage a self-referral to a provider for care. They may offer a safe and nonstigmatizing "first point of contact" for those who do not make initial direct contact with a service provider or clinic. In addition to anonymous screening, computing and information technology can provide options for delivering psychoeducational information, providing "common sense" advice, and promoting peer-group interaction. Such approaches may help to address the numerous challenges that exist for the DoD and the VA with regard to the growing need for health services in the military and veteran populations.

The Integrated Mental Health Strategy was launched in September 2010 to review computing and information technology resources and included more than 290 publically accessible technology resources in several categories: DoD, VA, and commercial websites; social media applications; mobile applications; and call centers. Each of those has advantages and gaps. Some more detailed examples of mobile applications and websites that offer screening or self-assessment for PTSD or related symptoms are described below.

- *afterdeployment.org*. This website was created and is maintained by the National Center for Telehealth and Technology, a component of the Defense Centers of Excellence for Psychological Health and Traumatic Brain Injury and part of the Military Health System. Its primary mission is to provide wellness resources for the military community. It provides extensive resources on posttraumatic stress, depression, TBI, family and friendships, and sleep. The screening section is extensive, with self-assessments covering 29 domains, including PTSD, depression, caregiver stress, mild-TBI symptom management, and sleep. The site uses the military version of the PCL to screen for PTSD, and users are given their scores following completion with recommendations for next steps (DCoE, 2012a).

- *PTSD Coach*. This free mobile application was created by the VA's National Center for PTSD and the DoD's National Center for Telehealth and Technology and is specifically designed for veterans and current service members who have or may have PTSD. It is available for both iPhone and Android smartphones and provides validated information about PTSD and its treatment and interactive tools for self-assessment, managing and tracking of symptoms (relaxation skills and coping techniques), and finding support. Any information entered is as secure as the device, but users may share data and are able to customize the tool content to integrate their own contacts, photographs, and music. This application is not intended to diagnose or treat PTSD and should not replace professional care. A PTSD Family Coach is under development (VA, 2012b).
- *My HealtheVet*. Screening for PTSD and other mental health conditions is available for all veterans through the VA's My Health*e*Vet website (VA, 2012c). The site allows all registered users of VA health care services to access their clinical records and provides a number of wellness and health-enhancement options. On the website (Researching Your Health—Mental Health Section), any veteran (even if not registered as a user of VA services) can complete the 17 questions of the PCL, have his or her score immediately displayed and, if the screen suggests a possible problem, be advised about seeing a VA mental health professional.
- *braveheartveterans.org*. A number of private foundations and organizations have been involved in outreach to aid service members and veterans in accessing mental health services. The Robert R. McCormick Foundation has joined with Major League Baseball Charities to support the national Welcome Back Veterans program. BraveHeart: Welcome Back Veterans Southeast Initiative launched a website aimed at outreach to veterans in Alabama, Georgia, and South Carolina. The website uses an avatar to help users to assess themselves for PTSD and then provides assistance in finding services through a ZIP code locator (Atlanta Braves and Emory University, 2011).

Biologic Screening

Much recent discussion concerning screening for and diagnosis of PTSD has centered on the many types of potential biologic markers. Some literature has suggested that startle responses and heart rate may be useful for screening for PTSD. No validated, accurate biologic screening test for

PTSD is currently available. A more complete discussion of biomarkers can be found in Chapter 3.

DIAGNOSIS

The diagnosis of PTSD rests on the ability of a trained professional to establish rapport with a patient and conduct a thorough clinical interview. Supplementary information can be obtained with self-rating scales for PTSD, suicidality, depression, quality of life, disability, and resilience. Several structured interviews have been validated for the diagnosis of PTSD; these scales vary in the time needed for administration. This section describes the components of the diagnostic process mentioned earlier.

Clinical Diagnostic Assessment

The diagnosis of PTSD ultimately rests on a careful and comprehensive clinical evaluation performed by a qualified professional (a psychologist, a social worker, a psychiatrist, or a psychiatric nurse practitioner) under conditions of privacy and confidentiality (DoD, 2007; IOM, 2006). It may take some time to elicit the information necessary to conclude that a person does or does not have PTSD. As discussed in Chapter 2, many pretraumatic factors have been found to be associated with development of PTSD, and the interview should obtain these and other important details, including chief complaints; lifetime history of exposures to trauma and experience of physical injury to self or others; frequency and severity of symptoms of PTSD and other morbidity; level of function (disability); quality of life and ongoing life stressors; medical history and present health; prior psychiatric diagnosis and treatment; details of family, recreations, and supports; personal strengths and vulnerabilities; styles of coping with stress; and experiences in the military. Obtaining all that information may not be straightforward and can be accompanied by the expression of strong affect by the patient, so it may be necessary to plan more than a single intake interview. The process can be facilitated by using information from screening scales and other ratings, such as scales to measure all main PTSD symptoms, such related problems as depression, other axis I conditions (for example panic disorder, social phobia, and generalized anxiety disorder), patterns of alcohol and substance use, disability, quality of life, and resilience. In some situations, more comprehensive personality and neurocognitive assessments might be indicated. It is important to determine whether the goal is to identify and assess pathologic conditions (the severity of diagnosable disorders, such as PTSD, and common comorbid conditions, such as depression and TBI), to assess functioning, or both. If assessing pathologic conditions, the clinician must be able to rule out some conditions that could also cause the symptoms and determine whether more than one disorder is present.

Besides helping to make an initial diagnosis, rating scales can serve as a measure of PTSD severity and as a benchmark against which future progress can be measured. For instance, use of the PCL can provide a measure of the extent of improvement during treatment, serve as a marker of remission, and highlight symptoms that may persist when others have improved.

Diagnostic Interviews

The *DSM-IV* criteria for PTSD have been given previously (Chapter 2). There are a number of well-tested and valid structured interviews for the diagnosis of PTSD, although in general they are unlikely to be adopted in routine clinical practice, where the benchmark continues to remain a thorough clinical interview. All of these structured interviews are primarily research tools that can be used for clinical assessment in situations where the diagnosis in not clear. The shortest assessments take 15–30 minutes to complete, and the longer ones take 45–60 minutes. However, there is considerable variability in the time needed to complete the assessment. It depends on the choice of scale, the complexity of the case, the number and type of traumas, and the subject's level of knowledge about PTSD. Although the VA/DoD guideline specifically mentions the use of the CAPS for diagnosis, they also state that "diagnosis of PTSD should be obtained based on a comprehensive clinical interview that assesses all the symptoms that characterize PTSD." Table 6-3 lists the structured interviews that can be used to diagnose PTSD.

TABLE 6-3 Structured Interviews for Assessment of PTSD

Instrument	Reference
Clinician-Administered PTSD Scale (CAPS)[a]	Blake et al., 1995
Structured Clinical Interview for *DSM-IV*[a]	Spitzer et al., 1992
Composite International Diagnostic Interview[b]	Robins et al., 1988
PTSD Symptom Scale—Interview Version[a]	Foa et al., 1993
Structured Interview for PTSD[a]	Davidson et al., 1997a
Diagnostic Interview Schedule[b]	Cottler, 2009; Robins et al., 1997
Mini-International Neuropsychiatric Interview[a]	Sheehan et al., 1998

[a] Indicates instruments that can be used to inform clinical assessment.
[b] Indicates instruments that are used for epidemiologic and treatment outcome research.

Among the many structured interviews, the CAPS (Blake et al., 1995), the Structured Clinical Interview for *DSM-IV* (First et al., 1995; Spitzer et al., 1992), PTSD Symptom Scale—Interview Version (PSS-I) (Foa et al., 1993), Structured Interview for PTSD (SIP) (Davidson et al., 1997a), Diagnostic Interview Schedule (DIS-IV) (Cottler, 2009; Robins et al., 1997), and Composite International Diagnostic Interview (CIDI) (Robins et al., 1988) have been noted in previous Institute of Medicine reports as potentially informing professional judgment, although they are used more often in epidemiologic or treatment-outcome research rather than clinical assessments. The widely used Mini-International Neuropsychiatric Interview (MINI) assesses most major diagnoses, including PTSD (Sheehan et al., 1998). All the above except the CAPS, PSS-I, and SIP assess multiple diagnoses. The PSS-I and SIP can be completed in 20–30 minutes. The DIS-IV can be administered either by a trained clinician or a lay interviewer or in a computerized format; the CIDI can also be administered by a trained professional or layperson. The Short PTSD Rating Interview (SPRINT) and the extended version (SPRINT-E) are not structured interviews, but they provide a more global overview of PTSD, disability, general health, depression, and suicide risk and can be used as brief interview-based diagnostic screens (Connor and Davidson, 2001; Norris et al., 2008). For most of these instruments, the respondent must be able to identify the most bothersome trauma and link it to many of the key PTSD symptoms.

Self-Rating Symptom Scales

Among the various self-rating scales for PTSD are the PCL (Blanchard et al., 1996; Weathers et al., 1991) and the Mississippi Scale (Keane et al., 1988; McFall et al., 1990), both of which exist in civilian and military or combat versions. Additional scales include the Impact of Event Scale (Horowitz et al., 1979), which antedates *DSM-III*, and its revised form, which accommodates all the *DSM-IV* symptoms (Weiss and Marmar, 1997); the MMPI-Keane PTSD Scale (Keane et al., 1984); the Hovens Self Rating Inventory for PTSD (Hovens et al., 2002); the PTSD Diagnostic Scale (Foa et al., 1997); the Davidson Trauma Scale (Davidson et al., 1997b); the War Zone Related PTSD subscale from the SCL-90 (Derogatis and Cleary, 1977); the Los Angeles Symptom Checklist (King et al., 1995); the 26-item Penn Inventory (Hammarberg, 1992); and the 22-item Self-Rating Scale for PTSD, developed by Carlier et al. (1998) from the SIP (Davidson et al., 1997a). These scales are summarized in Table 6-4. The shortest contains 17 items, and the longest contains 49.

All scales have been tested, albeit in different populations, and there is some variability with respect to their reliability and validity. Within the VA system, the PCL is perhaps the most often used severity scale. None of the

TABLE 6-4 Symptom-Severity Instruments for PTSD

Scale Name	Reference
PTSD Checklist—civilian and military versions	Blanchard et al., 1996 (civilian); Weathers et al., 1991 (military)
Mississippi Scale—civilian and combat versions	Keane et al., 1988, McFall et al., 1990
Impact of Event Scale updated for *DSM-IV*	Horowitz et al., 1979; Weiss and Marmar, 1997
MMPI-Keane PTSD Scale	Keane et al., 1984
Hovens Self Rating Inventory for PTSD	Hovens et al., 2002
PTSD Diagnostic Scale	Foa et al., 1997
Davidson Trauma Scale	Davidson et al., 1997b
War Zone Related PTSD subscale from the Symptom Checklist 90—Revised	Derogatis and Cleary, 1977
Los Angeles Symptom Checklist	King et al., 1995
26-item Penn Inventory	Hammarberg, 1992
22-item Self-Rating Scale for PTSD	Carlier et al., 1998, from the SIP (Davidson et al., 1997a)
Reactions to Stressful Experiences Scale	Johnson et al., 2011
PTSD Symptom Scale—Self Report Version	Foa et al., 1993

scales is intended to replace a clinical assessment, but they can constitute a useful supplement to information obtained in the face-to-face encounter.

QUALITY OF LIFE, DISABILITY, AND RESILIENCE MEASURES

Several instruments have been developed that measure quality of life, functioning and disability, and resilience and are shown in Table 6-5. Among the main quality of life scales that may be used in assessing people who have PTSD are the Quality of Life Experiences Scale (Endicott et al., 1993), the EURO-QOL (EuroQol, 1990), the 100-question World Health Organization Quality of Life Assessment and an abbreviated form (WHOQOL-BREF) (Harper et al., 1998), the Quality of Life Inventory (Frisch et al., 1992), and the Manchester Short Assessment of Quality of Life (Priebe et al., 1999).

Functioning can be assessed with the Medical Outcomes Study Short Form 36-item and shorter versions (such as SF-12) (McHorney et al., 1994),

TABLE 6-5 Quality of Life, Disability, and Resilience Measures

Instrument	Reference
Medical Outcomes Study Short Form 36	Ware and Sherbourne, 1992
Medical Outcomes Study Short Form 12	Ware et al., 1996
Quality of Life Experiences Scale	Endicott et al., 1993
Sheehan Disability Scale	Sheehan et al., 1996
World Health Organization Quality of Life Assessment	WHO, 1998
Manchester Short Assessment of Quality of Life	Priebe et al., 1999
Resilience Scale	Wagnild and Young, 1993
Resilience Scale for Adults	Friborg et al., 2003
Connor Davidson Resilience Scale, 25-, 10-, and 2-item versions	Connor and Davidson, 2003 (25 item); Campbell-Sills and Stein, 2007 (10 item); Vaishnavi et al., 2007 (2 item)
Quality of Life Inventory	Frisch et al., 1992
Dispositional Resilience Scale, 45-, 30-, and 15-item forms	Bartone et al., 2008
EURO-QOL	EuroQoL, 1990

the Global Assessment of Function (APA, 1994), and the Sheehan Disability Scale (Sheehan, 1983).

Resilience has become the focus of greater attention in recent years, and there are a number of psychometrically valid scales that measure this construct. They include the brief five-item scale of Smith et al. (2008), the 2-, 10-, and 25-item versions of the Connor-Davidson Resilience Scale (Campbell-Sills and Stein, 2007; Connor and Davidson, 2003; Vaishnavi et al., 2007), the 25- and 14-item versions of the Resilience Scale (Wagnild and Young, 1993), the Resilience Scale for Adults (Friborg et al., 2003), and the 45-, 30-, and 15-item forms of the Dispositional Resilience Scale (Bartone et al., 2008). As is the case with the PTSD symptom scales and measures of quality of life and disability, studies have shown that resilience can improve as the result of treatment (Lavretsky et al., 2010).

SUMMARY

Screening for PTSD is essential for identifying those who need treatment. Issues including stigma and timing of screening should be considered, in addition to the venue of screening (DoD, VA, and nonmilitary settings). Many types of screening instruments exist, but only a few are used by the DoD and the VA. Some are based on exposure to trauma and others are symptom-based. Screening instruments may be self-administered or clinician-administered. Although screening is useful for identifying potential PTSD cases, a diagnosis can be made only on the basis of a comprehensive clinical evaluation performed by a qualified professional. Several structured interviews and symptom-based rating scales may be used for diagnosis and to determine severity of symptoms. The next chapter describes the different treatments that have been found to be effective in treating persons who have a diagnosis of PTSD.

REFERENCES

Air Force Medical Operations Agency. 2011. *Primary behavioral health care services: Practice manual.* Lackland AFB, TX: Airforce Medical Operations Agency (AFMOA), Mental Health Division/SGHW.

APA (American Psychiatric Association). 1994. *Diagnostic and statistical manual of mental disorders: DSM-IV.* 4th ed. Washington, DC: American Psychiatric Association.

Armed Forces Health Surveillance Center (U.S.). 2011. *Deployment health assessments: U.S. Armed Forces.* Silver Spring, MD: Armed Forces Health Surveillance Center.

Atlanta Braves, and Emory University. 2011. *Braveheart: Welcome back veterans southeast initiative.* http://braveheartveterans.org/ (accessed January 24, 2012).

Bartone, P. T., R. R. Roland, J. J. Picano, and T. Williams. 2008. Psychological hardiness predicts success in US Army special forces candidates. *International Journal of Selection and Assessment* 16(1):78-81.

Batres, A. R. 2011. *Readjustment counseling service.* Paper presented to the Committee on the Assessment of Ongoing Efforts in the Treatment of PTSD, Washington, DC, April 21.

Bernstein, D. P., J. A. Stein, M. D. Newcomb, E. Walker, D. Pogge, T. Ahluvalia, J. Stokes, L. Handelsman, M. Medrano, D. Desmond, and W. Zule. 2003. Development and validation of a brief screening version of the childhood trauma questionnaire. *Child Abuse & Neglect* 27(2):169-190.

Blake, D. D., F. W. Weathers, L. M. Nagy, D. G. Kaloupek, F. D. Gusman, D. S. Charney, and T. M. Keane. 1995. The development of a clinician-administered PTSD scale. *Journal of Traumatic Stress* 8(1):75-90.

Blanchard, E. B., J. Jones-Alexander, T. C. Buckley, and C. A. Forneris. 1996. Psychometric properties of the PTSD checklist (PCL). *Behaviour Research & Therapy* 34(8):669-673.

Bliese, P. D., K. M. Wright, A. B. Adler, J. L. Thomas, and C. Hoge. 2007. Timing of post-combat mental health assessments. *Psychological Services* 4(3):141-148.

Boscarino, J. A., S. Larson, I. Ladd, E. Hill, and S. J. Paolucci. 2010. Mental health experiences and needs among primary care providers treating OEF/OIF veterans: Preliminary findings from the Geisinger Veterans Initiative. *International Journal of Emergency Mental Health* 12(3):161-170.

Breslau, N., E. L. Peterson, R. C. Kessler, and L. R. Schultz. 1999. Short screening scale for DSM-IV posttraumatic stress disorder. *American Journal of Psychiatry* 156(6):908-911.

Brewin, C. R. 2005. Systematic review of screening instruments for adults at risk of PTSD. *Journal of Traumatic Stress* 18(1):53-62.

Brewin, C. R., S. Rose, B. Andrews, J. Green, P. Tata, C. McEvedy, S. Turner, and E. B. Foa. 2002. Brief screening instrument for post-traumatic stress disorder. *British Journal of Psychiatry* 181:158-162.

Calhoun, P. S., S. D. McDonald, V. S. Guerra, A. M. Eggleston, J. C. Beckham, and K. Straits-Troster. 2010. Clinical utility of the primary care—PTSD screen among U.S. veterans who served since September 11, 2001. *Psychiatry Research* 178(2):330-335.

Campbell-Sills, L., and M. B. Stein. 2007. Psychometric analysis and refinement of the Connor-Davidson resilience scale (CD-RISC): Validation of a 10-item measure of resilience. *Journal of Traumatic Stress* 20(6):1019-1028.

Carlier, I. V. E., R. D. Lamberts, A. J. Van Uchelen, and B. P. R. Gersons. 1998. Clinical utility of a brief diagnostic test for posttraumatic stress disorder. *Psychosomatic Medicine* 60(1):42-47.

Cigrang, J. A., A. C. Dobmeyer, M. E. Becknell, R. A. Roa-Navarrete, and S. R. Yerian. 2006. Evaluation of a collaborative mental health program in primary care: Effects on patient distress and health care utilization. *Primary Care & Community Psychiatry* 11(3):121-127.

Cohen, S., T. Kamarck, and R. Mermelstein. 1983. A global measure of perceived stress. *Journal of Health and Social Behavior* 24(4):385-396.

Connor, K. M., and J. R. Davidson. 2001. SPRINT: A brief global assessment of post-traumatic stress disorder. *International Clinical Psychopharmacology* 16(5):279-284.

Connor, K. M., and J. R. Davidson. 2003. Development of a new resilience scale: The Connor-Davidson resilience scale (CD-RISC). *Depression & Anxiety* 18(2):76-82.

Cottler, L. 2009. *C DIS-IV: Computerized diagnostic interview schedule version IV.* http://epi.wustl.edu/CDISIV/C-DIS-IV_Brochure.pdf (accessed November 22, 2011).

Davidson, J. R. 2002. *SPAN addendum to DTS manual.* North Tonawanda, NY: Multi-Health Systems Inc.

Davidson, J. R., M. A. Malik, and J. Travers. 1997a. Structured interview for PTSD (SIP): Psychometric validation for DSM-IV criteria. *Depression & Anxiety* 5(3):127-129.

Davidson, J. R. T., S. W. Book, J. T. Colket, L. A. Tupler, S. Roth, D. David, M. Hertzberg, T. Mellman, J. C. Beckham, R. D. Smith, R. M. Davison, R. Katz, and M. E. Feldman. 1997b. Assessment of a new self-rating scale for posttraumatic stress disorder. *Psychological Medicine* 27(1):153-160.

DCoE (Defense Centers of Excellence). 2012. *Afterdeployment.org.* http://www.afterdeployment.org/ (accessed January 24, 2012).

Derogatis, L. R., and P. A. Cleary. 1977. Factorial invariance across gender for the primary symptom dimensions of the SCL-90. *British Journal of Clinical Psychology* 16(4):347-356.

DoD (Department of Defense). 1998. *Subject: Policy for pre- and post-deployment health assessments and blood samples.* HA Policy 99000002. Washington, DC: DoD.

DoD. 2005. *Subject: Post-deployment health reassessment.* HA Policy 05-011. Washington, DC: DoD.

DoD. 2007. *An achievable vision: Report of the Department of Defense Task Force on Mental Health.* Falls Church, VA: Defense Health Board.

DoD. 2011. Welcome to the RESPECT-MIL program. *RESPECT-Mil Newsletter* Fall. http://www.pdhealth.mil/respect-mil/index1.asp (accessed January 30, 2012).

Endicott, J., J. Nee, W. Harrison, and R. Blumenthal. 1993. Quality of life enjoyment and satisfaction questionnaire: A new measure. *Psychopharmacology Bulletin* 29(2):321-326.

Engel, C. C., T. Oxman, C. Yamamoto, D. Gould, S. Barry, P. Stewart, K. Kroenke, J. W. Williams, Jr., and A. J. Dietrich. 2008. RESPECT-MIL: Feasibility of a systems-level collaborative care approach to depression and post-traumatic stress disorder in military primary care. *Military Medicine* 173(10):935-940.

EuroQol Group. 1990. EuroQol—A new facility for the measurement of health-related quality of life. *Health Policy* 16(3):199-208.

First, M. B., R. L. Spitzer, M. Gibbon, and J. B. W. Williams. 1995. The structured clinical interview for DSM-III-R personality-disorders (SCID-II). 1. Description. *Journal of Personality Disorders* 9(2):83-91.

Fitzgerald, L. F., V. J. Magley, F. Drasgow, and C. R. Waldo. 1999. Measuring sexual harassment in the military: The sexual experiences questionnaire (SEQ-DOD). *Military Psychology* 11(3):243-263.

Foa, E. B., D. S. Riggs, C. V. Dancu, and B. O. Rothbaum. 1993. Reliability and validity of a brief instrument for assessing posttraumatic-stress-disorder. *Journal of Traumatic Stress* 6(4):459-473.

Foa, E. B., L. Cashman, L. Jaycox, and K. Perry. 1997. The validation of a self-report measure of posttraumatic stress disorder: The posttraumatic diagnostic scale. *Psychological Assessment* 9(4):445-451.

Forbes, D., M. Creamer, J. I. Bisson, J. A. Cohen, B. E. Crow, E. B. Foa, M. J. Friedman, T. M. Keane, H. S. Kudler, and R. J. Ursano. 2010. A guide to guidelines for the treatment of PTSD and related conditions. *Journal of Traumatic Stress* 23(5):537-552.

Friborg, O., O. Hjemdal, J. H. Rosenvinge, and M. Martinussen. 2003. A new rating scale for adult resilience: What are the central protective resources behind healthy adjustment? *International Journal of Methods in Psychiatric Research* 12(2):65-76.

Frisch, M. B. C., J., M. Villanueva, and P. Retzlaff. 1992. Clinical validation of the quality of life inventory: A measure of life satisfaction for use in treatment planning and outcome assessment. *Psychological Assessment* 4(1):92-101.

GAO (U.S. Government Accountability Office). 2008. *DoD health care: Mental health and traumatic brain injury screening efforts implemented, but consistent pre-deployment medical records review needed.* Washington, DC: GAO.

Gaynes, B. N., J. DeVeaugh-Geiss, S. Weir, H. B. Gu, C. MacPherson, H. C. Schulberg, L. Culpepper, and D. R. Rubinow. 2010. Feasibility and diagnostic validity of the M-3 checklist: A brief, self-rated screen for depressive, bipolar, anxiety, and post-traumatic stress disorders in primary care. *Annals of Family Medicine* 8(2):160-169.

Gebhart, R. J., and F. L. Neeley. 1996. Primary care and PTSD. *National Center for PTSD Clinical Quarterly* 6(4):72, 74.

Gilbody, S., T. Sheldon, and S. Wessely. 2006. Health policy—should we screen for depression? *British Medical Journal* 332(7548):1027-1030.

Goldberg, D. P. 1972. *The detection of psychiatric illness by questionnaire: A technique for the identification and assessment of non-psychotic psychiatric illness.* Institute of Psychiatry. Maudsley Monographs. London, UK: Oxford University Press.

Gore, K. L., C. C. Engel, M. C. Freed, X. Liu, and D. W. Armstrong. 2008. Test of a single-item posttraumatic stress disorder screener in a military primary care setting. *General Hospital Psychiatry* 30(5):391-397.

Hammarberg, M. 1992. Penn inventory for posttraumatic stress disorder: Psychometric properties. *Psychological Assessment* 4(1):67-76.

Harper, A., M. Power, and Working Group. 1998. Development of the World Health Organization WHOQOL-BREF quality of life assessment. *Psychological Medicine* 28(3):551-558.

Hendrix, C., and W. Schumm. 1990. Reliability and validity of the abusive violence scale. *Psychological Reports* 66(3):1251-1258.

Hollifield, M., V. Eckert, T. D. Warner, J. Jenkins, B. Krakow, J. Ruiz, and J. Westermeyer. 2005. Development of an inventory for measuring war-related events in refugees. *Comprehensive Psychiatry* 46(1):67-80.

Horowitz, M. J., N. Wilner, and W. Alvarez. 1979. *Impact of event scale: A measure of subjective stress.* Emmitsburg, MD: National Emergency Training Center.

Hovens, J. E., I. Bramsen, and H. M. van der Ploeg. 2002. Self-Rating Inventory for Posttraumatic Stress Disorder: Review of the psychometric properties of a new brief Dutch screening instrument. *Perceptual & Motor Skills* 94(3 Pt 1):996-1008.

Hyams, K. C. 2006. Mental health screening before troop deployment: Is not supported by current evidence. *British Medical Journal* 333(7576):979-980.

IOM (Institute of Medicine). 2006. *Posttraumatic stress disorder diagnosis and assessment.* Washington, DC: The National Academies Press.

Janes, G. R., J. Goldberg, S. A. Eisen, and W. R. True. 1991. Reliability and validity of a combat exposure index for Vietnam era veterans. *Journal of Clinical Psychology* 47(1):80-86.

Johnson, D. C., M. A. Polusny, C. R. Erbes, D. King, L. King, B. T. Litz, P. P. Schnurr, M. Friedman, R. H. Pietrzak, and S. M. Southwick. 2011. Development and initial validation of the response to stressful experiences scale. *Military Medicine* 176(2):161-169.

Keane, T. M., P. F. Malloy, and J. A. Fairbank. 1984. Empirical development of an MMPI subscale for the assessment of combat-related posttraumatic stress disorder. *Journal of Consulting and Clinical Psychology* 52(5):888-891.

Keane, T. M., J. M. Caddell, and K. L. Taylor. 1988. Mississippi scale for combat-related posttraumatic stress disorder—3 studies in reliability and validity. *Journal of Consulting and Clinical Psychology* 56(1):85-90.

Keane, T. M., J. A. Fairbank, J. M. Caddell, R. T. Zimering, K. L. Taylor, and C. A. Mora. 1989. Clinical evaluation of a measure to assess combat exposure. *Psychological Assessment* 1(1):53-55.

Kessler, R. C., A. Sonnega, E. Bromet, M. Hughes, and C. B. Nelson. 1995. Posttraumatic stress disorder in the national comorbidity survey. *Archives of General Psychiatry* 52(12):1048-1060.

Kessler, R. C., G. Andrews, L. J. Colpe, E. Hiripi, D. K. Mroczek, S. L. T. Normand, E. E. Walters, and A. M. Zaslavsky. 2002. Short screening scales to monitor population prevalences and trends in non-specific psychological distress. *Psychological Medicine* 32(6):959-976.

Kimerling, R., A. E. Street, J. Pavao, M. W. Smith, R. C. Cronkite, T. H. Holmes, and S. M. Frayne. 2010. Military-related sexual trauma among Veterans Health Administration patients returning from Afghanistan and Iraq. *American Journal of Public Health* 100(8):1409-1412.

King, D., L. King, G. Leskin, and D. W. Foy. 1995. The Los Angeles symptom checklist: A self-report measure of posttraumatic stress disorder. *Assessment* 2:1-17.

King, D., L. King, and D. Vogt. 2003. *Manual for the Deployment Risk and Resilience Inventory (DRRI): A collection of scales for studying deployment-related experiences in military veterans.* Boston, MA: National Center for Post-Traumatic Stress Disorder.

Kirchner, J. E. 2011. *Mental Health QUERI Center Strategic Plan.* North Little Rock, AR: VA, Quality Enhancement Research Initiative (QUERI). December.

Kroenke, K., R. L. Spitzer, and J. B. Williams. 2001. The PHQ-9: Validity of a brief depression severity measure. *Journal of General Internal Medicine* 16(9):606-613.

Kroenke, K., R. L. Spitzer, and J. B. Williams. 2003. The patient health questionnaire-2: Validity of a two-item depression screener. *Medical Care* 41(11):1284-1292.

Lang, A. J., and M. B. Stein. 2005. An abbreviated PTSD checklist for use as a screening instrument in primary care. *Behaviour Research and Therapy* 43(5):585-594.

Lavretsky, H., P. Siddarth, and M. R. Irwin. 2010. Improving depression and enhancing resilience in family dementia caregivers: A pilot randomized placebo-controlled trial of escitalopram. *American Journal of Geriatric Psychiatry* 18(2):154-162.

Leskin, G., and D. Westrup. 1999. *PTSD brief screen: Posttraumatic stress disorder implications for primary care.* Department of Defense/EES.

McClure, G. 2007. *Solider wellness assessment pilot program (SWAPP)*. PowerPoint slides. Fort Lewis, WA: Soldier Wellness Service.

McFall, M. E., D. E. Smith, D. K. Roszell, D. J. Tarver, and K. L. Malas. 1990. Convergent validity of measures of PTSD in Vietnam combat veterans. *American Journal of Psychiatry* 147(5):645-648.

McHorney, C. A., J. E. Ware, J. F. R. Lu, and C. D. Sherbourne. 1994. The MOS 36-item short-form health survey (SF-36). Tests of data quality, scaling assumptions, and reliability across diverse patient groups. *Medical Care* 32(1):40-66.

Means-Christensen, A. J., C. D. Sherbourne, P. P. Roy-Byrne, M. G. Craske, and M. B. Stein. 2006. Using five questions to screen for five common mental disorders in primary care: Diagnostic accuracy of the anxiety and depression detector. *General Hospital Psychiatry* 28(2):108-118.

Milliken, C. S., J. L. Auchterlonie, and C. W. Hoge. 2007. Longitudinal assessment of mental health problems among active and reserve component soldiers returning from the Iraq war. *Journal of the American Medical Association* 298(18):2141-2148.

Mollica, R. F., Y. Caspi-Yavin, P. Bollini, T. Truong, S. Tor, and J. Lavelle. 1992. The Harvard Trauma Questionnaire. Validating a cross-cultural instrument for measuring torture, trauma, and posttraumatic stress disorder in Indochinese refugees. *Journal of Nervous and Mental Disease* 180(2):111-116.

Mori, D. L., J. F. Lambert, B. L. Niles, J. D. Orlander, M. Grace, and J. S. LoCastro. 2003. The BAI-PC as a screen for anxiety, depression, and PTSD in primary care. *Journal of Clinical Psychology in Medical Settings* 10(3):187-192.

Morrison, A. S. 1992. *Screening in chronic disease, Monographs in epidemiology and biostatistics*. New York: Oxford University Press.

Nevin, R. L. 2009. Low validity of self-report in identifying recent mental health diagnosis among U.S. Service members completing pre-deployment health assessment (PREDHA) and deployed to Afghanistan, 2007: A retrospective cohort study. *BMC Public Health* 9:376.

Norris, F. H., J. L. Hamblen, L. M. Brown, and J. A. Schinka. 2008. Validation of the short posttraumatic stress disorder rating interview (expanded version, SPRINT-E) as a measure of postdisaster distress and treatment need. *American Journal of Disaster Medicine* 3(4):201-212.

O'Donnell, M. L., M. C. Creamer, R. Parslow, P. Elliott, A. C. N. Holmes, S. Ellen, R. Judson, A. C. McFarlane, D. Silove, and R. A. Bryant. 2008. A predictive screening index for posttraumatic stress disorder and depression following traumatic injury. *Journal of Consulting and Clinical Psychology* 76(6):923-932.

Patient-Centered Primary Care Collaborative. 2007. *Joint principles of the patient centered medical home*. http://www.pcpcc.net/content/joint-principles-patient-centered-medical-home (accessed January 30, 2012).

Priebe, S., P. Huxley, S. Knight, and S. Evans. 1999. Application and results of the Manchester Short Assessment of Quality of Life (MANSA). *International Journal of Social Psychiatry* 45(1):7-12.

Prins, A., P. Ouimette, R. Kimerling, R. P. Cameron, D. S. Hugelshofer, J. Shaw-Hegwer, A. Thrailkill, F. D. Gusman, and J. I. Sheikh. 2003. The primary care PTSD screen (PC-PTSD): Development and operating characteristics. *Primary Care Psychiatry* 9(1):9-14.

Prins, A., P. Ouimette, R. Kimerling, R. P. Cameron, D. S. Hugelshofer, J. Shaw-Hegwer, A. Thrailkill, F. D. Gusman, and J. I. Sheikh. 2004. The primary care PTSD screen (PC-PTSD): Corrigendum. *Primary Care Psychiatry* 9(151).

Robins, L. N., J. Wing, H. U. Wittchen, J. E. Helzer, T. F. Babor, J. Burke, A. Farmer, A. Jablenski, R. Pickens, D. A. Regier, N. Sartorius, and L. H. Towle. 1988. The composite international diagnostic interview. An epidemiologic instrument suitable for use in conjunction with different diagnostic systems and in different cultures. *Archives of General Psychiatry* 45(12):1069-1077.

Robins, L. N., L. Cottler, K. Bucholz, and W. Compton. 1997. *Diagnostic interview schedule for the DSM-IV (DIS-IV)*. St. Louis, MO: Washington University School of Medicine.

Rona, R. J., K. C. Hyams, and S. Wessely. 2005. Screening for psychological illness in military personnel. *Journal of the American Medical Association* 293(10):1257-1260.

Rona, R. J., R. Hooper, M. Jones, L. Hull, T. Browne, O. Horn, D. Murphy, M. Hotopf, and S. Wessely. 2006. Mental health screening in armed forces before the Iraq war and prevention of subsequent psychological morbidity: Follow-up study. *British Medical Journal* 333(7576):991.

Sandweiss, D. A., D. J. Slymen, C. A. Leardmann, B. Smith, M. R. White, E. J. Boyko, T. I. Hooper, G. D. Gackstetter, P. J. Amoroso, and T. C. Smith. 2011. Preinjury psychiatric status, injury severity, and postdeployment posttraumatic stress disorder. *Archives of General Psychiatry* 68(5):496-504.

Schnurr, P. P., and M. K. Jankowski. 1999. Physical health and post-traumatic stress disorder: Review and synthesis. *Seminars in Clinical Neuropsychiatry* 4(4):295-304.

Schoenhard, W. Statement to the Senate Committee on Veterans' Affairs. July 14, 2011.

Sheehan, D. V. 1983. *The anxiety disease*. New York: Scribner.

Sheehan, D. V., A. B. Raj, K. H. Sheehan, and S. Soto. 1990. Is buspirone effective for panic disorder? *Journal of Clinical Psychopharmacology* 10(1):3-11.

Sheehan, D. V., K. Harnett-Sheehan, and B. A. Raj. 1996. The measurement of disability. *International Clinical Psychopharmacology* 11:89-95.

Sheehan, D. V., Y. Lecrubier, K. Harnett-Sheehan, P. Amorim, J. Janavs, E. Weiller, T. Hergueta, R. Baker, and G. C. Dunbar. 1998. The Mini-International Neuropsychiatric Interview (MINI): The development and validation of a structured diagnostic psychiatric interview for DSM-IV and ICD-10. *Journal of Clinical Psychiatry* 59:22-33.

Skinner, K. M., N. Kressin, S. Frayne, T. J. Tripp, C. S. Hankin, D. R. Miller, and L. M. Sullivan. 2000. The prevalence of military sexual assault among female Veterans' Administration outpatients. *Journal of Interpersonal Violence* 15(3):291-310.

Smith, B. W., J. Dalen, K. Wiggins, E. Tooley, P. Christopher, and J. Bernard. 2008. The brief resilience scale: Assessing the ability to bounce back. *International Journal of Behavioral Medicine* 15(3):194-200.

Spitzer, R. L., J. B. Williams, M. Gibbon, and M. B. First. 1992. The structured clinical interview for DSM-III-R (SCID). I: History, rationale, and description. *Archives of General Psychiatry* 49(8):624-629.

Stein, M. B., J. R. Walker, A. L. Hazen, and D. R. Forde. 1997. Full and partial posttraumatic stress disorder: Findings from a community survey. *American Journal of Psychiatry* 154(8):1114-1119.

Sutker, P. B., M. Uddo, K. Brailey, J. J. Vasterling, and P. Errera. 1994. Psychopathology in war-zone deployed and nondeployed Operation-Desert-Storm troops assigned graves registration duties. *Journal of Abnormal Psychology* 103(2):383-390.

Unger, W. S., R. A. Gould, and M. Babich. 1998. The development of a scale to assess war-time atrocities: The war events scale. *Journal of Traumatic Stress* 11(2):375-383.

U.S. Air Force. 2011. *Primary behavioral health care services: Practice manual*. Lackland AFB, TX: Airforce Medical Operations Agency (AFMOA), Mental Health Division/SGHW.

U.S. Preventive Services Task Force, A. O. Berg, J. D. Allan, P. S. Frame, C. J. Homer, M. S. Johnson, J. D. Klein, T. A. Lieu, C. D. Mulrow, C. T. Orleans, J. F. Peipert, N. J. Pender, A. L. Siu, S. M. Teutsch, C. Westhoff, S. H. Woolf, and Agency for Healthcare Research and Quality Publications Cleaninghouse. 2002. Screening for depression: Recommendations and rationale. *Annals of Internal Medicine* 136(10):760-764.

VA (Department of Veterans Affairs). 2002. *Post-traumatic stress disorder: Implications for primary care.* Washington, DC: VA Employee Education System: The National Center for PTSD.

VA. 2005. *Implementation of the national clinical reminder for Afghan and Iraq post-deployment screening.* Washington, DC: VA.

VA. 2010. *Programs for veterans with post-traumatic stress disorder (PTSD).* Washingon, DC: Veterans Health Administration.

VA. 2012a. *Primary Care PTSD Screen.* http://www.ptsd.va.gov/professional/pages/assessments/pc-ptsd.asp (accessed March 26, 2012).

VA. 2012b. *Mobile app: PTSD coach.* http://www.PTSD.va.gov/public/pages/PTSDCoach.asp (accessed 24 January, 2012).

VA. 2012c. *My HealtheVet—the gateway to veteran health and wellness.* https://www.myhealth.va.gov/index.html (accessed January 30, 2012).

VA and DoD. 2010. *VA/DOD clinical practice guideline for management of post-traumatic stress.* Washington, DC: VA/DoD.

Vaishnavi, S., K. Connor, and J. R. T. Davidson. 2007. An abbreviated version of the Connor-Davidson Resilience Scale (CD-RISC), the CD-RISC2: Psychometric properties and applications in psychopharmacological trials. *Psychiatry Research* 152(2-3):293-297.

Wagnild, G. M., and H. M. Young. 1993. Development and psychometric evaluation of the resilience scale. *Journal of Nursing Measurement* 1(2):165-178.

Walker, E. A., E. Newman, D. J. Dobie, P. Ciechanowski, and W. Katon. 2002. Validation of the PTSD checklist in an HMO sample of women. *General Hospital Psychiatry* 24(6):375-380.

Ware, J. E., and C. D. Sherbourne. 1992. The MOS 36-item short-form health survey (SF-36). 1. Conceptual-framework and item selection. *Medical Care* 30(6):473-483.

Ware, J. E., M. Kosinski, and S. D. Keller. 1996. A 12-item short-form health survey—construction of scales and preliminary tests of reliability and validity. *Medical Care* 34(3):220-233.

Warner, C. H., G. N. Appenzeller, T. A. Grieger, S. Belenkly, J. Breitback, J. Parker, C. M. Warner, and C. W. Hoge. 2011. Importance of anonymity to encourage honest reporting in mental health screening after combat deployment. *Archives of General Psychiatry* 68:1065-1071.

Watson, C. G., T. Kucala, V. Manifold, P. Vassar, and M. Juba. 1988. Differences between posttraumatic stress disorder patients with delayed and undelayed onsets. *Journal of Nervous and Mental Disease* 176(9):568-572.

Weathers, F., J. Huska, and T. M. Keane. 1991. *The PTSD checklist military version (PCL-M).* http://www.metrowestneurofeedback.com/files/62410952_ptsd_checklist.pdf?PHPSESSID=d54732beed6cdaf5955a28feee0bdc17 (accessed 2011).

Weinick, R. M., E. B. Beckjord, C. M. Farmer, L. T. Martin, E. M. Gillen, J. D. Acosta, M. P. Fisher, J. Garnett, G. C. Gonzalez, T. C. Helmus, L. Jaycox, K. A. Reynolds, N. Salcedo, and D. M. Scharf. 2011. *Programs addressing psychological health and traumatic brain injury among U.S. military servicemembers and their families.* Santa Monica, CA: RAND Corporation.

Weiss, D. S., and C. Marmar. 1997. The impact of event scale—revisited. In *Assessing psychological trauma and PTSD*, edited by J. P. Wilson and T. M. Keane. New York: Guilford Press. Pp. 399-411.

WHO (World Health Organization). The World Health Organization Quality of Life Assessment (WHOQOL): Development and general psychometric properties. 1998. *Social Science & Medicine* 46(12):1569-1585.

Wilson, J., and G. Krause. 1980. *The Vietnam era stress inventory*. Cleveland, OH: Cleveland State University.

Wilson, J. M. G., and G. Jungner. 1968. *Principles and practice of screening for disease, Public health papers*. Geneva, Switzerland: World Health Organization.

Wolfe, J., P. Brown, J. Furey, and K. Levin. 1993. Development of a wartime stressor scale for women. *Psychological Assessment* 5(3):330-335.

Zeiss, A. M., and B. E. Karlin. 2008. Integrating mental health and primary care services in the Department of Veterans Affairs health care system. *Journal of Clinical Psychology in Medical Settings* 15:73-78.

7

Treatment

This chapter provides critical reviews of the various approaches to treatment for chronic posttraumatic stress disorder (PTSD), that is, PTSD lasting more than 3 months, although many of the treatments may be used with patients who suffer from acute PTSD (lasting more than 1 month and less than 3 months) and even those who have symptoms within 2 weeks after a traumatic event. The chapter begins with a description of the many psychosocial therapies whose efficacy is supported by an established evidence base—randomized controlled trials (RCTs). Among the psychosocial treatments discussed are exposure therapy, cognitive therapy, and group therapy. That is followed by a discussion of treatments that have been studied in open trials and for which RCTs have not been conducted. The efficacy of pharmacotherapy for PTSD is then considered, including the use of antidepressants—serotonin reuptake inhibitors (SRIs) and others—and the use of multiple drugs for PTSD and comorbid conditions. The efficacy of combinations of cognitive behavioral therapy and pharmacotherapy for PTSD is also discussed. The committee then looks at emerging treatments that are being used or being considered for use in the management of PTSD. These include manualized treatments (that is, those that have a manual of instructions) such as couple psychotherapy in which one or both persons have PTSD, and complementary and alternative medicine (CAM) treatments, most of which do not have a structured manual, such as yoga, acupuncture, and animal-assisted therapy. A synopsis of the many PTSD treatment guidelines is then given, including the Department of Veterans Affairs (VA)/Department of Defense (DoD) guideline for the management of posttraumatic stress that might assist the health care provider in selecting a treatment plan for a patient with PTSD.

There are numerous interventions for chronic PTSD, and not all of them have a robust database to support their efficacy for ameliorating PTSD symptoms. Not having RCTs supporting a particular treatment does not necessarily mean that it is not effective. The committee believes it is prudent to offer treatment supported by robust evidence before offering treatments that are not so supported. It should be noted that many of the treatments discussed in this chapter, even those with a robust body of evidence, may not have been tested specifically on military personnel who had PTSD, but in the absence of a well-reasoned argument against it, it is safe to hypothesize that treatments that were effective in well-controlled studies of a variety of civilian populations that had PTSD will also be effective in military personnel.

Not all people who have PTSD respond satisfactorily to initial treatment, and many remain treatment-resistant to varied degrees. Some guidelines offer recommendations on levels of care or stages of treatment in the event that the first evidence-based approaches fail to produce a satisfactory response. There is no widely accepted definition of what constitutes satisfactory response. Some studies use at least a 50% reduction in PTSD symptoms to indicate a satisfactory response; another indicator of a satisfactory response is a score of 15 on the Posttraumatic Stress Diagnostic Inventory to indicate subclinical PTSD severity and a score of 10 to indicate remission (Foa et al., 1993). On the Clinician-Assisted PTSD Scale (CAPS), subclinical PTSD is indicated by a score of 50, and remission by a score of 20 or less (Tucker et al., 2001). The percentage of responders varies among studies, types of traumas, definitions of response, magnitudes of intent to treat, and completer analyses. Depending on the specific cognitive behavioral treatment and the study sample, the percentage of responders can be as high as 90% and as low as 50% (Kar, 2011), and treatment outcomes are stable over time (e.g., Foa et al., 2005).

The evidence base for the best second- and third-line line treatment approaches for PTSD falls substantially, and more reliance is placed on expert opinion rather than empirical information. Examples of those treatments are antidepressants or use of an antipsychotic drug with a selective serotonin reuptake inhibitor (SSRI) in cases of partial SSRI response, watchful waiting for the first 4 weeks after trauma for those who have mild symptoms, but brief cognitive behavioral therapy (CBT) even within the first month in more severe cases.

PSYCHOSOCIAL TREATMENTS FOR CHRONIC PTSD

This section describes the psychosocial treatments whose efficacy has been examined in RCTs. A review of treatments whose efficacy has been examined in open trials follows, and finally, treatments that have been suggested but whose efficacy has not been examined are briefly described.

Treatments Supported in Randomized Controlled Trials

The vast majority of treatments that have been examined via RCT are in the general group of psychosocial therapies called cognitive behavioral therapy. They include exposure therapies, stress inoculation training or anxiety-management programs, and cognitive therapies. Many treatment programs combine components of each of those general treatment groups, and CBT has become an overarching concept that includes variants of exposure therapy, stress inculcation training, cognitive therapies, and their combinations.

Exposure Therapies

Exposure therapies are designed to reduce PTSD symptoms and related problems (such as depression, anger, and guilt) by helping patients to confront their trauma-related situations, memories, and feelings. Exposure interventions include imaginal exposure, which consists of repeated revisiting of the traumatic memory, and in vivo exposure, which involves confronting feared situations that are objectively safe. Treatment programs that include both kinds of exposure, such as prolonged exposure (PE), tend to produce better outcomes than programs that consist of only one of the components (e.g., Bryant et al., 2008).

Many RCTs have consistently shown that several exposure therapy protocols for PTSD are effective, and they have been recommended as a first-line treatment for PTSD by several treatment guidelines, such as the National Institute for Health and Clinical Excellence (NICE) and Australian National Health and Medical Research Council guidelines.

The most commonly used exposure protocol is PE (Foa et al., 2007). PE is based on emotional-processing theory (Foa and Kozak, 1986), which posits that anxiety disorders, including PTSD, reflect specific pathologic fears of places, situations, or objects that are safe but are perceived as dangerous, and therefore, are avoided (Foa and Cahill, 2001). PE is designed to modify PTSD sufferers' typical erroneous perceptions that "The world is an utterly dangerous place" and "I am completely incompetent and unable to cope with stress." The central components of PE are in vivo exposure and imaginal exposure. In vivo exposure consists of having the patient gradually and systematically approach situations, places, and people that he or she has been avoiding. Through repeated exposure to those stimuli, the dysfunctional, unrealistic expectations of harm are disconfirmed, and the patient experiences a reduction in the associated fear response. Imaginal exposure involves revisiting the memory in imagination and recounting the traumatic event in a way that promotes emotional engagement with the trauma memory and then processing the revisiting experience. Processing provides an opportunity for patients to examine their beliefs related to the trauma memory and to gain a new perspective on the trauma. Like in vivo exposure, repeated, prolonged imaginal exposure provides information that disconfirms dysfunctional erroneous cognitions and reduces the distress associated with confronting the memory. Psychoeducation and controlled-breathing exercises play a secondary role in PE. Psychoeducation comprises a discussion about what maintains PTSD and the reactions that commonly follow a trauma; controlled-breathing training is designed to lower a person's baseline level of anxiety, which might have become heightened in part by rapid and shallow breathing. Treatment commonly consists of 8 to 12 sessions of 60–90 minutes each.

Many RCTs—the largest number of such trials of any psychosocial treatment for PTSD—indicate that PE effectively reduces PTSD symptoms in a variety of populations (such as female rape survivors, male and female veterans, and refugees; see Cahill et al., 2009, for a full review). PE is effective for both chronic PTSD (e.g., Foa et al., 1999a, 2005; Resick et al., 2002) and acute stress disorder (Bryant et al., 1999; Foa et al., 1995, 2006). Patients treated with PE generally maintain their gains at follow-ups of a year or more (e.g., Foa et al., 2005; Resick et al., 2002). In addition, PE consistently has been associated with rapid change and maintenance of large effect sizes over time (e.g., Foa et al., 2005). A recently published long-term follow-up study of civilians treated with cognitive processing therapy and PE indicated about 80% of participants were treated to the point of remission at the posttreatment point and remained in remission for 5–10 years after the end of treatment (Resick et al., 2011).

PE produces significantly greater pretreatment to posttreatment reductions in PTSD symptoms than supportive counseling (Bryant et al., 2003; Schnurr et al., 2007), relaxation training (Marks et al., 1998; Taylor et al., 2003; Vaughan et al., 1994), and treatment-as-usual, including pharmacotherapy (Asukai et al., 2010), nonexposure-based individual psychotherapy (Boudewyns and Hyer, 1990), and combinations of psychopharmacology, counseling, and group therapy (e.g., Nacasch et al., 2010).

A similar protocol that includes both imaginal and in vivo exposure was developed by Marks et al. (1998). Imaginal exposure is conducted in the first half of the treatment and in vivo exposure in the second half. Only two RCTs used this protocol: Marks et al. (1998) and Taylor et al. (2003).

Because of the similarity between the Foa et al. and Marks et al. protocols, the committee does not distinguish between them in this section.

Other Forms of Exposure Therapy

Variations of exposure therapy have been shown to be efficacious in RCTs. For example, Resick et al. (2008) compared cognitive processing therapy (CPT), which includes cognitive therapy and written exposure, with written exposure of the traumatic memory only and without the cognitive component of CPT without writing (see "Cognitive Therapies" section). Written exposure consisted of two preparatory sessions followed by five 2-hour sessions in which the patient was asked to write for about 60 minutes alone about his or her experienced trauma and then to read the narrative to the therapist, who provided unstructured supportive feedback. The written-exposure group did nearly as well as the group that had CPT with and without writing; at the 6-month follow-up, there was no significant difference between the groups. Van Emmerik et al. (2008) also found that structured writing therapy was as efficacious as cognitive therapy in treatment for PTSD.

Exposure in the context of a broader narration of the patient's life also has empirical support. For example, narrative exposure therapy, a brief manualized treatment, has been shown to be efficacious for treating PTSD in war-ravaged refugee populations (Neuner et al., 2008). A variation of this treatment is testimony therapy, which is a brief nonmanualized individual intervention designed for survivors of war; however, the only RCT found no difference between this treatment and wait list (WL) both soon after and 11 months after treatment (Igreja et al., 2006).

Blanchard et al. (2003) developed CBT–MVA (motor vehicle accident), a short-term manualized exposure therapy protocol that targets victims of motor vehicle incidents who have PTSD. CBT–MVA includes in vivo exposure, progressive muscle relaxation, cognitive restructuring, one session of couple therapy (if the patient has a spouse) and one session focusing on anger or existential issues stemming from the incident. In an RCT, patients who received CBT–MVA reported greater reductions in PTSD symptoms than patients who received supportive psychotherapy, who in turn reported greater reductions in PTSD than those on WL. Gains made in the two treatment groups were maintained at 3 months.

Imagery rescripting (Smucker et al., 1995) is another exposure therapy protocol that has been examined in RCTs both as an addendum to PE and as a stand-alone therapy for victims of childhood sexual abuse. The patient first engages in an imaginal exposure, immediately followed by a rescripting, in which the patient is encouraged to revisit the trauma while developing mastery imagery by imagining himself or herself as an adult entering the room during the trauma and rescuing and protecting the vulnerable child (Cukor et al., 2009). An RCT compared imaginal exposure coupled with imagery rescripting with imagery rescripting alone and found that both groups experienced improvement in PTSD symptoms with those on WL. There were no differences between the two treatment groups (Arntz et al., 2007).

McLean and Foa (2011) reviewed the evidence base for exposure therapy. Several meta-analyses of exposure therapy (e.g., Bradley et al., 2005) have found that it is far more effective than WL or supportive therapy and as effective as SSRIs in the short-term with lower dropout rates, but data on long-term effects are sparse (Van Etten and Taylor, 1998). Other meta-analyses have shown that exposure therapy is more effective than "non–trauma-focused" treatments or WL in reducing PTSD symptoms, but the differences in outcomes among the different exposure therapies was not significant (Bisson and Andrew, 2007; Seidler and Wagner, 2006). A recent meta-analysis of 13 PE studies found a large effect size for PE compared with WL or psychological placebo immediately after treatment that was maintained at follow-up (Powers et al., 2010). Studies have also shown that PE leads to significantly greater pretreatment to posttreatment reductions in PTSD symptoms than supportive counseling (Bryant et al., 2003; Schnurr et al., 2007), relaxation (Marks et al., 1998; Taylor et al., 2003; Vaughan et al., 1994), and treatment-as-usual (Asukai et al., 2010; Boudewyns and Hyer, 1990; Cooper and Clum, 1989; Nacasch et al., 2010). Furthermore, comparative treatment studies have found PE to be of at least comparable efficacy with other forms of CBTs, such as stress inoculation training (SIT), CPT, cognitive therapy (CT), and eye movement and desensitization reprocessing (EMDR) (Bryant et al., 2003, 2008; Foa et al., 1991, 1999a, 2005; Marks et al., 1998; Paunovic and Ost, 2001; Power et al., 2002; Resick et al., 2002, 2008; Rothbaum et al., 2005; Schnurr et al., 2001; Tarrier et al., 1999; van Emmerik et al., 2008; see Powers et al., 2010, for meta-analytic review of these findings). Finally, adding SIT or CT to PE has little benefit (Foa et al., 1999a, 2005).

In a comprehensive review of RCTs for exposure therapy for PTSD, an Institute of Medicine (IOM) committee looked at 23 studies, 8 of which met the committee's quality criteria for inclusion in its assessment. These studies demonstrated a statistically significant improvement in patients receiving exposure therapy based on a primary PTSD scale or loss of a diagnosis of PTSD. The committee found that "the evidence is sufficient to conclude the efficacy of exposure therapies in the treatment of PTSD" (IOM, 2008).

In conclusion, there is strong evidence of the efficacy and effectiveness of variants of exposure therapy, in particular PE, in different trauma populations on the basis of studies conducted in independent centers around the world. Treatment benefits have been maintained at 5–10 years follow-up

(Resick et al., 2011). Exposure therapy has also been successfully disseminated among community therapists in individual clinics in the United States and other countries and in large mental health systems, such as that of the VA.

Cognitive Therapies

CT (Beck et al., 2005) is a treatment protocol in which the therapist helps the patient to identify and modify the negative thoughts and beliefs that are considered to underlie pathologic emotions and behaviors. In PTSD treatment, the target is thoughts and beliefs related to a traumatic experience (for example, survival guilt, self-blame for causing the trauma, feelings of personal inadequacy, or worries about the future) with the goal of modifying them to reduce PTSD symptoms and improve mood and functioning. In several RCTs, CT alone has been shown to be an effective intervention for patients who have PTSD with significant reductions in PTSD symptoms (Cottraux et al., 2008; Marks et al., 1998; Resick et al., 2008; Tarrier et al., 1999).

CPT (Resick et al., 2002) is a manualized treatment that combines aspects of CT and PE. It consists of four components: education about specific PTSD symptoms and how the treatment can be beneficial, increasing the patient's awareness of his or her thoughts and feelings, learning skills to help patients question or challenge maladaptive thoughts, and understanding that experiencing a trauma can change a person's beliefs about the world and relationships. The aim of CPT is to help patients find a better balance between the beliefs they had before and after their trauma. The treatment program consists of 12 1-hour sessions delivered over 6 weeks. The original protocol included an exposure component in the form of repeated writing of the traumatic memory and reading of it to the therapist.

Resick et al. (2008) disentangled the effects of the cognitive component of CPT and the component of writing and reading of the traumatic memory by comparing three groups: full CPT protocol, CT without writing, and writing alone. Although patients in all three groups showed substantial improvement, CT alone showed greater reduction in PTSD symptoms than writing alone. However, at the end of treatment there was no superiority to CPT with and without writing, and writing and reading alone were almost as efficacious as the other two protocols. The writing and reading protocol requires much less therapist training than CPT and seems to be less expensive. Resick is examining the efficacy of group and individual CPT in military personnel.

Elhers and Clark (2000) have developed a CT protocol for PTSD that is based on their cognitive model of PTSD. The protocol focuses on modifying negative thoughts about the trauma and its consequences, reducing re-experiencing by elaboration of the trauma memories and identification of triggers, and encouraging patients to stop dysfunctional behaviors and cognitive strategies. CT also uses in vivo and imaginal exposure. This treatment has been evaluated in two RCTs (Ehlers et al., 2003, 2005), both of which found it to be efficacious.

Kubany et al. (2003) developed a specific CT protocol for female victims of spousal violence. Cognitive trauma therapy for battered women who have PTSD is a manualized short-term treatment that includes a number of treatment elements adapted from other CBTs for PTSD—including psychoeducation about PTSD, stress management (including relaxation training), and exposure—and other techniques, including reducing irrational guilt-related beliefs and negative self-talk by the women about guilt and shame. Two RCTs that compared cognitive trauma therapy for battered women to WL found that patients who received the treatment experienced large reductions in PTSD symptoms, depression, and guilt, and increases in self-esteem (Kubany et al., 2003, 2004).

In conclusion, variants of CT have received support for their efficacy through well-controlled studies. However, the number of studies of each treatment program is small compared with exposure therapy.

Eye Movement Desensitization and Reprocessing

EMDR (Shapiro, 1989a,b) is a manualized treatment to assist patients in accessing and processing traumatic memories while bringing them to an adaptive resolution (Shapiro, 2001). The patient is asked to access a disturbing image associated with the traumatic event, solicit the experience of body sensations associated with the image, identify a negative self-referring belief, and identify a preferred positive belief to replace the negative belief. The patient is then asked to hold the disturbing image, sensations, and the negative belief or thought in mind while tracking the clinician's moving finger back and forth in front of his or her visual field for about 20 seconds. This process is repeated until the patient has no negative associations with the targeted image.

Results of four RCTs suggest that EMDR is an efficacious treatment for PTSD. Lee et al. (2002) and Power et al. (2002) found that its results were equivalent to those of CBT. Taylor et al. (2003) found PE to be more effective than EMDR and relaxation training; moreover, PE, but not EMDR, was significantly more efficacious than relaxation (the control condition). Rothbaum et al. (2005) found that in a 6-month follow-up a significantly larger fraction of patients who received PE were responders than of those who received EMDR.

Several studies (e.g., Davidson and Parker, 2001; Spates et al., 2009) have examined the relative contribution of the eye-movement component and found no effects of its efficacy. Consequently, some PTSD treatment experts posit that the efficacy of EMDR is due to the exposure component that it shares with other existing, successful treatments, such as PE. An IOM committee that critically assessed four RCTs for EMDR concluded that the evidence was inadequate to determine its efficacy for the treatment of PTSD (IOM, 2008).

Imagery Rehearsal Therapy

Imagery rehearsal therapy (IRT) targets the nightmares that are a common symptom of PTSD by changing the content of a patient's nightmares to promote mastery over the content threat, thereby altering the meaning and importance of and orientation to the nightmares. In a small RCT, Krakow et al. (2001) compared IRT and WL and found that among treatment completers, participants who received IRT had a larger reduction in self-reported PTSD severity at the 3-month follow-up, the impact of their nightmares was reduced, and their sleep quality improved. However, a recent large RCT comparing IRT with a group nightmare-management treatment in Vietnam veterans with PTSD found that neither treatment produced significant or sustainable improvement in overall PTSD symptom severity, nightmare frequency, or sleep quality (Cook et al., 2010). Thus, although IRT has empirical support as being an effective treatment for nightmares, its efficacy as a treatment for PTSD is questionable.

Psychodynamic Psychotherapy

Brom et al. (1989) conducted an RCT to compare the efficacy of Horowitz's (1976) brief psychodynamic therapy, which focuses on solving intrapsychic conflicts that result from a traumatic experience, with hypnotherapy, trauma desensitization, and a WL control group. Not all study participants met the criteria for PTSD. Re-experiencing and avoidance symptoms improved significantly in all treatment groups but not in the WL group; no differences were found among the three treatments.

Brief Eclectic Psychotherapy

Gersons et al. (2000) developed manualized brief eclectic psychotherapy, which includes imaginal exposure combined with relaxation, writing assignments, use of mementos of the traumatic experience, exploration of meaning, a farewell ritual, and psychoeducation. Significant reductions in PTSD symptoms and anxiety symptoms were detected compared with the result of WL in an RCT of 42 police officers after the 16 sessions and at 3-month follow-up. It is unclear which of the several treatment components are responsible for the improved outcomes. Lindauer et al. (2005) conducted an RCT with 24 patients and found that brief eclectic psychotherapy resulted in a reduction in PTSD and symptoms of general anxiety compared with WL.

Hypnosis

Hypnosis is defined as a heightened state of relaxation during which a health professional or researcher guides a person with suggestions for experiencing changes in sensations, perceptions, thoughts, or behaviors (Everly and Lating, 2004). Hypnotic techniques have been used as an adjunctive therapy focusing on nightmares and insomnia in PTSD (Kirsch, 1999; Spiegel and Spiegel, 1987). Brom et al. (1989) found hypnosis to decrease intrusive symptoms more than WL, but not all research participants met the criteria for PTSD. Abramowitz et al. (2008) compared hypnotherapy with the use of zolpidem in an RCT of veterans who had combat PTSD and insomnia. All patients were already taking an SSRI. Hypnotherapy improved PTSD symptoms, sleep quality, and ability to concentrate more than zolpidem did.

Relaxation

Three RCTs have examined the efficacy of relaxation used in control groups in the study of imaginal exposure, EMDR, PE, or CT (Marks et al., 1998; Taylor et al., 2003; Vaughan et al., 1994). The results of the studies suggest that relaxation has at best a moderate effect on PTSD symptoms, but it is not as effective as exposure or cognitive therapy.

Stress Inoculation Training

SIT (Meichenbaum, 1974) was developed as an anxiety-management treatment and has been modified to treat rape victims (Kilpatrick et al., 1982). SIT includes relaxation training, breathing retraining, positive thinking and self-talk, assertiveness training, and thought stopping (Foa et al. 1999b). Some SIT protocols also include cognitive restructuring and exposure therapy. Two studies have compared the efficacy of SIT in the treatment of female sexual assault victims who had PTSD with the efficacy of PE, supportive counseling, and WL (Foa et al., 1991) and with the efficacy of SIT plus PE (Foa et al., 1999a). Both studies found SIT to be more effective than WL in reducing PTSD and related symptoms and to be of comparable efficacy to PE on some measures. Chemtob et al. (1997) found that SIT was more effective than anger management and treatment-as-usual in reducing anger and re-experiencing of symptoms.

Interpersonal Therapy

Interpersonal therapy (IPT) is a manualized time-limited structured psychotherapy. Targeted IPT interventions seek to improve distressing interpersonal problems (role conflict, role transition, and loss) and thus to lead to greater social support with consequent benefits regarding mood and anxiety. Because PTSD is often accompanied by problems with intimate familial relationships, it has been hypothesized that treatment that focuses on interpersonal concerns would lead to amelioration of PTSD symptoms.

A single RCT compared individual IPT with WL in a small sample of Sudanese refugees living in Cairo, Egypt (Meffert et al., 2011). The authors used conservative intent-to-treat analyses and found that IPT predicted a significant decrease in symptoms of PTSD, state anger, and depression.

Skills Training in Affect and Interpersonal Regulation

Cloitre et al. (2002) developed a two-phase treatment consisting of eight sessions of skills training in affect and interpersonal regulation (STAIR) followed by eight sessions of imaginal exposure. The two-phase combined treatment was more effective than WL in increasing emotional regulation and reducing PTSD. Imaginal exposure but not STAIR reduced PTSD symptoms; moreover, imaginal exposure increased emotional regulation as much as did STAIR despite being delivered at the second stage of treatment. In a follow-up study, Cloitre et al. (2010) compared the combination of STAIR and imaginal exposure with counseling and imaginal exposure. There was a tendency for STAIR and imaginal exposure to produce more recovery from PTSD, but the difference was not significant.

Behavior Activation

In small RCTs (Jakupcak et al., 2010; Wagner et al., 2007) and open trials (Nixon and Nearmy, 2011), behavioral activation has been shown to be an effective CBT intervention for PTSD, although more well-controlled studies are needed to determine efficacy. The primary goal of this model is to assist people in accessing their emotions and experiences while focusing on living a fulfilling life as opposed to avoiding and escaping pain (Hayes et al., 2006). The treatment is implemented in both groups and individuals. Five specific themes shape the manualized program: escape does not work effectively and leads to "creative helplessness," efforts to control pain create struggles, people are separate from their thoughts, moving beyond the struggle for control is central, and moving toward a commitment to action that is consistent with world views and values. The model has been evaluated for its efficacy in several anxiety disorders, but at present there is no evidence of its efficacy for PTSD (Pull, 2009).

Group Therapy

A number of group-based treatments for PTSD that draw on efficacious individual therapies are associated with symptom improvement. One benefit of group treatments over individual treatment is the efficiency in provision of treatment; another is the potential of group members to give social support to each other, which is key for people who have PTSD, inasmuch as lack of social support is a known risk factor for PTSD (e.g., Brewin et al., 2000; Ozer et al., 2003).

Six RCTs have examined the efficacy of CBT group therapy approaches. Schnurr et al. (2003) investigated trauma-focused group therapy in male Vietnam veterans in a large and rigorous study. Trauma-focused group therapy is a manualized treatment (30 sessions) consisting of education about PTSD, coping resource assessment, and self-management of symptoms; writing of premilitary autobiographies; war zone scene identification, exposure, and cognitive restructuring; and relapse prevention. One-third of the sessions are devoted to individual work (Foy et al., 2002). In Schnurr et al. (2003), trauma-focused group therapy was compared with present-centered group therapy, an approach designed to provide nonspecific factors of support and interpersonal connection inherent in group treatment. The investigators found that both groups experienced significant modest pretreatment to posttreatment improvement in PTSD, which was maintained at 12 months. No differences between the groups were detected.

Rogers et al. (1999) compared a single session of flooding-based exposure group therapy with a single session of group EMDR in 12 Vietnam veterans in an inpatient setting. No differences were found between groups in PTSD symptoms after treatment, and both groups showed significant improvements.

Beck et al. (2009) randomized people who had motor vehicle incident-related PTSD to group CBT or a minimal-contact comparison group. The group CBT was a 14-week treatment adaptation of individual exposure-based CBT to a group setting. After treatment, group CBT had resulted in significantly greater reductions in PTSD symptoms in those who completed treatment. Furthermore, 88.3% of patients who received group CBT no longer had a diagnosis of PTSD compared with 31.3% of the patients in the minimal-contact group.

Two RCTs have compared different types of group CBT with WL, all involving female populations. Zlotnick et al. (1997) randomly assigned female survivors of childhood sexual abuse to either 15 weekly 2-hour group dialectical behavior therapy group sessions or WL. The group sessions comprised education and practice of various affect-management skills, including emotion identification, anger management, self-soothing, and distress tolerance. The group treatment resulted in significant reductions in self-reported PTSD severity and dissociation, compared with no change in the WL group. Finally, multiple channel exposure therapy—which incorporates PE, CPT, and interoceptive exposure for panic disorder—was found to be superior to a control group in women who have PTSD and comorbid panic attacks (Falsetti et al., 2005).

Two RCTs have examined non-CBT approaches with WL in women who had PTSD related to sexual abuse. Comparison of a WL group with a trauma-focused group and a present-focused group, both based on psychodynamic principles, showed no differences between either treatment and the WL group (Spiegel et al., 2004). However, Krupnick et al. (2008) conducted an RCT to compare group-based interpersonal treatment with WL and found that the treatment was significantly more effective in treating symptoms of PTSD and depression than was WL.

In summary, several studies of group therapy found it to be efficacious in reducing PTSD, but the reduction was modest. An IOM committee that reviewed four studies of group therapy concluded that the evidence was inadequate to determine the efficacy of group therapy formats for the treatment of PTSD, primarily due to the lack of well-designed studies comparing group and individual formats with an appropriate control group (IOM, 2008).

Treatments Studied in Open Trials

Virtual-Reality Exposure

Virtual-reality exposure (VRE) therapy uses real-time computer graphics and head-mounted visual displays as a tool to deliver PE. Users are provided with a relevant multisensory controlled-stimulus environment, and the clinician can systematically control the presence or absence of provocative stimuli delivered in the VR simulation to pace the level of exposure. Proponents of VRE assert that the use of VR in the context of PE can increase activation and modification of the fear structure more than can imaginal exposure without VR. They also assert that some patients who have "grown up digital" may be more likely to seek PE delivered in a technology–media format that they are familiar with from video games. To date, there is no evidence of the superiority of PE plus VRE to PE alone in patients who have PTSD, although preliminary data in support of the assertion that some patients are likely to seek PE when it is accompanied by VRE have been reported (Reger et al., 2009). Case studies suggest that the use of VRE is effective in reducing PTSD (Difede and Hoffman, 2002;

Rothbaum and Hodges, 1999; Rothbaum et al., 2001) and more effective than WL (Difede et al., 2007), but no RCT has compared the efficacy of PE alone with that of VRE alone.

The virtual Iraq/Afghanistan VRE application (Rizzo et al., 2011) consists of a series of virtual scenarios that are designed to resemble the general contexts that most service members experience during deployment to Iraq or Afghanistan and that are used as digital contexts for delivering PE. Two early case reports showed positive results of the system (Gerardi et al., 2008; Reger and Gahm, 2008). Following those, an open clinical trial with 24 active-duty soldiers produced significant pretreatment to posttreatment reductions in PTSD Checklist–Military version scores with a large treatment effect size (Reger et al., 2011). After an average of seven sessions, 46% of those treated no longer screened positive for PTSD, and 62% had reliably improved. In a second open clinical trial, 20 active-duty Operation Enduring Freedom (OEF) and Operation Iraqi Freedom (OIF) service members, who had previously received PTSD treatments (such as PE, group counseling, EMDR, and medication) without benefit, received an average of 11 VRE sessions. Of the treatment completers, 80% showed both statistically and clinically meaningful reductions in PTSD, anxiety, and depression symptoms. Patients reported improvements in their everyday life that were maintained at 3-months posttreatment (Rizzo et al., 2011). In contrast, a study that used a combined sample of active-duty soldiers who had undergone either VR or imaginal PE therapy showed only modest pretreatment to posttreatment gains on the CAPS although changes in functional magnetic resonance imaging brain responses to emotional stimuli suggest a positive response to treatment (Roy et al., 2010).

The U.S. Army is currently evaluating the efficacy of VRE compared with PE in RCTs, but no results have been reported at this time. Until the results from the four ongoing RCTs are available, there is insufficient evidence for the efficacy of the virtual Iraq/Afghanistan VRE in reducing PTSD symptoms.

Acceptance and Commitment Therapy

Acceptance and commitment therapy (ACT) is a behavior-based treatment that is grounded in the concept that suffering emerges from avoidance of pain rather than from a direct experience of pain. It is used in many VA medical centers to treat chronic PTSD. Walser and Westrup (2007) have published an ACT manual for the treatment of PTSD. Support for ACT is limited to a single case study by Twohig (2009), who treated a woman who had PTSD and depression and initially received 20 sessions of CBT that included written exposure and cognitive restructuring. The patient received 21 sessions of ACT and showed significant reduction in PTSD, depression, and anxiety in response to trauma-related thoughts by the end of treatment.

Helping to Overcome PTSD with Empowerment

Helping to Overcome PTSD with Empowerment (HOPE) is a short-term CBT treatment for battered women who have PTSD and are in domestic violence shelters (Johnson and Zlotnick, 2009). It is a manualized 9–12-session treatment that addresses the women's needs (such as establishing safety, self-care, and protection; remembrance and mourning; and reconnection) while including such CBT components as cognitive restructuring and psychoeducation.

Metacognitive Therapy

Metacognitive therapy (Wells and Sembi, 2004a) is a brief, manualized, cognitive-based treatment that includes mindfulness and strategies to shift attention away from rumination and worry. Wells and Sembi (2004b) provided metacognitive therapy to five women and one man and found improvements in general emotion and specific PTSD measures that were maintained at follow-up (18–41 months).

Trauma Management Therapy

Trauma management therapy (Frueh et al., 1996) is a mixed individual and group therapy for veterans who have combat-related PTSD that focuses on such PTSD symptoms as social withdrawal, numbing, expression of anger, and interpersonal difficulties. The therapy combines intensive individual exposure therapy, programmed practice, and structured social and emotional skills training groups. In individual counseling sessions, psychoeducation and exposure therapy are given, followed by programmed practice at home that consists of exercises for controlling one's own exposure; after this, a social and emotional rehabilitation phase begins. The latter phase is conducted in small groups of two to five veterans, and includes social skills training, anger management, and training on how to communicate to civilians about military issues. In one study of 15 veterans, Frueh et al. (1996) found that the 11 veterans who completed the program experienced significant improvement in anxiety, flashbacks, nightmares, sleep difficulty, heart rate reactivity, and overall social functioning.

Trauma Incident Reduction

Gerbode (1995) developed trauma incident reduction, in which the patient is initially instructed to revisit the traumatic event mentally without verbalizing it, and only then to follow it with a verbalization of the memory. Trauma incident reduction appears to be very similar to imaginal exposure. Support for trauma incident reduction for people who have PTSD consists mostly of case studies or case series (Carbonell and Figley, 1999; Figley et al., 1999).

PHARMACOTHERAPY

Medication has long been an integral part of the treatment for chronic PTSD. Sargant et al. (1972) noted that in the 1960s that tricyclic and monoamine oxidase inhibitor (MAOI) antidepressants were the most effective, and clinical trials have confirmed the accuracy of these observations. The authors saw medication as playing a primarily supportive role in which control of symptoms permitted patients to mobilize their own coping mechanisms. More recent neurobiological studies of PTSD and related disorders have indicated the relevance of various neurotransmitter systems—such as noradrenergic, dopaminergic, serotonergic, glutamatergic and GABAergic (producing gamma-aminobutyric acid) pathways—and the different drug groups that are now used to treat the disorders act mostly through these systems.

The main recommendations for the use of pharmacotherapy to treat chronic PTSD are based on whether medication is a first-line treatment for PTSD. The choice of a drug depends on the evidence base to support the choice and studies that support the treatment for specific problems in PTSD such as smoking cessation, sleep disturbances, and irritability.

The VA/DoD, International Society for Traumatic Stress Studies (ISTSS), American Psychiatric Association (APA), British Association of Psychopharmacology, World Federation of Societies of Biological Psychiatry, and International Psychopharmacology Algorithm Project (IPAP) guidelines (discussed later in this chapter) all recommend the use of an SSRI (such as paroxetine or sertraline) or the serotonin norepinephrine reuptake inhibitor (SNRI) antidepressant venlafaxine extended-release as a first choice, giving them the same status as psychotherapy. The UK and Australian guidelines recommend drug therapy only as a second choice unless the patient declines psychotherapy or manifests particular clinical features. An IOM report (2008) on treatments for PTSD concluded that neither SRIs nor any other drugs could be considered effective for treatment for PTSD although the committee's conclusion was not unanimous. A Cochrane review (Stein et al., 2006) found that there was good evidence for SSRI and SNRI drugs in chronic PTSD as both short-term and maintenance treatment, and a subsequent meta-analysis of pharmacotherapies for PTSD also found that medication reduced PTSD symptom severity (Ipser and Stein, 2011). A meta-analysis of the effectiveness of pharmacotherapy compared with psychotherapy for the treatment of combat-related PTSD found that pharmacotherapy resulted in a significantly greater decrease in PTSD symptoms from baseline than did psychotherapy within a 6-month timeframe, based on standardized scores (Stewart and Wrobel, 2009). Based on this analysis, the authors suggest that pharmacotherapy be considered as a first-line treatment for veterans who have combat-related PTSD, particularly those with severe symptoms. The following sections discuss the evidence supporting the use of various pharmacotherapies for PTSD.

Antidepressants

Tricyclics and Monoamine Oxidase Inhibitors (MAOIs)

Although these drugs are now perhaps underused, the first placebo-controlled RCTs of medication for PTSD found that the tricyclic drugs amitriptyline and imipramine, and the MAOI phenelzine, were more effective than placebo in veterans of World War II and Vietnam (Davidson et al., 1990; Kosten et al., 1991). Given the later difficulty of showing the efficacy of antidepressants in veteran populations, those positive findings deserve to be emphasized, especially because amitriptyline and imipramine, broad-spectrum drugs, also help to restore sleep and reduce pain. One study of desipramine was negative, but the treatment dose and duration may have been insufficient (Reist et al., 1989) and the drug's selective effect only on norepinephrine may have been a limitation. Studies of the reversible MAOI class A have been disappointing (Baker et al., 1995; Katz et al., 1994).

Selective Serotonin Reuptake Inhibitors

Because of their greater safety and tolerability, SSRIs have largely replaced the older antidepressants in clinical practice, and there is reasonably strong evidence to support their use in PTSD on the basis of numerous placebo-controlled RCTs. Two drugs, sertraline (Brady et al., 2000, 2005; Davidson et al., 2001; Friedman et al., 2007) and paroxetine immediate-release (Marshall et al., 2001; Stein et al., 2003; Tucker et al., 2001), have been approved in the United States and some other countries for PTSD, and these two SSRIs have been the most extensively studied (e.g., Ipser and Stein, 2011; Stein et al., 2006; Zhang and Davidson, 2007) and cited in PTSD guidelines (APA, 2004; British Association of Psychopharmacology et al., 2005; IPAP, 2005; NCCMH and NICE, 2005). Ipser and Stein (2011) found evidence of efficacy for two of four SSRIs, sertraline and paroxetine, in their meta-analysis of pharmacotherapy for PTSD, with paroxetine being significantly more effective than the other SSRIs ($P = 0.0001$).

Although the VA/DoD guideline recommends SRIs as first-line treatment, this committee is unaware of any positive trials of this class of drugs conducted in U.S. veterans only. However, two placebo-controlled studies in foreign veterans demonstrated efficacy of SRI treatment for PTSD. In Bosnian War veterans, fluoxetine was substantially better than placebo (Martenyi et al., 2002b). An additional placebo-controlled RCT showed greater benefit of sertraline than of placebo in Iranian veterans of the Iran–Iraq war (Panahi et al., 2011). In a trial of sertraline compared with placebo exclusively in U.S. veterans, there was no difference between treatments (Friedman et al., 2007). In the main paroxetine reports (Marshall et al., 2001; Stein et al., 2003; Tucker et al., 2001), analysis of response by trauma type found that combat-related PTSD responded better to the drug than to placebo; however, the number of cases of combat-related PTSD in these studies was small, less than 10% of the total number of patients in each RCT.

There have been no placebo-controlled trials of the SSRIs fluvoxamine or escitalopram. There has been one negative trial of citalopram (Tucker et al., 2003), and although the VA/DoD guideline (2010) initially recommended its use, the VA and the DoD have recently issued a warning against using citalopram for persons with risks or predisposition to specific comorbid heart conditions. One other SSRI, fluoxetine, has been extensively studied. Efficacy was demonstrated in some (Connor et al., 1999; Vanderkolk et al., 1994) but not all studies. A fixed-dose trial of fluoxedine at 20 mg and 40 mg failed to differ from placebo in a large group of women who had PTSD (Martenyi et al., 2007). Trials of fluoxetine in U.S. veterans have been negative (Hertzberg et al., 2000; Vanderkolk et al., 1994), and one in Bosnian War veterans was positive (Martenyi et al., 2002b). It is possible that the full benefits of SSRI drugs are not detected in standard RCTs; nevertheless, many clinicians in the VA and DoD health care systems still favor their use.

Serotonin-Norepinephrine Reuptake Inhibitors

There have been two positive trials of venlafaxine versus placebo: one in the United States (Davidson et al., 2006b) and one in other countries (Davidson et al., 2006a). In the U.S. study, sertraline was adopted as an active control and had the same results as the placebo. In the international study, the period of double-blind treatment extended to 6 months, and rates of remission increased further between 12 and 24 weeks: there was a significant drug effect on resilience. In a report of pooled data from the two studies, there was no difference between drug and placebo in subjects who had combat-related PTSD (Rothbaum et al., 2008a).

Other Antidepressants

Nefazodone had greater benefit than placebo in one study of U.S. veterans (Davis et al., 2004), and mirtazapine was found to be superior to placebo in nonveterans (Davidson et al., 2003). In veterans, bupropion was no different from placebo in PTSD, although it helped in achieving greater smoking cessation (Becker et al., 2007; Hertzberg et al., 2001). It may be relevant that the first two drugs affect both serotonin and norepinephrine and improve sleep, whereas bupropion, a selective dopamine and norepinephrine modulator, has minimal benefit on sleep.

Anticonvulsants

Four placebo-controlled trials have failed to show the benefit of lamotrigine, tiagabine, topiramate, or divalproex (Davidson et al., 2007; Davis et al., 2008a; Hertzberg et al., 1999; Tucker et al., 2007) for PTSD. The studies of lamotrigine and divalproex were conducted in veterans.

Antipsychotics

Monotherapy trials of atypical antipsychotic therapy versus placebo have yielded mixed results. They include a small negative trial of olanzapine in veterans (Butterfield et al., 2001) and two partially positive studies of risperidone in women who had PTSD stemming from childhood abuse (Padala et al., 2006; Reich et al., 2004): in one of these (Reich et al., 2004), almost half the sample were receiving other drugs. Quetiapine was found to be superior to placebo in a two-site trial of 80 veterans who had PTSD (Canive et al., 2009).

Several small initial augmentation RCTs of the antipsychotic drugs risperidone and olanzapine in veterans and civilians showed that the drugs reduced some symptoms of PTSD, particularly sleep disturbance (Bartzokis et al., 2005; Hamner et al., 2003; Monnelly et al., 2003; Rothbaum et al., 2008b; Stein et al., 2002), but the largest RCT, a 6-month study of risperidone in veterans with combat-related PTSD was negative on the primary and most secondary outcome measures (Krystal et al., 2011). In the latter trial, differences favored risperidone for re-experiencing and hyperarousal symptoms, but according to the investigators, the size of this difference was not clinically meaningful. Questions remain about the effect of atypical antipsychotic augmentation in PTSD and whether between-drug differences are important. As with all treatments, side effects should be taken into account, and the issues surrounding the metabolic syndrome and abnormal movements are a concern with regard to antipsychotic drugs.

Benzodiazepines and Other GABAergic Drugs

One small study of alprazolam in people who have various types of trauma showed no advantage over placebo (Braun et al., 1990), and another small crossover study of clonazepam versus placebo in combat-related PTSD was also negative (Cates et al., 2004). However, Pollack et al. (2011) found a short-term improvement in overall PTSD severity and associated sleep disturbances in a small RCT of the non-benzodiazepine hypnotic drug eszopiclone in 24 civilians.

Benzodiazepines and some other drugs, such as beta blockers, might have the potential to impair positive coping after trauma or interfere with extinction of fear responses. However, the data have demonstrated through animal studies (Bouton et al., 1990) or single dose use in close proximity to psychotherapy that this is difficult to translate into everyday clinical situations.

Antiadrenergic Drugs

The alpha-1 adrenergic blocker prazosin has been shown to be more effective than placebo for reducing PTSD-associated sleep disturbances in three trials, two in veterans with combat-related chronic PTSD (Raskind et al., 2003, 2007) and one in civilians with PTSD (Taylor et al., 2006), all of whom had prominent sleep disruption or nightmares. More information is needed concerning the optimal dose of prazosin and interactions that may result from the concurrent use of other drugs. In a study of the antiadrenergic drug guanfacine, no benefit was found, but the population was not selected according to criteria of sleep disturbance (Neylan et al., 2006). A second study (Davis et al., 2008b) also failed to show a benefit of guanfacine over placebo. In animal studies, beta blockers such as propranolol have been shown to reduce the consolidation of aversive memories significantly (for example, see Rodriguez-Romaguera et al., 2009). On the basis of those findings, the use of propranolol for the prevention of PTSD has been explored and has had mostly negative results (Pitman et al., 2002; Stein et al., 2007). Question remain about the use of antiadrenergic agents in the prevention of and treatment for PTSD.

Other Drugs

Negative studies have been published for the use of monotherapy with D-cycloserine (DCS) and inositol in chronic PTSD (Heresco-Levy et al., 2002; Kaplan et al., 1996).

Special Considerations in Pharmacotherapy for PTSD

There are two issues that merit consideration when prescribing pharmacotherapy for PTSD: polypharmacy, the use of multiple drugs for PTSD symptoms; and maintenance of drug therapy and its implications for relapse. Both of these concerns are discussed in this section.

Polypharmacy

Treatment for PTSD can be complicated, and there is a place for various classes of drug treatment beyond antidepressants (Pfeiffer et al., 2011), sometimes involving drug combinations, including those for which high-grade evidence is lacking. Polypharmacy for PTSD is addressed by Davidson et al. (2005a) as part of the IPAP.

Studies of the VA National Registry for Depression and the VA Drug Benefit Management System cast light on the issues of polypharmacy and off-label drug use for PTSD. In a survey of the VA National Registry in 2001, Valenstein et al. (2004) reported that benzodiazepines were prescribed to 36% of patients, mostly on a long term basis. Of those who had PTSD, 43% received a benzodiazepine. In the overall sample of depressives, 41% had two psychiatric diagnoses, and 46% had three or more.

In a large national sample of veterans who had PTSD, VA drug benefit data from October 2003 to September 2004 showed that psychotropic drugs were prescribed for 80% of the patients. Of those receiving psychotropic drugs, 89% received an antidepressant, 61% an anxiolytic or hypnotic, and 34% a first-generation or second-generation antipsychotic (Mohamed and Rosenheck, 2008). Rates of comorbidity were high and encompassed a wide array of other disorders, including those for which the different drug groups were indicated (for example, an antipsychotic for bipolar disorder). However, off-label prescribing was also common.

From these studies, it is clear that the majority of veterans who have PTSD and receive care at the VA are being prescribed more than one psychotropic drug, including about 80% of them being given an SSRI antidepressant. Other drugs are used extensively, some of which may be appropriate for the diagnosis or targeted at particular symptoms. Thus, there is a clear place for rational and carefully conducted polypharmacy, but risks need to be minimized and case records should explain the basis of such practices. Those injunctions apply not only to combining psychotropics, but also to the use of psychotropics with medicines from other categories that have a potential for adverse drug interactions. Given that some drugs carry the potential for abuse or are not known to be effective for PTSD when given alone (such as benzodiazepines, narcotics, and some hypnotics), there needs to be justification for their use and adequate monitoring.

Maintenance Treatment and Risk of Relapse

Given the chronicity of both full and partial PTSD (see Chapter 2) many OEF and OIF veterans will require long-term treatment to ameliorate their symptoms. There have been five trials of long-term maintenance or relapse prevention in people who responded to short-term treatment with antidepressants or anticonvulsants in PTSD. Two placebo-controlled relapse-prevention studies found that fluoxetine maintenance led to a lower chance of relapse than placebo over 1 year (Davidson et al., 2005b; Martenyi et al., 2002a), and similar findings were reported for sertraline over a longer period (Davidson et al., 2001). No maintenance benefit was obtained with tiagabine over placebo (Connor et al., 2006), and a large relapse-prevention trial of paroxetine versus placebo failed to show differences—both groups had an unusually low rate of relapse over 1 year—and called into question the nature of the original sample (NCCMH and NICE, 2005). Ipser and Stein (2011) noted although there are a number of studies supporting the use of SSRIs and the SNRI venlafaxine for the treatment of PTSD, less is known about how long patients should be treated and the optimal treatment duration to prevent relapse. The relapse rate for PTSD once medication is discontinued is about 40% to 50% and for those who continue on medication, about 15% to 20%, although most studies do not follow outcomes for more than about 15 months.

Although there is debate about antidepressants as a treatment for PTSD (for example, see IOM [2008], NICE, and Australian guidelines), a Cochrane review (Stein et al., 2006) found that response rates in 13 studies were greater for drug than for placebo (the number needed to treat was 4.85, 95% CI 3.85–6.25; n = 1272). The review found that medication was superior to placebo in reducing the severity of PTSD symptom clusters, comorbid depression, and disability, but that it was less well tolerated than placebo. The authors concluded that their results support recommending SSRIs as first-line pharmacotherapy for PTSD for short-term and long-term treatment. A follow-up report by the same group has updated the findings to some extent (Ipser and Stein, 2011) and contains some useful recommendations, including reference to the treatment needs of refractory patients, for whom augmentation or combination approaches may be required. They stated studies of the addition of antipsychotics to ongoing treatment with

SSRIs for refractory PTSD "appear to support the efficacy of this strategy, at least with respect to combat-related traumas." It concluded that war trauma, dose of drug, and sex were not as important in determining the effect of drug treatment as were the size of the study sample and the duration of PTSD.

COMBINED PSYCHOTHERAPY AND PHARMACOTHERAPY APPROACHES

There are two primary strategies for combining pharmacotherapy and psychotherapy for PTSD (Rothbaum, 2008). The additive model combines two effective interventions on the assumption that the benefits would be cumulative. Although some studies suggest there is no advantage in combining traditional psychiatric medications with CBT for any other anxiety disorder (Foa et al., 2002; Gerardi et al., 2009), other studies indicate positive outcomes (Barlow et al., 2000; Blanco et al., 2010).

DCS is an *n*-methyl-d-aspartate (NMDA) partial agonist that has been found to facilitate the extinction of fear (Davis et al., 2006). It is used in a direct attempt at chemical stimulation of the NMDA-glutamate synapses—thought to be the critical nerve-cell mechanisms that support short-term learning and memory (Bear, 1996; Newcomer and Krystal, 2001)—at the same moment that exposure therapy is helping the patient to learn new behaviors (Davis et al., 2006). DCS alone has no beneficial effect on PTSD (Heresco-Levy et al., 2002); however, combination strategies that involve acute administration of DCS during exposure therapy are being studied (for example, Ressler et al., 2004). In such trials, the medication is expected not to be as effective as the monotherapy but to have an augmenting or facilitating effect in the psychotherapy.

Only one study used both medication and psychotherapy from the outset for the treatment of PTSD (Schneier et al., 2012). The researchers found benefits with combined therapy of 10 weeks of paroxetine and prolonged imaginal exposure in adult survivors of the World Trade Center attacks of September 11, 2001, compared with PE and placebo. However, the benefits of combined therapy at 10 weeks disappeared after an additional 12 weeks of follow-up medication, that is response rates at 22 weeks were similar to placebo. The data are insufficient to determine whether there are additive or interactive effects (or both) of simultaneously administered pharmacotherapy and psychotherapy for PTSD.

In the first published RCT of combined treatment for PTSD, male and female civilian outpatients who had PTSD were treated with open-label sertraline (up to 200 mg) and then were randomly assigned to receive continuation with sertraline alone or augmentation with PE (Rothbaum et al., 2006). Overall, the additional 5 weeks of sertraline alone was not associated with further improvement on measures of PTSD severity, depression, or general anxiety. However, among partial responders to medication in the first phase, augmentation with PE was associated with further reduction in PTSD severity only (Choi, 2010). In a combination trial that mirrored the Rothbaum et al. (2006) study design, participants first received eight sessions of PE over 4–6 weeks and then were randomly assigned to receive five additional sessions of PE plus either controlled-release paroxetine or placebo (Simon et al., 2008). PE was associated with the largest reductions in PTSD symptoms, and there were no significant differences between placebo and paroxetine in the augmentation phase. Thus, in those two trials, PE enhanced the medication effects in weak medication responders, but medication did not appear to add to the PE effects. In a pilot study of 10 female Cambodian refugees randomly assigned to treatment with open-label sertraline alone or the combination of open-label sertraline and 10 sessions of group CBT, medium to large effect sizes were reported in the combined group (Otto et al., 2003).

INTEGRATIVE COLLABORATIVE CARE

Three large-scale randomized effectiveness trials have successfully used collaborative care models to target and reduce PTSD symptoms in civilian patients presenting at primary care and acute care medical settings (Craske et al., 2011; Zatzick et al., 2004, 2012). Collaborative care is a disease-management model that integrates general medical providers and mental health providers in the treatment of patients who have PTSD and comorbid medical conditions. Collaborative care combines care management with evidence-based psychotherapy (for example, CBT) or pharmacotherapy targeting PTSD. A large series of randomized trials have established the effectiveness of collaborative care that integrates care management, evidence-based pharmacotherapy, and CBT in the treatment of primary care patients who have depression (Bower et al., 2006; Bruce et al., 2004; Dobscha et al., 2009; Gilbody et al., 2006; Katon et al., 1999, 2001, 2010; Kroenke et al., 2009; Miranda et al., 2003; Unutzer et al., 2002; Von Korff, 2004; Wells et al., 2000). However, collaborative care for PTSD has received much less investigative attention. Collaborative care may be useful for the integration of psychotherapy and pharmacotherapy targeting PTSD in nonspecialty mental health settings such as primary care (see also Chapters 6, 8, and 9). Collaborative care may be particularly useful in the integration of new treatment delivery technologies that dismantle or combine elements of established evidence-based practices (Geiss Trusz et al., 2011).

EMERGING THERAPIES FOR PTSD

In this section, the committee considers PTSD treatments that are being used for individuals who have PTSD or for couples and families that have a member who has PTSD. Although a number of studies are being conducted by the DoD, VA, and private researchers on these treatments (see Chapter 4), particularly alternative treatments such as yoga, tai chi, and thought field therapy, to date there is not a substantial evidence base by which to judge their efficacy. It may be difficult to distinguish between alternative treatments that may prove to be efficacious in future studies and those that will not, that is to "differentiate snake oil from penicillin" (Peterson et al., 2011). The committee has heard from numerous service members that such treatments as yoga are helping them, so it is appropriate to discuss these treatments in this report. Furthermore, the committee was specifically asked by Congress to examine these often innovative treatments. The committee expects phase 2 will include more studies on which to base a discussion of the efficacy of these treatments, particularly CAM treatments.

Couple and Family Therapy

Couple Therapy

Cognitive-behavioral conjoint therapy (CBCT) is one couple-based treatment model that focuses on treatment for PTSD and has some evidence to support its efficacy although other couple-based therapy models are undergoing different levels of systematic empirical review.

CBCT for PTSD is a manualized couple-based treatment that has three stages: psychoeducation and safety-building; confronting avoidance, enhancing relationship satisfaction, and improving communication; and cognitive interventions addressing relationship problems and symptoms of PTSD, focusing on maladaptive thoughts around the trauma (Monson et al., 2004, 2008).

In an open trial of CBCT, Monson et al. (2004) treated seven pairs of male Vietnam veterans and their spouses. After treatment, patients experienced significant improvement in PTSD scores based on clinician and spouse ratings but not patient ratings. Spouses expressed slightly improved relationship satisfaction, and veterans reported improvements in depression and anxiety. In another uncontrolled trial, seven couples participated in an uncontrolled trial of CBCT for PTSD (Monson et al., 2011). Among the six couples who completed the treatment, five of the patients no longer met the criteria for PTSD, and there were across-treatment effect-size improvements in patients' total PTSD symptoms according to independent clinician assessment and reports from the patients and partners. Three of the four couples who had distressed relationships before treatment expressed satisfaction in their relationships after treatment. Patients reported nonsignificant moderate to large improvements in relationship satisfaction and nonsignificant improvements in depression and associated symptoms of anger; however, their partners reported statistically significant, large effect-size improvements in relationship satisfaction. Although there are findings related to moderation of PTSD symptoms, improvements in relationship satisfaction proved to be uneven. Limitations of this study include the small sample size and the absence of a control sample (Monson et al., 2011).

One RCT examined marital adjustment of Middle East combat veterans who had been diagnosed with PTSD (Ahamdy et al., 2009). Impaired marital adjustment and chronic marital distress are considered among the most common manifestations of PTSD. The researchers randomized 60 PTSD veterans who had low degrees of marital adjustment into intervention and control groups. Both groups were evaluated with the ENRICH scale for marital adjustment before and after intervention. The research team concluded that marital adjustment is high in veterans who have PTSD (43%) after the intervention and that the efficacy of CBCT was significant in both the veterans and their spouses.

Although additional couple-therapy approaches are being used with service members, veterans, and their families, data on their efficacy are lacking.

Family Therapy

Sherman et al. (2005) studied access to and use of family and individual treatment for female partners of Vietnam veterans with combat-related PTSD. Of the 89 women surveyed, 64% said access to individual therapy to help with coping was very important and 78% said involvement in family therapy was important for the veteran and his partner, but only 28% of the women had received mental health care in the past 6 months.

The Reaching Out to Educate and Assist Caring, Healthy Families (REACH) program at the Oklahoma City VA Medical Center is a 9-month psychoeducation program for families of veterans with PTSD (Sherman et al., 2009). As assessment of 294 veterans with PTSD who had a family member willing to meet the REACH staff for motivational interviewing sessions, found that 50% of the veterans (and a family member) were willing to learn about the psychoeducation model in spite of the need to overcome such barriers as a more than 15-minute time commitment, the need to relate to a new therapist, and fear of stigma.

Khaylis et al. (2011) conducted a study that used an anonymous self-reported questionnaire aimed at assessing PTSD symptoms, relationship issues, and treatment preference, including interest in family-focused interventions using a sample of 100 National Guard soldiers recently returned from Iraq. A majority of married or partnered soldiers expressed concerns about getting along with their partners and about child-rearing capacities. PTSD symptoms were significantly associated with the degree of relationship concerns. Finally, soldiers revealed a surprising preference for family-based interventions over individual treatment and attached higher importance to family-based interventions tailored to address mental health problems and co-occurring family problems.

Complementary and Alternative Medicine

In response to the committee's charge to look at CAM therapies for PTSD, it conducted an extensive literature search to identify open-label and RCTs of CAM (also called complementary and integrative medicine) in subjects who had PTSD-related conditions. The evidence base for the use of the therapies for PTSD management is summarized below. The committee will consider CAM treatments for PTSD in greater detail in phase 2 of this study. Many of the studies included in this section were small and case studies or anecdotal reports, but the committee has included them in this report because they illustrate the wide variety of approaches that are being used. The CAM therapies discussed below are not exhaustive. Many CAM approaches are being used by people with PTSD as reported in the popular press, but these approaches are not necessarily being formally studied to assess their efficacy.

As noted in Chapter 4, the use of CAM by military personnel ranges from about 37% (Smith et al., 2007) to about 72% (McPherson and Schwenka, 2004). To examine this widespread use of CAM, the VA, as part of its evidence-based synthesis program, looked at the efficacy of CAM therapies for PTSD (Strauss et al., 2011). Three types of CAM were considered: mind–body techniques such as acupuncture, yoga, and meditation; manipulative and body-base techniques such as spinal manipulation and massage; and movement-based or energy therapies. The VA found that there was insufficient evidence to support the use of meditation versus active treatment, relaxation versus control or active treatment, massage versus control, and movement-based and energy therapies versus control. There was also insufficient evidence to support the use of meditation versus usual care or acupuncture versus group CBT, but there was moderate evidence for acupuncture versus control, based on one RCT.

Yoga

Yoga is a type of mind–body therapy that aims to improve control over the body and mind through the practice of physical positions, breathing, and meditation (Strauss et al., 2011). Iyengar yoga, which uses props to achieve proper body alignment (Shapiro et al., 2007), has been reviewed by Brown and Gerbarg (2005) in which they cite three studies of this form of yoga. In one study, eight Vietnam veterans who had PTSD received 6 weeks of Iyengar yoga instruction; depression, but not anger or insomnia, improved. In a second study of Vietnam veterans, the Iyengar yoga poses for anxiety failed to benefit eight veterans and were discontinued. A third study of eight patients assessed a complex of different approaches and found that breathing techniques, such as Ham Su, provided greater benefit in many core PTSD symptoms.

Sudarshan Kriya yoga (SKY) combines elements of CBT and psychoeducation, so it is hard to determine the relative contributions of conventional PTSD therapies and yoga therapy. Brown and Gerbarg (2009) described further work with yoga in PTSD, citing (with few details) open and uncontrolled trials in survivors of Hurricane Katrina, in Australian Vietnam veterans, and in patients who had PTSD associated with sexual abuse. Descilo et al. (2010) obtained beneficial results with SKY in a nonrandomized controlled trial with 183 survivors of the 2004 Asian tsunami; SKY alone and SKY followed by 3–8 hours of exposure therapy were both more effective than a 6-week WL. In a WL-controlled study of 30 Australian veterans, SKY significantly improved PTSD symptoms (Carter and Byrne, 2006).

A randomized WL-controlled trial of 22 flood survivors showed benefit for Patanjali yoga, which emphasized a set series of stretching, postures, breathing, and relaxation (Telles et al., 2010).

Contemplative Approaches

Transcendental meditation, Vipassana meditation, mantram repetition, mindfulness, and mind–body skills approaches have all been studied. Transcendental meditation showed greater improvement than treatment-as-usual in a nonrandomized trial with veterans who had PTSD (Brooks and Scarano, 1985). Five veterans of OEF and OIF responded to 12 weeks of transcendental meditation in an uncontrolled trial by Rosenthal et al. (2011).

Vipassana meditation, a practice of self-observation, failed to improve PTSD in incarcerated people with comorbid substance use disorder and PTSD (Simpson et al., 2007).

Eight weeks of mindfulness training through meditation-based stress reduction was found to result in small but statistically significant improvement in PTSD at 24 weeks in 21 women who had survived child-abuse trauma (Kimbrough et al., 2010).

An uncontrolled trial of frequent mantram repetition, the chanting of a spiritually significant word or phrase to promote focus, calmness, relaxation, or balance (Strauss et al., 2011), resulted in modest but statistically significant improvement in 62 VA outpatients who had PTSD (Bormann et al., 2005). One RCT that compared mantram repetition with WL in 33 veterans who had PTSD showed a significant advantage for the treatment group (Bormann et al., 2008).

Levine et al. (2005) randomized 181 survivors of breast cancer to receive 12 sessions of a CAM program consisting of meditation, imagery, yoga, and a support group with lectures on health, or a standard supportive treatment of weekly psychoeducation. The authors concluded that standard treatment was preferable to CAM on the grounds of cost in that CAM required the services of several professionals.

In an uncontrolled observational study of 25 community-clinic psychiatric patients who received individualized CAM programs for trauma symptoms (massage, acupuncture, Reiki, or Healing Touch), Collinge et al. (2005) noted a mean improvement of 8.6 on a 10-point self-rating scale.

Acupuncture

Acupuncture seeks to improve health and wellness by stimulating the body and mind with the insertion and manipulation of needles placed in particular anatomic points. Hollifield et al. (2007) conducted a three-arm 12-week RCT of acupuncture, CBT, and WL control in civilian patients, most of whom had PTSD stemming from trauma experienced in childhood or adolescence. Both acupuncture and CBT outperformed WL in reducing PTSD. Zhang et al. (2011) conducted a 1-week trial of CBT alone versus CBT plus acupoint electrostimulation in earthquake survivors. Both treatments produced improvement, but the combined CBT–acupuncture group performed significantly better.

Emotional Freedom Technique and Thought Field Therapy

The emotional freedom technique (EFT) uses manual stimulation of acupuncture energy points combined with the patient's focusing on the traumatic event (Karatzias et al., 2011). In a small pilot study with nine veterans who had combat trauma, 5 days of EFT sessions resulted in lower scores on the PTSD Checklist–Military version immediately after treatment as well as 30 and 90 days after treatment (Church, 2010). A small randomized study with 46 civilians who had PTSD compared EFT with EMDR. Both treatments were effective in lowering CAPS scores immediately after treatment, but at a 90-day follow-up, EMDR resulted in more substantial clinical improvement (Karatzias et al., 2011).

Thought field therapy is a tapping sequence that has been used to treat a variety of mental health problems including phobias, anxiety, trauma, depression, fatigue, attention deficit hyperactivity disorder, learning difficulties, compulsions, obsessions, eating disorders, anger, and physical pain (Callahan 2001a,b). However, there are no empirical studies to support its effectiveness.

Neurofeedback

Neurofeedback—also known as neurotherapy, neurobiofeedback, and EEG biofeedback—uses electroencephalography or functional magnetic resonance imaging to monitor brain activity and the state of a person's physiological functioning (Othmer and Othmer, 2009). The technique combines systematic desensitization, temperature biofeedback, guided imagery, constructed visualizations, rhythmic breathing, and autogenic training incorporating alpha-theta (3–7 Hz) brainwave neurofeedback therapy. One study conducted in 20 Vietnam combat veterans who had PTSD and comorbid alcohol abuse found significant improvement after treatment that was maintained at 30 months (Peniston, 1998; Peniston and Kulkosky, 1991).

Qigong and T'ai Chi

Qigong and t'ai chi are traditional Chinese practices that encourage gentle movement of the body to achieve better focus and improved flow of bodily energy (Strauss et al., 2011). Grodin et al. (2008) described four subjects who had PTSD and who benefited from 15 minutes of qigong and t'ai chi before and after 1-hour psychotherapy sessions.

Herbal and Dietary Supplements

Shams et al. (2007) described positive results with the addition of 200 mg of *Ginkgo biloba* in subjects who had PTSD from an earthquake and who had partially responded to conventional drug therapy. Southwick et al. (1999) reported on four people who had PTSD and experienced worsening panic and anxiety from yohimbine. There have been no PTSD studies of the widely used herbs St. John's wort and kava, which have been studied extensively in anxiety and depression (Sarris and Kavanagh, 2009).

Two preliminary reports of fish oil did not suggest any benefit in PTSD (Kaplan et al., 2005; Matsuoka et al., 2010), but this treatment has not been adequately studied.

Homeopathy

Homeopathy seeks to treat disease by stimulating the body with serial dilutions of substances that cause similar symptoms of particular disease in healthy people (National Center for Complementary and Alternative Medicine, 2010). Three brief case reports of patients who had PTSD symptoms after sexual trauma and responded to homeopathy were identified (Coll, 2002; Katz, 1996; Morrison and National Center for Homeopathy, 1993). There is no other literature on homeopathy for PTSD.

Art Therapy

Art therapy encourages creative expression as an outlet for emotional processing and expression to facilitate psychologic health. Avrahami (2005) described two cases of veterans with combat PTSD that responded to visual-art therapy. The DoD National Intrepid Center of Excellence at Walter Reed National Military Medical Center has developed the Healing Arts Program, which seeks to treat psychologic health issues through creative avenues including art therapy (Cronk, 2012).

Animal-Assisted Therapy

The use of animals for therapeutic purposes for patients suffering from chronic or acute illness has been documented since the 1800s (Velde et al., 2005). In 1986, the U.S. Army surgeon general appointed a human–animal bond adviser, who has implemented numerous animal-assisted activities and animal-assisted therapy in the DoD. Only animal-assisted therapy specifies the animal as a crucial part of the therapy aimed at improving patient function and has been well documented and evaluated. Animal-assisted therapy programs are run through volunteer organizations or through the support of Vet Centers and are available in diverse locations. Therapy dogs are used in combat and operational stress control activities and also as service animals for wounded service members and veterans. Several organizations, including the Walter Reed Army Medical Center Warrior Transition Battalion, encourage returned service members to train dogs as service animals for other veterans. The presence of a service animal encourages socialization and comforts the patient, disrupting the emotional numbing, hyperarousal, and avoidance that are common symptoms of PTSD, but there are also benefits to the trainer, including learning new skills, developing an emotional bond with the animal, and fulfilling the "warrior ethos" of helping fellow service members who are in need (Ritchie, 2011).

Other animals have also been used for psychotherapy. Horses have been used for animal-assisted activities and animal-assisted therapy, and there is growing evidence of their effectiveness as adjuvants to mental health care in equine-facilitated or equine-assisted psychotherapy. However, very few papers have reviewed equine-facilitated or equine-assisted psychotherapy in the treatment of PTSD, and no RCTs have evaluated its use (Cantin and Marshall-Lucette, 2011; Lentini and Knox, 2009). Dolphins have also been used in animal-facilitated therapy to treat depression and anxiety, but not PTSD specifically. Antonioli and Reveley (2005) conducted an RCT comparing animal-facilitated therapy with dolphins (education, interaction, and care of the dolphins) with an outdoor nature program control group. The dolphin care program resulted in significantly higher decreases in the Beck depression inventory and the Hamilton rating scale for depression than the control program.

Other Somatic Treatments

Electroconvulsive Therapy

Electroconvulsive therapy uses electricity to induce seizures in the brain of an anesthetized patient (Rudorfer et al., 2003). Two reports in the VA/DoD guideline suggest its benefit in PTSD. One open-label outpatient trial of 20 patients who had treatment-refractory PTSD found that a course of six bilateral treatments achieved a 40% reduction in PTSD symptom severity that was maintained at 6-month follow-up (Margoob et al., 2010). A retrospective chart review found that 12 patients who had PTSD and depression responded partially, that is, depressive but not PTSD symptoms improved after electroconvulsive therapy (Watts, 2007).

Repetitive Transcranial Magnetic Stimulation (rTMS)

In repetitive transcranial magnetic stimulation (rTMS), electromagnets are used to induce cortical neurons in the brain to fire (Cohen et al., 2004). Four studies have assessed rTMS in patients who had PTSD. Three were RCTs, but they used rTMS at different doses, varied laterality (left or right sides of the brain), and varied numbers of treatment applications. Also, few of the subjects were veterans.

In the first RCT, a three-group, 30-patient, double-blind, sham-controlled trial, right- and left-sided 20-Hz rTMS applied to the dorsolateral prefrontal cortex both outperformed the control immediately and at a 3-month follow-up, and right-sided TMS was significantly better than left-sided TMS. Further, it was not associated with worsening of cognitive function (Boggio et al., 2010). In another RCT, Cohen et al. (2004) administered 10-Hz rTMS and found significantly greater benefit than control in re-experiencing and avoidance symptoms. Such et al. (2009) administered either 5-Hz rTMS or placebo in a randomized crossover design in which rTMS was given in combination with exposure therapy and antidepressants to nine patients. In this small and underpowered sample, rTMS showed improvement only in hyperarousal symptoms. In an open-label and non-controlled trial, Rosenberg et al. (2002) reported a benefit of rTMS only for depression in 12 patients who also had PTSD.

On the basis of those findings, the VA/DoD guideline concludes there is sufficient evidence to recommend use of rTMS in treatment for PTSD. It is not known which frequency produces the best response, whether the laterality of treatment (right or left) is important, and what the optimal number of treatments is.

Vagal Nerve Stimulation

There is a single report on vagal nerve stimulation, whereby the brain stem is stimulated through electric current applied to the vagus nerve in the neck (George and Aston-Jones, 2010). Vagal nerve stimulation was given as open-label treatment to two patients that were treatment resistant (George et al., 2008). Four years after implantation, one of the patients was still receiving vagal nerve stimulation and had sustained improvement compared with baseline. Although there was some evidence of acute and long-term improvement in these patients, no recommendation can be made regarding vagal nerve stimulation for PTSD.

Hyperbaric Oxygen

A preliminary study of low-pressure hyperbaric oxygen therapy (HBOT) was conducted in 16 veterans who had chronic blast-induced mild to moderate traumatic brain injury and PTSD. HBOT is administered in a total-body chamber in which the patient breathes pure oxygen at greater than atmospheric pressure, encouraging the dissolution of oxygen in the body's fluids and tissues to aid healing (Harch et al., 2007). Results indicated that 40 therapy sessions in 1 month were safe and that there were significant improvements in both postconcussive syndrome and PTSD symptoms (Harch et al., 2012). Those findings, however, must be viewed within the context of the history of HBOT in the treatment of other central nervous system conditions.

Over the past 40 years, small clinical series and individual practitioner experiences have variously led to claims that HBOT was beneficial in the treatment of stroke, dementia, anoxic encephalopathy, multiple sclerosis, and other conditions (for example, Barnes et al., 1987). However, clinical trials have failed to substantiate the claims (for example, Kindwall et al., 1991). Conversely, substantial evidence documents the benefit of HBOT in the delayed treatment of central nervous system decompression sickness (Kizer, 1982). Notwithstanding the challenges in conducting controlled clinical trials of HBOT, such studies will be essential for determining whether this treatment is effective for PTSD.

Conclusions Regarding Other Somatic Treatments

The VA/DoD guideline indicates that electroconvulsive therapy may be considered as an alternative in chronic, severe, medication- and psychotherapy-resistant PTSD—level of evidence II-3 and II-2, fair quality of evidence, and strength of recommendation B. The level of evidence supporting the use of rTMS varies between I and III—generally fair or good quality of evidence and the strength of recommendation B.

GUIDELINES FOR TREATMENT OF PTSD

A number of treatment guidelines for PTSD have been published, some aiming at informing clinicians in general in a given country (such as the United States, the United Kingdom, or Australia), others aiming to inform practice in a specific health system (such as the VA and DoD). This section reviews guidelines issued by the VA and the DoD, the APA, the UK NICE, the Australian National Health and Medical Research Council (NHMRC), and the ISTSS. Table 7-1 (at the end of this section) provides a visual comparison of treatment recommendations of those guidelines with their levels of evidence or rating systems. A summary of the rating systems used by various organizations for PTSD treatment may be found in the review by Forbes et al. (2010). The committee did not evaluate the rating system or evidence base for each guideline. At the very least, the committee believes mental health care providers in the DoD and the VA should adhere to their own guideline for the management of PTSD in service members and veterans, respectively.

VA/DoD Clinical Practice Guideline for Management of Post-Traumatic Stress

This guideline, issued in 2010, constitutes an update of the 2004 guideline (VA and DoD, 2004, 2010). The VA Office of Quality Performance and the Office of Patient Care Services and the DoD Army Medical Command selected clinical leaders in primary care, psychiatry, psychology, internal medicine, pharmacology, nursing, and social work to be members of the working group that developed the guideline. The working group supervised a literature review of all PTSD treatment studies from January 2002 to August 2009 and used the results of the review and the ISTSS and APA guideline to come up with the 2010 guideline.

A five-point rating system—*A, B, C, D,* and *I*—was used to indicate the strength of recommendations; the ratings were based on the literature review and on expert consensus. *A* was the highest rating and indicated there was good evidence that the intervention in question improved outcomes. A rating of *B* indicated a fair amount of evidence supported the use of the intervention in question. A rating of *C* indicated that the working group did not make a recommendation for or against the routine use of the intervention inasmuch as the benefit–risk ratio was too close to make a general recommendation. A rating of *D* indicated the presence of evidence that either the intervention was harmful or the risks outweighed the benefits offered by it. Finally, *I* indicated evidence was lacking, of insufficient quality, or conflicting; therefore, a recommendation could not be made for or against providing the treatment routinely. The working group also included a set of algorithms oriented to the initial point of contact being a primary care or a mental health setting in a VA or DoD context.

The working group recommended that initial treatment include both psychotherapy and pharmacotherapy. It also cautioned against the use of psychologic debriefing immediately after a traumatic event.

The guideline recommends evidence-based psychotherapeutic interventions for PTSD that are most strongly supported by RCTs: those interventions are broadly categorized as trauma-focused psychotherapy or stress inoculation training (VA and DoD, 2010). Trauma-focused psychotherapies commonly involve exposure or cognitive restructuring (for example, PE, CPT, and EMDR), and they may be combined with anxiety management, stress reduction skills, and psychoeducation. The guideline states that other CBT interventions that are not trauma focused are less effective. The working group noted that therapy provided in clinical trial settings differs from therapy practiced in day-to-day care, and the recommendations in the guideline represent the techniques and protocols as reported in the RCTs.

Although benzodiazepines have historically been used as effective treatments for anxiety and insomnia, the guideline recommends against their use as preventive measures "due to lack of evidence for effectiveness and risks that may outweigh potential benefits." Studies with propranolol have had mixed results, and overall the VA/DoD guideline concluded that despite some positive results, "the size and weak study designs of the investigations do not allow for definitive conclusions regarding the value of these medications in preventing the development of PTSD symptoms after traumatic events."

The VA/DoD 2010 guideline states that "there is insufficient evidence to draw concrete conclusions or make specific recommendations regarding the use of pharmacological agents for prevention of PTSD." The guideline further concludes that there is insufficient evidence to recommend the use of CAM approaches as a first-line treatment for PTSD; however, it states that CAM approaches may be considered as adjunctive treatments for specific symptoms of PTSD such as relaxation techniques (for example, yoga and massage) for hyperarousal and for comorbid conditions, such as using acupuncture for the management of chronic pain.

The committee notes that new policy guidance on assessment and treatment of PTSD issued by the U.S. Army (2012) on the use of atypical antipsychotics and benzodiazepines requires that health care providers who prescribe these drugs must clearly document their rationale for using them in the patient's medical record and must obtain informed consent from the patient. The guidance also states that clinicians should use the 2010 VA/DoD guideline when treating patients with symptoms of traumatic stress.

American Psychiatric Association Guideline

The APA published *Practice Guideline for the Treatment of Patients with Acute Stress Disorder and Posttraumatic Stress Disorder* in October 2004 and followed it with a *Guideline Watch* in March 2009, which updated the research review of PTSD treatments. The guideline was developed by a work group that consisted primarily of psychiatrists. In a review of the different PTSD guidelines, Forbes et al. (2010) noted that although the group developed evidence tables that summarized studies, it did not present clear concluding statements for each of the treatments that it assessed.

The work group used a three-point coding system—*I*, *II*, and *III*—to identify treatments. *I* indicated a recommendation with substantial clinical confidence; *II*, with moderate clinical confidence; and *III*, on the basis of individual circumstances. The ratings were based on a review of the treatment literature and expert consensus.

The APA guideline and the *Guideline Watch* recommend three potential treatment approaches for PTSD, either alone or in combination: education and support, psychotherapy, and pharmacotherapy. The guideline states that "the therapist should first exhaust the treatments for which there is the best evidence of efficacy before trying more novel treatments." Furthermore, the response to treatment may be affected by trauma type and timing of the treatment after the traumatic event.

The guideline recommends CBT as an effective treatment for core symptoms of acute and chronic PTSD. Other recommended psychotherapies include EMDR, stress inoculation, imagery rehearsal, and PE for treatment of PTSD and PTSD-associated symptoms such as anxiety and avoidance. The guideline notes that all of these treatments share an element of controlled exposure and that this may be the critical intervention.

The APA guideline (APA, 2004; Benedek et al., 2009) recommend SSRI and SNRI antidepressants as the drugs of first choice on the grounds that they reduce all core symptom clusters of PTSD and important associated symptoms (such as suicidality, impulsivity, and aggression) and several common comorbid disorders (such as panic and depression). The guideline mentions, however, a series of five negative SSRI–SNRI trials in U.S. samples of combat veterans. Only one small study of nefazodone proved positive. The tricyclic drugs imipramine and amitryptline and the MAOI phenelzine are recommended as backup approaches, but these drugs have greater toxicity. The three positive trials of these drugs were all carried out in U.S. World War II and Vietnam veterans who had combat-related PTSD, and this suggests a possible role for the older antidepressants in nonresponders.

UK National Institute of Health and Clinical Excellence Guideline

The UK NICE guideline for PTSD was developed by the National Collaborating Center for Mental Health and issued in 2005 (NECMH and NICE, 2005). The guideline development group was focused on informing policy and practice primarily through evidence-based recommendations, and thus, considered treatments that had demonstrated efficacy. The group first developed a scope document that set out specific criteria for the guideline (such as population to be focused on and types of treatments to review), so the final guideline would be applicable to the British National Health System as a whole and cover generally available therapies. A set of research questions was developed (for example, "For adults with PTSD, does any psychological intervention confer any advantage over other psychological interventions?") to determine the current state of evidence supporting specific PTSD interventions. Using the questions as guidance, a group separate from the guideline development group reviewed RCTs and conducted formal meta-analyses. Effect sizes for clinical effectiveness were determined, as were relative risk ratios to represent clinically significant differences. The guideline development group then used that information to produce evidence statements.

The guideline development group established a four-point rating system—*A*, *B*, *C*, and *GPP*—that was based on the level of empirical support available for a given treatment. An *A* rating indicated the intervention was supported by a consistent body of evidence, including at least one RCT. A *B* rating indicated the treatment was supported by well-conducted clinical trials but that no RCTs had tested the intervention. A *C* rating indicated the treatment was supported by expert committee reports or opinion but that good clinical studies were absent. Finally, a *GPP* (good practice point) rating indicated the treatment was considered good practice by the guideline development group.

The guideline development group also recommended that a trauma-focused psychotherapeutic intervention be considered initially, not pharmacologic interventions. And it recommended against single-session psychotherapy interventions that focus on the trauma in the aftermath of a trauma.

The guideline states that using the criterion for a clinically important effect, the drug treatments were disappointing. Although there are a number of RCTs that met the inclusion criteria, they had relatively small samples and needed to be interpreted with some caution. These RCTs suggest there may be a clinically important effect for mirtazapine, amitriptyline, and the MAOI antidepressants phenelzine and brofaromine. The guideline recommends paroxetine on the basis of robust data although it did not meet the criterion of a clinically significant effect. The guideline is similar to the Australian guideline with respect to recommendations for pharmacotherapy for PTSD and essentially reaches the same conclusions, albeit with some differences in the specific drugs that are recommended.

Australian National Health and Medical Research Council Guidelines

The *Australian Guidelines for the Treatment of Adults with Acute Stress Disorder and Posttraumatic Stress Disorder* were published by the Australian Centre for Posttraumatic Mental Health (NHMRC, 2007). The guideline development group consisted of trauma experts in Australia who worked in consultation with a multidisciplinary group consisting of professionals who worked with people who had PTSD. In an approach similar to that of the group that developed the NICE guideline, the group started with a series of 18 research questions (for example, "For adults with PTSD, is the combination of individual therapy and group therapy more effective than either alone?") that an outside group, Adelaide Health Technology Assessment, used as the basis of a systematic review of RCTs. The guideline development group also drew on the reviews conducted by NICE (2005) and by the VA and the DoD (2004). Again, as in the case of the NICE guidelines, formal meta-analyses were conducted, effect sizes for clinical effectiveness were determined, and relative risk ratios were calculated to represent clinically significant differences.

The guideline development group made recommendations based on a five-point scale—*A*, *B*, *C*, *D*, and *GPP*—with *A* indicating that a treatment had the strongest evidence supporting its use and *D* indicating that a treatment had very weak evidence supporting its use. Treatments deemed to be effective on the basis of expert consensus opinion despite lacking empirical evidence were rated *GPP* (good practice point). Like the NICE guideline group, the Australian group recommended that a trauma-focused psychotherapeutic intervention be considered the first line of treatment, not pharmacologic interventions. The group also recommended against offering psychologic debriefing and other structured psychosocial interventions in the wake of a traumatic event. Although this guideline favors psychotherapy as the first-line treatment for PTSD, it outlines a number of clinical scenarios in which use of an antidepressant is warranted and indicates a preference for SSRIs in such circumstances.

In interpreting the Australian guideline, it is important to point out that the guideline development committee used idiosyncratic criteria to define remission (which was regarded as synonymous with failing to meet the diagnostic criteria for PTSD) and then failed to include response or remission rates as an outcome even though these have traditionally been key measures in psychopharmacology studies.

International Society for Traumatic Stress Studies Guidelines

A group of PTSD treatment experts developed a set of PTSD treatment guidelines, *Effective Treatments for PTSD: Second Edition*, for ISTSS, a group of practitioners in different disciplines, which were issued in 2009. The focus of the guidelines was on identifying any evidence available to support the use of numerous psychotherapeutic and psychopharmacologic treatments for PTSD that were currently in use. Different working groups focused on specific intervention categories and developed evidence summaries. Forbes et al. (2010) note that although some working groups included evidence tables, information on the methods used to review the literature, and treatment effect sizes, this was not done uniformly by all the groups.

The working groups used a six-point scale—*A*, *B*, *C*, *D*, *E*, and *F*—to grade the strength of evidence available for each intervention. A grade of *A* indicated that evidence for a particular treatment was based on RCTs, *B* indicated evidence was based on well-designed studies without randomization or placebo comparison, *C* indicated evidence was based on naturalistic clinical studies and clinical observations, *D* indicated evidence was based on long-standing and widespread clinical practice that had yet to be tested empirically, *E* indicated evidence was based on long-standing practice by a selected group of clinicians that had not been tested empirically, and *F* indicated a treatment was new and had not been tested empirically.

Although the authors of the guidelines did not provide recommendations on which treatments should be considered first-line, they did recommend that psychopharmacologic treatment should be considered if CBT were not available or should be used in combination with CBT. Furthermore, the ISTSS guidelines did not recommend psychologic debriefing immediately after a traumatic event.

Summary of Guidelines

There are many similarities among the recommendations of the reviewed guidelines as shown in Table 7-1. All the guidelines strongly support the use of trauma-focused psychologic treatment for PTSD in adults and children with an emphasis on trauma-focused CBT, such as PE and CT. All but one of the guidelines recommended against the use of psychologic debriefing soon after exposure to trauma.

TABLE 7-1 Treatment Guideline Categorizations for PTSD

Treatment Modality	VA/DoD	APA	NICE	NHMRC	ISTSS
Psychotherapy					
Exposure therapy	A	I			A
Prolonged exposure	A	I		A	A
Virtual reality exposure					
Other exposure therapies					
Cognitive-based therapies	A	I	A	A	A
Trauma-focused cognitive	A			A	A
Behavioral therapy	I				
Cognitive processing therapy					
Internet-based	I				
Eye movement desensitization and reprocessing	A	II	A	A (with in vivo exposure)	A
Stress inoculation training	A	II			A
Group therapy	C	III			
Hypnosis	C				
Imagery rehearsal therapies	C	II			
Psychodynamic psychotherapy	C	II		C (stress management)	D
Patient education	C				
Relaxation	C				
Dialectic behavioral Therapy	I				
Acceptance and commitment therapy	I				
Family therapy	I				

TABLE 7-1 Continued

Treatment Modality	VA/DoD	APA	NICE	NHMRC	ISTSS
Pharmacotherapy					
Antidepressants					
SSRI	A	I	B	B	A
SNRI	A	I			A
	B	II	B	B	A
	B	III	B	B	A
	D				A
Tricyclic and MOAIs					
Mirtazapine					
Nefazodone					
Anticonvulsants	D	III			Not efficacious
Antipsychotics					
Conventional	I				
Atypical	B (as adjunct) I (as monotherapy)	III			A (as adjunct) C (quetiapine)
Benzodiazepines and GABAerigic drugs	D (benzodiazepine)	III			Not efficacious
Antiadrenergic drugs		III			
Prazosin	B (for sleep); C (for global PTSD)				
Guanfacine					
Clonidine	D				Not efficacious
	I				
Other drugs					
Busprione	I				
Nonbenzodiazepine hypnotics	I				
Bupropion	I	Not endorsed		C	
Trazodone	I			C	
Gabapentin	I			Not efficacious	
Lamotrigine	I				
Propranolol	I	II		Not efficacious	
D-cycloserine					
Complementary and alternative medicines	I				

NOTE: See discussion of each guideline for an explanation of category codes and specific therapies in each treatment modality. MAOI = monoamine oxidase inhibitor; SNRI = serotonin norepinephrine reuptake inhibitor; SSRI = selective serotonin reuptake inhibitor.

Key differences among the guidelines are the extent to which expert consensus contributed to the strength of the recommendation rating and the kind of the literature reviewed (only RCTs vs. all PTSD-treatment studies). Some guidelines were more stringent in what studies were allowed in their review (NICE and NHMRC examined only RCTs) and gave high recommendations to a small number of treatments (predominantly trauma-focused psychotherapies). Other guidelines (such as ISTSS, APA, and VA/DoD) were more expansive in their review of the literature and incorporated clinical consensus into their recommendations; this resulted in more (admittedly muted) recommendations for other types of therapy, such as IRT in the case of VA/DoD and APA.

One example of the variation in the guidelines assessment of a specific therapy is EMDR. EMDR was given the highest rating in all but one of the guidelines. The APA guideline was the only one that did not accord EMDR the highest rating, instead giving it a second-tier rating. Forbes et al. (2010) noted that what contributed to that difference was how the absence of support for the use of eye movements in EMDR was addressed. The other guidelines used effect sizes to determine the effectiveness and significance of EMDR, but the APA work group took into account the lack of empirical support for the use of eye movements when determining their recommendations. The NHMRC guidelines stated that EMDR should be considered a first-line treatment only if it included in vivo exposure. Forbes et al. (2010) note that such an approach questions when it is justified to engage in focused analyses and whether it is unfair to subject one type of intervention and not another to such analysis.

Other Organizational Reviews of Pharmacotherapy for PTSD

Institute of Medicine Report

The 2008 IOM report on treatment for PTSD concluded that the evidence was inadequate to determine the efficacy of SSRIs and all other drug categories in PTSD. However, one committee member (the expert in psychopharmacology) dissented from that view and indicated that, in his opinion, the evidence in favor of SSRI monotherapy was suggestive of efficacy in the general population, but not male veterans, with chronic PTSD. For atypical antipsychotics, he believed the evidence was also suggestive of efficacy for this add-on treatment.

The committee further found there was sufficient evidence on the basis of RCTs of the efficacy of exposure therapy to treat PTSD, but that there was inadequate evidence for the efficacy of EMDR, cognitive restructuring, and coping skills training. The committee also concluded there was inadequate evidence on the efficacy of therapy delivered in a group format.

International Psychopharmacology Algorithms

In 2005, an international group of PTSD academicians prepared an evidence-based set of stepwise clinical decisions for PTSD with specific reference to different clinical situations, such as suicidal patients, substance abusers, people who had bipolar disorder, pregnant women, and litigation. It recommended medications and dosing (Connor and Stein, 2005; Davidson et al., 2005a; IPAP, 2005; Stowe and Newport, 2005). The algorithms are unique in addressing whether, when, and how to stop a drug, switch drugs, augment or change a dosage, and manage PTSD in women of childbearing potential.

Other Authorities

The British Association of Psychopharmacology (2005), the World Federation of Societies of Biological Psychiatry (2008), and the Canadian Psychiatric Association (2006) all recommend the choice of an SSRI or SNRI antidepressant as first-line therapy if pharmacotherapy is to be used for chronic PTSD. The drugs are fluoxetine, paroxetine, sertraline, and venlafaxine-extended release.

SUMMARY

There are numerous psychosocial treatments for PTSD, many of which are variants of evidence-based treatments, such as exposure therapy and cognitive therapy. On a whole, the efficacy of these treatments has been limited to pretreatment and posttreatment self-reported assessments, which makes interpretation of the outcomes difficult. The frequent lack of control groups in efficacy studies means that reductions in PTSD symptoms may be due to factors unrelated to the treatment under investigation such as repeated assessment, passage of time, and expectation that being in a treatment is helpful. There are also several effective pharmacotherapies for treating PTSD, particularly SSRIs.

Overall, group-based CBT treatment for individuals diagnosed with PTSD is associated with improvements in symptoms of PTSD, but in general, the outcome is not as good as that found in individual therapy (Schnurr et al., 2003). One study is examining the efficacy of group versus individual CPT in active-duty military personnel, but results are not yet available. Although cognitive behavioral treatments have been studied extensively in the treatment of PTSD, there are still areas that need to be investigated. These areas include how to increase the immediate and long-term efficacy and efficiency of existing treatments; how to deliver effective treatments in fewer sessions; the use of pharmacological agents such as DCS to enhance inhibitory learning during exposure; and the use of other agents such as yohimbine as possible adjuncts to exposure therapies. Researchers are also challenged by the fact that some patients who improved with CBT have shown various degrees of relapse, and this suggests that treatments do not eradicate the trauma memories. Other areas for research include ways to improve the training in and use of recommended PTSD treatments throughout the DoD and the VA.

Currently, there is a lack of empirical evidence that supports CAM approaches to treat for PTSD. The most substantial evidence comes from studies of yoga, contemplative treatments, and acupuncture, but there are still few RCTs. Where the evidence is suggestive, as for yoga and acupuncture, there is considerable debate as to what particular approach is most effective. There is a considerable amount of work being done to find new approaches for delivering evidence-based treatments for PTSD to service members, veterans, and their families, including group and couple therapy and telemental health and Internet-based therapies. If these treatment delivery methods are beneficial, they may be used to reach service members and veterans who might otherwise not have access to mental health care because of location, timing, or other concerns. In Chapter 9 the committee discusses barriers for disseminating effective treatments and possible ways to overcome them.

REFERENCES

Abramowitz, E. G., Y. Barak, I. Ben-Avi, and H. Y. Knobler. 2008. Hypnotherapy in the treatment of chronic combat-related PTSD patients suffering from insomnia: A randomized, zolpidem-controlled clinical trial. *International Journal of Clinical and Experimental Hypnosis* 56(3):270-280.

Ahamdy, K., G. Karami, S. Noohi, A. Mokhtari, H. Gholampour, and A.-A. Rahimi. 2009. The efficacy of cognitive behavioral couple's therapy (CBCT) on marital adjustment of PTSD–diagnosed combat veterans. *Europe's Journal of Psychology* 5(2).

Antonioli, C., and M. A. Reveley. 2005. Randomised controlled trial of animal facilitated therapy with dolphins in the treatment of depression. *British Medical Journal* 331(7527): 1231-1234.

APA (American Psychiatric Association). 2004. *Practice guideline for the treatment of patients with acute stress disorder and posttraumatic stress disorder.* Washington, DC: American Psychiatric Association.

Arntz, A., M. Tiesema, and M. Kindt. 2007. Treatment of PTSD: A comparison of imaginal exposure with and without imagery rescripting. *Journal of Behavior Therapy & Experimental Psychiatry* 38(4):345-370.

Asukai, N., A. Saito, N. Tsuruta, J. Kishimoto, and T. Nishikawa. 2010. Efficacy of exposure therapy for Japanese patients with posttraumatic stress disorder due to mixed traumatic events: A randomized controlled study. *Journal of Traumatic Stress* 23(6):744-750.

Avrahami, D. 2005. Visual art therapy's unique contribution in the treatment of post-traumatic stress disorders. *Journal of Trauma & Dissociation* 6(4):5-38.

Baker, D. G., B. I. Diamond, G. Gillette, M. Hamner, D. Katzelnick, T. Keller, T. A. Mellman, E. Pontius, M. Rosenthal, P. Tucker, B. A. vander Kolk, and R. Katz. 1995. A double-blind, randomized, placebo-controlled, multi-center study of brofaromine in the treatment of post-traumatic stress disorder. *Psychopharmacology* 122(4):386-389.

Barlow, D. H., J. M. Gorman, M. K. Shear, and S. W. Woods. 2000. Cognitive-behavioral therapy, imipramine, or their combination for panic disorder: A randomized controlled trial. *Journal of the American Medical Association* 283(19):2529-2536.

Barnes, M. P., D. Bates, N. E. F. Cartlidge, J. M. French, and D. A. Shaw. 1987. Hyperbaric-oxygen and multiple-sclerosis—final results of a placebo-controlled, double-blind trial. *Journal of Neurology Neurosurgery and Psychiatry* 50(11):1402-1406.

Bartzokis, G., P. H. Lu, J. Turner, J. Mintz, and C. S. Saunders. 2005. Adjunctive risperidone in the treatment of chronic combat-related posttraumatic stress disorder. *Biological Psychiatry* 57(5):474-479.

Bear, M. F. 1996. A synaptic basis for memory storage in the cerebral cortex. *Proceedings of the National Academy of Sciences of the United States of America* 93(24):13453-13459.

Beck, A. T., G. Emery, and R. L. Greenberg. 2005. *Anxiety disorders and phobias: A cognitive perspective.* 15th anniversary ed. Cambridge, MA: Basic Books.

Beck, J. G., S. F. Coffey, D. W. Foy, T. M. Keane, and E. B. Blanchard. 2009. Group cognitive behavior therapy for chronic posttraumatic stress disorder: An initial randomized pilot study. *Behavior Therapy* 40(1):82-92.

Becker, M. E., M. A. Hertzberg, S. D. Moore, M. F. Dennis, D. S. Bukenya, and J. C. Beckham. 2007. A placebo-controlled trial of bupropion-SR in the treatment of chronic posttraumatic stress disorder. *Journal of Clinical Psychopharmacology* 27(2):193-197.

Benedek, D., M. Friedman, D. Zatzick, and R. Ursano. 2009. *Guideline watch (March 2009): Practice guideline for the treatment of patients with acute stress disorder and posttraumatic stress disorder.* Washington, DC: American Psychiatric Association.

Bisson, J., and M. Andrew. 2007. Psychological treatments of post-traumatic stress disorder (PTSD). *Cochrane Database Systematic Reviews* 18(3).

Blanchard, E. B., E. J. Hickling, T. Devineni, C. H. Veazey, T. E. Galovski, E. Mundy, L. S. Malta, and T. C. Buckley. 2003. A controlled evaluation of cognitive behavioural therapy for posttraumatic stress in motor vehicle accident survivors. *Behaviour Research and Therapy* 41(1):79-96.

Blanco, C., R. G. Heimberg, F. R. Schneier, D. M. Fresco, H. Chen, C. L. Turk, D. Vermes, B. A. Erwin, A. B. Schmidt, H. R. Juster, R. Campeas, and M. R. Liebowitz. 2010. A placebo-controlled trial of phenelzine, cognitive behavioral therapy, and their combination for social anxiety disorder. *Archives of General Psychiatry* 67(3):286-295.

Boggio, P. S., M. Rocha, M. O. Oliveira, S. Fecteau, R. B. Cohen, C. Campanha, E. Ferreira-Santos, A. Meleiro, F. Corchs, S. Zaghi, A. Pascual-Leone, and F. Fregni. 2010. Non-invasive brain stimulation with high-frequency and low-intensity repetitive transcranial magnetic stimulation treatment for posttraumatic stress disorder. *Journal of Clinical Psychiatry* 71(8):992-999.

Bormann, J. E., T. L. Smith, S. Becker, M. Gershwin, L. Pada, A. H. Grudzinski, and E. A. Nurmi. 2005. Efficacy of frequent mantram repetition on stress, quality of life, and spiritual well-being in veterans: A pilot study. *Journal of Holistic Nursing* 23(4):395-414.

Bormann, J. E., S. Thorp, J. L. Wetherell, and S. Golshan. 2008. A spiritually based group intervention for combat veterans with posttraumatic stress disorder: Feasibility study. *Journal of Holistic Nursing* 26(2):109-116.

Boudewyns, P. A., and L. Hyer. 1990. Physiological-response to combat memories and preliminary treatment outcome in Vietnam veteran PTSD patients treated with direct therapeutic exposure. *Behavior Therapy* 21(1):63-87.

Bouton, M. E., F. A. Kennedy, and C. Rosengard. 1990. State-dependent fear extinction with two benzodiazepine tranquilizers. *Behavioral Neuroscience* 104(1):44-55.

Bower, P., S. Gilbody, D. Richards, J. Fletcher, and A. Sutton. 2006. Collaborative care for depression in primary care—making sense of a complex intervention: Systematic review and meta-regression. *British Journal of Psychiatry* 189:484-493.

Bradley, R., J. Greene, E. Russ, L. Dutra, and D. Westen. 2005. A multidimensional meta-analysis of psychotherapy for PTSD. *American Journal of Psychiatry* 162(2):214-227.

Brady, K., T. Pearlstein, G. M. Asnis, D. Baker, B. Rothbaum, C. R. Sikes, and G. M. Farfel. 2000. Efficacy and safety of sertraline treatment of posttraumatic stress disorder: A randomized controlled trial. *Journal of the American Medical Association* 283(14):1837-1844.

Brady, K. T., S. Sonne, R. F. Anton, C. L. Randall, S. E. Back, and K. Simpson. 2005. Sertraline in the treatment of co-occurring alcohol dependence and posttraumatic stress disorder. *Alcoholism: Clinical & Experimental Research* 29(3):395-401.

Braun, P., D. Greenberg, H. Dasberg, and B. Lerer. 1990. Core symptoms of posttraumatic-stress-disorder unimproved by alprazolam treatment. *Journal of Clinical Psychiatry* 51(6):236-238.

Brewin, C. R., B. Andrews, and J. D. Valentine. 2000. Meta-analysis of risk factors for post-traumatic stress disorder in trauma-exposed adults. *Journal of Consulting and Clinical Psychology* 68(5):748-766.

British Association of Psychopharmacology, D. S. Baldwin, I. M. Anderson, D. J. Nutt, B. Bandelow, A. Bond, J. R. T. Davidson, J. A. Den Boer, N. A. Fineberg, M. Knapp, J. Scott, and H. U. Wittchen. 2005. Evidence-based guidelines for the pharmacological treatment of anxiety disorders: Recommendations from the British Association for Psychopharmacology. *Journal of Psychopharmacology* 19(6):567-596.

Brom, D., R. J. Kleber, and P. B. Defares. 1989. Brief psychotherapy for posttraumatic stress disorders. *Journal of Consulting & Clinical Psychology* 57(5):607-612.

Brooks, J., and T. Scarano. 1985. Transcendental meditation in the treatment of post-Vietnam adjustment. *Journal of Counseling and Development* 64:212-215.

Brown, R. P., and P. L. Gerbarg. 2005. Sudarshan kriya yogic breathing in the treatment of stress, anxiety, and depression. Part II—clinical applications and guidelines. *Journal of Alternative & Complementary Medicine* 11(4):711-717.

Brown, R. P., and P. L. Gerbarg. 2009. Yoga breathing, meditation, and longevity. *Annals of the New York Academy of Sciences* 1172:54-62.

Bruce, M. L., T. R. Ten Have, C. F. Reynolds, I. I. Katz, H. C. Schulberg, B. H. Mulsant, G. K. Brown, G. J. McAvay, J. L. Pearson, and G. S. Alexopoulos. 2004. Reducing suicidal ideation and depressive symptoms in depressed older primary care patients—a randomized controlled trial. *Journal of the American Medical Association* 291(9):1081-1091.

Bryant, R. A., T. Sackville, S. T. Dang, M. Moulds, and R. Guthrie. 1999. Treating acute stress disorder: An evaluation of cognitive behavior therapy and supportive counseling techniques. *American Journal of Psychiatry* 156(11):1780-1786.

Bryant, R. A., M. L. Moulds, and R. V. D. Nixon. 2003. Cognitive behaviour therapy of acute stress disorder: A four-year follow-up. *Behaviour Research and Therapy* 41(4):489-494.

Bryant, R. A., M. L. Moulds, R. M. Guthrie, S. T. Dang, J. Mastrodomenico, R. D. V. Nixon, K. L. Felmingham, S. Hopwood, and M. Creamer. 2008. A randomized controlled trial of exposure therapy and cognitive restructuring for posttraumatic stress disorder. *Journal of Consulting and Clinical Psychology* 76(4):695-703.

Butterfield, M. I., M. E. Becker, K. M. Connor, S. Sutherland, L. E. Churchill, and J. R. Davidson. 2001. Olanzapine in the treatment of post-traumatic stress disorder: A pilot study. *International Clinical Psychopharmacology* 16(4):197-203.

Cahill, S. P., B. O. Rothbaum, P. A. Resick, and V. M. Follette. 2009. Cognitive behavioral therapy for adults. In *Effective treatments for PTSD: Practice guidelines from the International Society for Traumatic Stress Studies*, edited by E. B. Foa, T. M. Keane, M. J. Friedman, and J. A. Cohen, 2nd ed. New York: Guilford Press.

Callahan, R. J. 2001a. The impact of thought field therapy on heart rate variability. *Journal of Clinical Psychology* 57(10):1153-1170.

Callahan, R. J. 2001b. Raising and lowering of heart rate variability: Some clinical findings of thought field therapy. *Journal of Clinical Psychology* 57(10):1175-1186.

Canadian Psychiatric Association, R. P. Swinson, M. Antony, P. Bleau, P. Chokka, M. Craven, A. Fallu, M. Katzman, K. Kjernisted, R. A. Lanius, D. McIntosh, J. Plamondon, K. Rabheru, M. van Ameringen, and J. R. Walker. 2006. Clinical practice guidelines: Management of anxiety disorders. *Canadian Journal of Psychiatry* 51(Suppl 2).

Canive, J., M. Hamner, L. A. Calais, S. Robert, G. Villareal, V. L. Durkalski, Y. Zhai, and A. Smith. 2009. Quetiapine monotherapy in chronic PTSD: A randomized, double-blind, placebo-controlled trial. Paper read at Collegium Internationale Neuropsychopharmacologicum (CINP) Internationale Thematic Meeting, 24-27 April, Edinburgh, Scotland.

Cantin, A., and S. Marshall-Lucette. 2011. Examining the literature on the efficacy of equine assisted therapy for people with mental health and behavioural disorders. *Mental Health and Learning Disabilities Research and Practice* 8(1):51-61.

Carbonell, J. L., and C.R. Figley 1999. A systematic clinical demonstration of promising PTSD treatment approaches. *Traumatology* 5(1): article 4.

Carter, J. J., and G. G. Byrne. 2006. PTSD Australian Vietnam veterans: Yoga adjunct treatment, two RCT's: MCYI and SKY. Paper read at Proceedings World Conference Expanding Paradigms: Science, Consciousness and Spirituality Proceedings. New Delhi, India.

Cates, M. E., M. H. Bishop, L. L. Davis, J. S. Lowe, and T. W. Woolley. 2004. Clonazepam for treatment of sleep disturbances associated with combat-related posttraumatic stress disorder. *Annals of Pharmacotherapy* 38(9):1395-1399.

Chemtob, C. M., R. W. Novaco, R. S. Hamada, and D. M. Gross. 1997. Cognitive-behavioral treatment for severe anger in posttraumatic stress disorder. *Journal of Consulting and Clinical Psychology* 65(1):184-189.

Choi, D. C., B. O. Rothbaum, M. Gerardi, and K. J. Ressler. 2010. Pharmacological enhancement of behavioral therapy: Focus on posttraumatic stress disorder. *Current Topics in Behavioral Neuroscience* 2:279-299.

Church, D. 2010. The treatment of combat trauma in veterans using EFT (emotional freedom techniques): A pilot protocol. *Traumatology OnlineFirst* 16(1):55-65.

Cloitre, M., K. C. Koenen, L. R. Cohen, and H. Han. 2002. Skills training in affective and interpersonal regulation followed by exposure: A phase-based treatment for PTSD related to childhood abuse. *Journal of Consulting and Clinical Psychology* 70(5):1067-1074.

Cloitre, M., K. C. Stovall-McClough, K. Nooner, P. Zorbas, S. Cherry, C. L. Jackson, W. Gan, and E. Petkova. 2010. Treatment for PTSD related to childhood abuse: A randomized controlled trial. *American Journal of Psychiatry* 167(8):915-924.

Cohen, H., Z. Kaplan, M. Kotler, I. Kouperman, R. Moisa, and N. Grisaru. 2004. Repetitive transcranial magnetic stimulation of the right dorsolateral prefrontal cortex in posttraumatic stress disorder: A double-blind, placebo-controlled study. *American Journal of Psychiatry* 161(3):515-524.

Coll, L. 2002. Homeopathy in survivors of childhood sexual abuse. *Homeopathy: The Journal of the Faculty of Homeopathy* 91(1):3-9.

Collinge, W., R. Wentworth, and S. Sabo. 2005. Integrating complementary therapies into community mental health practice: An exploration. *Journal of Alternative & Complementary Medicine* 11(3):569-574.

Connor, K. M., and D. J. Stein. 2005. Clinical considerations at each stage of evaluation and treatment of trauma survivors and PTSD. *Psychiatric Annals* 35(11):903-909.

Connor, K. M., S. M. Sutherland, L. A. Tupler, M. L. Malik, and J. R. T. Davidson. 1999. Fluoxetine in post-traumatic stress disorder—randomised, double-blind study. *British Journal of Psychiatry* 175:17-22.

Connor, K. M., J. R. T. Davidson, R. H. Weisler, W. Zhang, and K. Abraham. 2006. Tiagabine for posttraumatic stress disorder: Effects of open-label and double-blind discontinuation treatment. *Psychopharmacology* 184(1):21-25.

Cook, J. M., G. C. Harb, P. R. Gehrman, M. S. Cary, G. M. Gamble, D. Forbes, and R. J. Ross. 2010. Imagery rehearsal for posttraumatic nightmares: A randomized controlled trial. *Journal of Traumatic Stress* 23(5):553-563.

Cooper, N. A., and G. A. Clum. 1989. Imaginal flooding as a supplementary treatment for PTSD in combat veterans—a controlled-study. *Behavior Therapy* 20(3):381-391.

Cottraux, J., I. Note, S. N. Yao, C. de Mey-Guillard, F. Bonasse, D. Djamoussian, E. Mollard, B. Note, and Y. H. Chen. 2008. Randomized controlled comparison of cognitive behavior therapy with Rogerian supportive therapy in chronic post-traumatic stress disorder: A 2-year follow-up. *Psychotherapy and Psychosomatics* 77(2):101-110.

Craske, M. G., M. B. Stein, G. Sullivan, C. Sherbourne, A. Bystritsky, R. D. Rose, A. J. Lang, S. Welch, L. Campbell-Sills, D. Golinelli, and P. Roy-Byrne. 2011. Disorder-specific impact of coordinated anxiety learning and management treatment for anxiety disorders in primary care. *Archives of General Psychiatry* 68(4):378-388.

Cronk, T. M. 2012. Therapist uses art to help troops heal. *American Forces Press Service*, March 8, 2012.

Cukor, J., J. Spitalnick, J. Difede, A. Rizzo, B. O. Rothbaum. 2009. Emerging treatments for PTSD. *Clinical Psychology Review* 29(8):715-726.

Davidson, J., H. Kudler, R. Smith, S. L. Mahorney, S. Lipper, E. Hammett, W. B. Saunders, and J. O. Cavenar. 1990. Treatment of posttraumatic-stress-disorder with amitriptyline and placebo. *Archives of General Psychiatry* 47(3):259-266.

Davidson, J., T. Pearlstein, P. Londborg, K. T. Brady, B. Rothbaum, J. Bell, R. Maddock, M. T. Hegel, and G. Farfel. 2001. Efficacy of sertraline in preventing relapse of posttraumatic stress disorder: Results of a 28-week double-blind, placebo-controlled study. *American Journal of Psychiatry* 158(12):1974-1981.

Davidson, J. R. T., R. H. Weisler, M. I. Butterfield, C. D. Casat, K. M. Connor, S. Barnett, and S. van Meter. 2003. Mirtazapine vs. placebo in posttraumatic stress disorder: A pilot trial. *Biological Psychiatry* 53(2):188-191.

Davidson, J., M. Bernik, K. M. Connor, M. J. Friedman, K. O. Jobson, Y. Kim, Y. Lecrubier, H. Ma, F. Njenga, D. J. Stein, and J. Zohar. 2005a. A new treatment algorithm for posttraumatic stress disorder. *Psychiatric Annals* 35(11):887-898.

Davidson, J. R., K. M. Connor, M. A. Hertzberg, R. H. Weisler, W. H. Wilson, and V. M. Payne. 2005b. Maintenance therapy with fluoxetine in posttraumatic stress disorder: A placebo-controlled discontinuation study. *Journal of Clinical Psychopharmacology* 25(2):166-169.

Davidson, J., D. Baldwin, D. J. Stein, E. Kuper, I. Benattia, S. Ahmed, R. Pedersen, and J. Musgnung. 2006a. Treatment of posttraumatic stress disorder with venlafaxine extended release—a 6-month randomized controlled trial. *Archives of General Psychiatry* 63(10):1158-1165.

Davidson, J., B. O. Rothbaum, P. Tucker, G. Asnis, I. Benattia, and J. J. Musgnung. 2006b. Venlafaxine extended release in posttraumatic stress disorder: A sertraline- and placebo-controlled study. *Journal of Clinical Psychopharmacology* 26(3):259-267.

Davidson, J. R., K. Brady, T. A. Mellman, M. B. Stein, and M. H. Pollack. 2007. The efficacy and tolerability of tiagabine in adult patients with post-traumatic stress disorder. *Journal of Clinical Psychopharmacology* 27(1):85-88.

Davidson, P. R., and K. C. H. Parker. 2001. Eye movement desensitization and reprocessing (EMDR): A meta-analysis. *Journal of Consulting and Clinical Psychology* 69(2):305-316.

Davis, L. L., M. E. Jewell, S. Ambrose, J. Farley, B. English, A. Bartolucci, and F. Petty. 2004. A placebo-controlled study of nefazodone for the treatment of chronic posttraumatic stress disorder—a preliminary study. *Journal of Clinical Psychopharmacology* 24(3):291-297.

Davis, L. L., J. R. T. Davidson, L. C. Ward, A. Bartolucci, C. L. Bowden, and F. Petty. 2008a. Divalproex in the treatment of posttraumatic stress disorder: A randomized, double-blind, placebo-controlled trial in a veteran population. *Journal of Clinical Psychopharmacology* 28(1):84-88.

Davis, L. L., C. Ward, A. Rasmusson, J. M. Newell, F. Frazier, and S. M. Southwick. 2008b. A placebo-controlled trial of guanfacine for the treatment of posttraumatic stress disorder in veterans. *Psychopharmacology Bulletin* 41(1):8-18.

Davis, M., K. Ressler, B. O. Rothbaum, and R. Richardson. 2006. Effects of d-cycloserine on extinction: Translation from preclinical to clinical work. *Biological Psychiatry* 60(4): 369-375.

Descilo, T., A. Vedamurtachar, P. L. Gerbarg, D. Nagaraja, B. N. Gangadhar, B. Damodaran, B. Adelson, L. H. Braslow, S. Marcus, and R. P. Brown. 2010. Effects of a yoga breath intervention alone and in combination with an exposure therapy for post-traumatic stress disorder and depression in survivors of the 2004 south-east Asia tsunami. *Acta Psychiatrica Scandinavica* 121(4):289-300.

Difede, J., and H. G. Hoffman. 2002. Virtual reality exposure therapy for World Trade Center post-traumatic stress disorder: A case report. *Cyberpsychology & Behavior* 5(6):529-535.

Difede, J., L. S. Malta, S. Best, C. Henn-Haase, T. Metzler, R. Bryant, and C. Marmar. 2007. A randomized controlled clinical treatment trial for World Trade Center attack-related PTSD in disaster workers. *Journal of Nervous & Mental Disease* 195(10):861-865.

Dobscha, S. K., K. Corson, N. A. Perrin, G. C. Hanson, R. Q. Leibowitz, M. N. Doak, K. C. Dickinson, M. D. Sullivan, and M. S. Gerrity. 2009. Collaborative care for chronic pain in primary care a cluster randomized trial. *Journal of the American Medical Association* 301(12):1242-1252.

Ehlers, A., and D. M. Clark. 2000. A cognitive model of posttraumatic stress disorder. *Behaviour Research & Therapy* 38(4):319-345.

Ehlers, A., D. M. Clark, A. Hackmann, F. McManus, M. Fennell, C. Herbert, and R. Mayou. 2003. A randomized controlled trial of cognitive therapy, a self-help booklet, and repeated assessments as early interventions for posttraumatic stress disorder. *Archives of General Psychiatry* 60(10):1024-1032.

Ehlers, A., D. M. Clark, A. Hackmann, F. McManus, and M. Fennell. 2005. Cognitive therapy for post-traumatic stress disorder: Development and evaluation. *Behaviour Research & Therapy* 43(4):413-431.

Everly, G. S., Jr., and J. M. Lating. 2004. *Personality-guided therapy for posttraumatic stress disorder: Personality-guided psychology.* Washington, DC: American Psychological Association.

Falsetti, S. A., H. S. Resnick, and J. Davis. 2005. Multiple channel exposure therapy—combining cognitive-behavioral therapies for the treatment of posttraumatic stress disorder with panic attacks. *Behavior Modification* 29(1):70-94.

Figley, C. R., J. L. Carbonell, J. A. Boscarino, and J. Chang. 1999. A clinical demonstration model for assessing the effectiveness of therapeutic interventions: An expanded clinical trials methodology. *International Journal of Emergency Mental Health* 1(3):155-164.

Foa, E. B., and S. P. Cahill. 2001. Psychological therapies: Emotional processing. In *International encyclopedia of the social and behavioral sciences*, edited by N. J. Smelser and P. B. Baltes. Amsterdam: Elsevier.

Foa, E. B., and M. J. Kozak. 1986. Emotional processing of fear—exposure to corrective information. *Psychological Bulletin* 99(1):20-35.

Foa, E. B., B. O. Rothbaum, D. S. Riggs, and T. B. Murdock. 1991. Treatment of posttraumatic stress disorder in rape victims: A comparison between cognitive-behavioral procedures and counseling. *Journal of Consulting and Clinical Psychology* 59(5):715-723.

Foa, E. B., D. S. Riggs, C. V. Dancu, and B. O. Rothbaum. 1993. Reliability and validity of a brief instrument for assessing posttraumatic-stress-disorder. *Journal of Traumatic Stress* 6(4):459-473.

Foa, E. B., D. Hearstikeda, and K. J. Perry. 1995. Evaluation of a brief cognitive-behavioral program for the prevention of chronic PTSD in recent assault victims. *Journal of Consulting and Clinical Psychology* 63(6):948-955.

Foa, E. B., C. V. Dancu, E. A. Hembree, L. H. Jaycox, E. A. Meadows, and G. P. Street. 1999a. A comparison of exposure therapy, stress inoculation training, and their combination for reducing posttraumatic stress disorder in female assault victims. *Journal of Consulting & Clinical Psychology* 67(2):194-200.

Foa, E. B., J. R. T. Davidson, and A. Frances. 1999b. The expert consensus guideline series: Treatment of posttraumatic stress disorder. *Journal of Clinical Psychiatry* 60(Suppl 16).

Foa, E. B., M. E. Franklin, and J. Moser. 2002. Context in the clinic: How well do cognitive-behavioral therapies and medications work in combination? *Biological Psychiatry* 52(10):987-997.

Foa, E. B., E. A. Hembree, S. P. Cahill, S. A. M. Rauch, D. S. Riggs, N. C. Feeny, and E. Yadin. 2005. Randomized trial of prolonged exposure for posttraumatic stress disorder with and without cognitive restructuring: Outcome at academic and community clinics. *Journal of Consulting and Clinical Psychology* 73(5):953-964.

Foa, E. B., L. A. Zoellner, and N. C. Feeny. 2006. An evaluation of three brief programs for facilitating recovery after assault. *Journal of Traumatic Stress* 19(1):29-43.

Foa, E. B., E. A. Hembree, and B. O. Rothbaum. 2007. *Prolonged exposure therapy for PTSD: Emotional processing of traumatic experiences: Therapist guide, Treatments that work.* New York: Oxford University Press.

Forbes, D., M. Creamer, J. I. Bisson, J. A. Cohen, B. E. Crow, E. B. Foa, M. J. Friedman, T. M. Keane, H. S. Kudler, and R. J. Ursano. 2010. A guide to guidelines for the treatment of PTSD and related conditions. *Journal of Traumatic Stress* 23(5):537-552.

Foy, D. W., J. I. Ruzek, S. M. Glynn, S. J. Riney, and F. D. Gusman. 2002. Trauma focus group therapy for combat-related PTSD: An update. *Journal of Clinical Psychology* 58(8):907-918.

Friedman, M. J., C. R. Marmar, D. G. Baker, C. R. Sikes, and G. M. Farfel. 2007. Randomized, double-blind comparison of sertraline and placebo for posttraumatic stress disorder in a Department of Veterans Affairs setting. *Journal of Clinical Psychiatry* 68(5):711-720.

Frueh, B. C., S. M. Turner, D. C. Beidel, R. F. Mirabella, and W. J. Jones. 1996. Trauma management therapy: A preliminary evaluation of a multicomponent behavioral treatment for chronic combat-related PTSD. *Behaviour Research and Therapy* 34(7):533-543.

Geiss Trusz, S., A. W. Wagner, J. Russo, J. Love, and D. F. Zatzick. 2011. Assessing barriers to care and readiness for cognitive behavioral therapy in early acute care PTSD interventions. *Psychiatry: Interpersonal and Biological Processes* 74(3):207-233.

George, M. S., and G. Aston-Jones. 2010. Noninvasive techniques for probing neurocircuitry and treating illness: Vagus nerve stimulation (VNS), transcranial magnetic stimulation (TMS) and transcranial direct current stimulation (TCDS). *Neuropsychopharmacology* 35(1):301-316.

George, M. S., H. E. Ward, P. T. Ninan, M. Pollack, Z. Nahas, B. Anderson, S. Kose, R. H. Howland, W. K. Goodman, and J. C. Ballenger. 2008. A pilot study of vagus nerve stimulation (VNS) for treatment-resistant anxiety disorders. *Brain Stimulation* 1(2):112-121.

Gerardi, M., B. O. Rothbaum, K. Ressler, M. Heekin, and A. Rizzo. 2008. Virtual reality exposure therapy using a virtual Iraq: Case report. *Journal of Traumatic Stress* 21(2):209-213.

Gerardi, M., K. Ressler, and B.O. Rothbaum. 2009. Combined treatment of anxiety disorders. In *Textbook of Anxiety Disorders*, edited by D. J. Stein, E. Hollander, and B. O. Rothbaum. Arlington, VA: American Psychiatric Association.

Gerbode, F. A. 1995. *Beyond psychology: An introduction to metapsychology*. 3rd ed. Menlo Park, CA: IRM Press.

Gersons, B. P. R., I. V. E. Carlier, R. D. Lamberts, and B. A. van der Kolk. 2000. Randomized clinical trial of brief eclectic psychotherapy for police officers with posttraumatic stress disorder. *Journal of Traumatic Stress* 13(2):333-347.

Gilbody, S., P. Bower, J. Fletcher, D. Richards, and A. J. Sutton. 2006. Collaborative care for depression—a cumulative meta-analysis and review of longer-term outcomes. *Archives of Internal Medicine* 166(21):2314-2321.

Grodin, M. A., L. Piwowarczyk, D. Fulker, A. R. Bazazi, and R. B. Saper. 2008. Treating survivors of torture and refugee trauma: A preliminary case series using qigong and t'ai chi. *Journal of Alternative & Complementary Medicine* 14(7):801-806.

Hamner, M. B., R. A. Faldowski, H. G. Ulmer, B. C. Frueh, M. G. Huber, and G. W. Arana. 2003. Adjunctive risperidone treatment in post-traumatic stress disorder: A preliminary controlled trial of effects on comorbid psychotic symptoms. *International Clinical Psychopharmacology* 18(1):1-8.

Harch, P. G., C. Kriedt, K. W. Van Meter, and R. J. Sutherland. 2007. Hyperbaric oxygen therapy improves spatial learning and memory in a rat model of chronic traumatic brain injury. *Brain Research* 1174:120-129.

Harch, P. G., S. R. Andrews, E. F. Fogarty, D. Amen, J. C. Pezzullo, J. Lucarini, C. Aubrey, D. V. Taylor, P. K. Staab, and K. W. Van Meter. 2012. A phase I study of low-pressure hyperbaric oxygen therapy for blast induced post-concussion syndrome and post-traumatic stress disorder. *Journal of Neurotrauma* 29(1):168-185.

Hayes, S. C., J. B. Luoma, F. W. Bond, A. Masuda, and J. Lillis. 2006. Acceptance and commitment therapy: Model, processes and outcomes. *Behaviour Research and Therapy* 44(1):1-25.

Heresco-Levy, U., I. Kremer, D. C. Javitt, R. Goichman, A. Reshef, M. Blanaru, and T. Cohen. 2002. Pilot-controlled trial of D-cycloserine for the treatment of post-traumatic stress disorder. *International Journal of Neuropsychopharmacology* 5(4):301-307.

Hertzberg, M. A., M. I. Butterfield, M. E. Feldman, J. C. Beckham, S. M. Sutherland, K. M. Connor, and J. R. T. Davidson. 1999. A preliminary study of lamotrigine for the treatment of posttraumatic stress disorder. *Biological Psychiatry* 45(9):1226-1229.

Hertzberg, M. A., M. E. Feldman, J. C. Beckham, H. S. Kudler, and J. R. Davidson. 2000. Lack of efficacy for fluoxetine in PTSD: A placebo controlled trial in combat veterans. *Annals of Clinical Psychiatry* 12(2):101-105.

Hertzberg, M. A., S. D. Moore, M. E. Feldman, and J. C. Beckham. 2001. A preliminary study of bupropion sustained-release for smoking cessation in patients with chronic posttraumatic stress disorder. *Journal of Clinical Psychopharmacology* 21(1):94-98.

Hollifield, M., N. Sinclair-Lian, T. D. Warner, and R. Hammerschlag. 2007. Acupuncture for posttraumatic stress disorder: A randomized controlled pilot trial. *Journal of Nervous & Mental Disease* 195(6):504-513.

Horowitz, M. J. 1976. *Stress response syndromes*. New York: J. Aronson.

Igreja, V., W. Kleijn, and A. Richters. 2006. When the war was over, little changed: Women's posttraumatic suffering after the war in Mozambique. *Journal of Nervous & Mental Disease* 194(7):502-509.

IOM (Institute of Medicine). 2008. *Treatment of posttraumatic stress disorder: An assessment of the evidence.* Washington, DC: The National Academies Press.

IPAP (International Psychopharmacology Algorithm Project). 2005. *IPAP post-traumatic stress disorder algorithm notes.* http://ipap.org/pdf/PTSD/en/IPAP_PTSDnotes_en.pdf (accessed January 30, 2012).

Ipser, J. C., and D. J. Stein. 2011. Evidence-based pharmacotherapy of post-traumatic stress disorder (PTSD). *International Journal of Neuropsychopharmacology* (July 29):1-16 [Epub ahead of print].

ISTSS (International Society for Traumatic Stress Studies). 2009. *Effective treatments for PTSD: Practice guidelines from the International Society for Traumatic Stress Studies.* Edited by E. B. Foa, T. M. Keane, M. J. Friedman, and J. A. Cohen, 2nd Ed. New York: Guilford Press.

Jakupcak, M., A. Wagner, A. Paulson, A. Varra, and M. McFall. 2010. Behavioral activation as a primary care-based treatment for PTSD and depression among returning veterans. *Journal of Traumatic Stress* 23(4):491-495.

Johnson, D. M., and C. Zlotnick. 2009. Hope for battered women with PTSD in domestic violence shelters. *Professional Psychology-Research and Practice* 40(3):234-241.

Kaplan, Z., M. Amir, M. Swartz, and J. Levine. 1996. Inositol treatment of post-traumatic stress disorder. *Anxiety* 2(1):51-52.

Kaplan, Z., M. Michael, K. Ram, and C. Hagit. 2005. Possible deleterious effects of adjunctive omega-3 fatty acids in post-traumatic stress disorder patients. *Journal of Neuropsychiatric Disease and Treatment* 1(2):187-190.

Kar, N. 2011. Cognitive behavioral therapy for the treatment of post-traumatic stress disorder: A review. *Journal of Neuropsychiatric Disease and Treatment* 7:167-181.

Karatzias, T., K. Power, K. Brown, T. McGoldrick, M. Begum, J. Young, P. Loughran, Z. Chouliara, and S. Adams. 2011. A controlled comparison of the effectiveness and efficiency of two psychological therapies for posttraumatic stress disorder: Eye movement desensitization and reprocessing vs. emotional freedom techniques. *Journal of Nervous & Mental Disease* 199(6):372-378.

Katon, W., M. Von Korff, E. Lin, G. Simon, E. Walker, J. Unutzer, T. Bush, J. Russo, and E. Ludman. 1999. Stepped collaborative care for primary care patients with persistent symptoms of depression: A randomized trial. *Archives of General Psychiatry* 56(12):1109-1115.

Katon, W., C. Rutter, E. J. Ludman, M. Von Korff, E. Lin, G. Simon, T. Bush, E. Walker, and J. Unutzer. 2001. A randomized trial of relapse prevention of depression in primary care. *Archives of General Psychiatry* 58(3):241-247.

Katon, W. J., E. H. Lin, M. Von Korff, P. Ciechanowski, E. J. Ludman, B. Young, D. Peterson, C. M. Rutter, M. McGregor, and D. McCulloch. 2010. Collaborative care for patients with depression and chronic illnesses. *New England Journal of Medicine* 363(27):2611-2620.

Katz, R. J., M. H. Lott, P. Arbus, L. Crocq, P. Herlobsen, O. Lingjaerde, G. Lopez, G. C. Loughrey, D. J. MacFarlane, R. McIvor, L. Mehlum, D. Nugent, S. W. Turner, L. Weisaeth, and W. Yule. 1994. Pharmacotherapy of post-traumatic stress disorder with a novel psychotropic brofaromine. *Anxiety* 1(4):169-174.

Katz, T. 1996. Adult survivors of sexual abuse. *British Homeopathic Journal* 85:214-220.

Khaylis, A., M. A. Polusny, C. R. Erbes, A. Gewirtz, and C. M. Rath. 2011. Posttraumatic stress, family adjustment, and treatment preferences among National Guard soldiers deployed to OEF/OIF. *Military Medicine* 176(2):126-131.

Kilpatrick, D. G., L. J. Veronen, and P. A. Resick. 1982. Psychological sequelae to rape: Assessment and treatment strategies. In *Behavioral medicine: Assessment and treatment strategies*, edited by D. M. Doleys, R. L. Meredith, and A. R. Ciminero. New York: Plenum Press.

Kimbrough, E., T. Magyari, P. Langenberg, M. Chesney, and B. Berman. 2010. Mindfulness intervention for child abuse survivors. *Journal of Clinical Psychology* 66(1):17-33.

Kindwall, E. P., M. P. Mcquillen, B. O. Khatri, H. W. Gruchow, and M. L. Kindwall. 1991. Treatment of multiple-sclerosis with hyperbaric-oxygen—results of a national registry. *Archives of Neurology* 48(2):195-199.

Kirsch, I. 1999. *Clinical hypnosis and self-regulation: Cognitive-behavioral perspectives*, 1st ed. Dissociation, trauma, memory, and hypnosis book series. Washington, DC: American Psychological Association.

Kizer, K. W. 1982. Delayed treatment of dysbarism a retrospective review of 50 cases. *Journal of the American Medical Association* 247(18):2555-2558.

Kosten, T. R., J. B. Frank, E. Dan, C. J. Mcdougle, and E. L. Giller. 1991. Pharmacotherapy for posttraumatic-stress-disorder using phenelzine or imipramine. *Journal of Nervous and Mental Disease* 179(6):366-370.

Krakow, B., M. Hollifield, L. Johnston, M. Koss, R. Schrader, T. D. Warner, D. Tandberg, J. Lauriello, L. McBride, L. Cutchen, D. Cheng, S. Emmons, A. Germain, D. Melendrez, D. Sandoval, and H. Prince. 2001. Imagery rehearsal therapy for chronic nightmares in sexual assault survivors with posttraumatic stress disorder: A randomized controlled trial. *Journal of the American Medical Association* 286(5):537-545.

Kroenke, K., M. J. Bair, T. M. Damush, J. W. Wu, S. Hoke, J. Sutherland, and W. Z. Tu. 2009. Optimized antidepressant therapy and pain self-management in primary care patients with depression and musculoskeletal pain: A randomized controlled trial. *Journal of the American Medical Association* 301(20):2099-2110.

Krupnick, J. L., B. L. Green, P. Stockton, J. Miranda, E. Krause, and M. Mete. 2008. Group interpersonal psychotherapy for low-income women with posttraumatic stress disorder. *Psychotherapy Research* 18(5):497-507.

Krystal, J. H., R. A. Rosenheck, J. A. Cramer, J. C. Vessicchio, K. M. Jones, J. E. Vertrees, R. A. Horney, G. D. Huang, and C. Stock. 2011. Adjunctive risperidone treatment for antidepressant-resistant symptoms of chronic military service-related PTSD: A randomized trial. *Journal of the American Medical Association* 306(5):493-502.

Kubany, E. S., E. E. Hill, and J. A. Owens. 2003. Cognitive trauma therapy for battered women with PTSD: Preliminary findings. *Journal of Traumatic Stress* 16(1):81-91.

Kubany, E. S., E. E. Hill, J. A. Owens, C. Iannce-Spencer, M. A. McCaig, K. J. Tremayne, and P. L. Williams. 2004. Cognitive trauma therapy for battered women with PTSD (CTT-BW). *Journal of Consulting and Clinical Psychology* 72(1):3-18.

Lee, C., H. Gavriel, P. Drummond, J. Richards, and R. Greenwald. 2002. Treatment of PTSD: Stress inoculation training with prolonged exposure compared to EMDR. *Journal of Clinical Psychology* 58(9):1071-1089.

Lentini, J., and M. Knox. 2009. A qualitative and quantitative review of equine facilitated psychotherapy (EFP) with children and adolescents. *Open Complementary Medicine Journal* 1:51-57.

Levine, E. G., J. Eckhardt, and E. Targ. 2005. Change in post-traumatic stress symptoms following psychosocial treatment for breast cancer. *Psycho-Oncology* 14(8):618-635.

Lindauer, R. J., B. P. Gersons, E. P. van Meijel, K. Blom, I. V. Carlier, I. Vrijlandt, and M. J. Olff. 2005. Effects of brief eclectic psychotherapy in patients with posttraumatic stress disorder: Randomized clinical trial. *Journal of Trauma Stress* 18(3):205-212.

Margoob, M. A., Z. Ali, and C. Andrade. 2010. Efficacy of ECT in chronic, severe, antidepressant- and CBT-refractory PTSD: An open, prospective study. *Brain Stimulation* 3(1):28-35.

Marks, I., K. Lovell, H. Noshirvani, M. Livanou, and S. Thrasher. 1998. Treatment of posttraumatic stress disorder by exposure and/or cognitive restructuring: A controlled study. *Archives of General Psychiatry* 55(4):317-325.

Marshall, R. D., K. L. Beebe, M. Oldham, and R. Zaninelli. 2001. Efficacy and safety of paroxetine treatment for chronic PTSD: A fixed-dose, placebo-controlled study. *American Journal of Psychiatry* 158(12):1982-1988.

Martenyi, F., E. B. Brown, H. Zhang, S. C. Koke, and A. Prakash. 2002a. Fluoxetine v. placebo in prevention of relapse in post-traumatic stress disorder. *British Journal of Psychiatry* 181:315-320.

Martenyi, F., E. B. Brown, H. Zhang, A. Prakash, and S. C. Koke. 2002b. Fluoxetine versus placebo in posttraumatic stress disorder. *Journal of Clinical Psychiatry* 63(3):199-206.

Martenyi, F., E. B. Brown, and C. D. Caldwell. 2007. Failed efficacy of fluoxetine in the treatment of posttraumatic stress disorder: Results of a fixed-dose, placebo-controlled study. *Journal of Clinical Psychopharmacology* 27(2):166-170.

Matsuoka, Y., D. Nishi, N. Yonemoto, K. Hamazaki, K. Hashimoto, and T. Hamazaki. 2010. Omega-3 fatty acids for secondary prevention of posttraumatic stress disorder after accidental injury: An open-label pilot study. *Journal of Clinical Psychopharmacology* 30(2):217-219.

McLean, C. P., and E. B. Foa. 2011. Prolonged exposure therapy for post-traumatic stress disorder: A review of evidence and dissemination. *Expert Reviews in Neurotherapeutics* 11(8):1151-1163.

McPherson, F., and M. A. Schwenka. 2004. Use of complementary and alternative therapies among active duty soldiers, military retirees, and family members at a military hospital. *Military Medicine* 169(5):354-157.

Meffert, S. M., A. O. Abdo, O. A. A. Alla, Y. O. M. Elmakki, A. A. Omer, S. Yousif, T. J. Metzler, and C. Marmar. 2011. A pilot randomized controlled trial of interpersonal psychotherapy for Sudanese refugees in Cairo, Egypt. *Psychological Trauma: Theory, Research, Practice, and Policy*. May 2.

Meichenbaum, D. 1974. *Cognitive behavior modification, university programs modular studies*. Morristown, NJ: General Learning Press.

Miranda, J., J. Y. Chung, B. L. Green, J. Krupnick, J. Siddique, D. A. Revicki, and T. Belin. 2003. Treating depression in predominantly low-income young minority women: A randomized controlled trial. *Journal of the American Medical Association* 290(1):57-65.

Mohamed, S., and R. A. Rosenheck. 2008. Pharmacotherapy of PTSD in the U.S. Department of Veterans Affairs: Diagnostic- and symptom-guided drug selection. *Journal of Clinical Psychiatry* 69(6):959-965.

Monnelly, E. P., D. A. Ciraulo, C. Knapp, and T. Keane. 2003. Low-dose risperidone as adjunctive therapy for irritable aggression in posttraumatic stress disorder. *Journal of Clinical Psychopharmacology* 23(2):193-196.

Monson, C. M., P. P. Schnurr, S. P. Stevens, and K. A. Guthrie. 2004. Cognitive-behavioral couple's treatment for posttraumatic stress disorder: Initial findings. *Journal of Traumatic Stress* 17(4):341-344.

Monson, C. M., S. J. Fredman, and K. C. Adair. 2008. Cognitive-behavioral conjoint therapy for posttraumatic stress disorder: Application to Operation Enduring and Iraqi Freedom veterans. *Journal of Clinical Psychology* 64(8):958-971.

Monson, C. M., S. J. Fredman, K. C. Adair, S. P. Stevens, P. A. Resick, P. P. Schnurr, H. Z. MacDonald, and A. Macdonald. 2011. Cognitive-behavioral conjoint therapy for PTSD: Pilot results from a community sample. *Journal of Traumatic Stress* 24(1):97-101.

Morrison, R., and National Center for Homeopathy. 1993. *Materia medica of PTSD panel discussion*. Alexandria, VA: National Center for Homeopathy.

Nacasch, N., E. B. Foa, J. D. Huppert, D. Tzur, L. Fostick, Y. Dinstein, M. Polliack, and J. Zohar. 2010. Prolonged exposure therapy for combat- and terror-related posttraumatic stress disorder: A randomized control comparison with treatment as usual. *Journal of Clinical Psychiatry* 72(9):1174-1180.

National Center for Complementary and Alternative Medicine. 2010. *Homeopathy: An introduction*. http://nccam.nih.gov/health/homeopathy/homeopathy.pdf (accessed January 30, 2012).

NCCMH (National Collaborating Centre for Mental Health) and NICE (National Institute for Clinical Excellence). 2005. *Post-traumatic stress disorder: The management of PTSD in adults and children in primary and secondary care, National clinical practice guideline*. Clinical Guideline 26. London, UK: Gaskell and the British Psychological Society.

Neuner, F., C. Catani, M. Ruf, E. Schauer, M. Schauer, and T. Elbert. 2008. Narrative exposure therapy for the treatment of traumatized children and adolescents (kidnet): From neurocognitive theory to field intervention. *Child & Adolescent Psychiatric Clinics of North America* 17(3):641-664, x.

Newcomer, J. W., and J. H. Krystal. 2001. NMDA receptor regulation of memory and behavior in humans. *Hippocampus* 11(5):529-542.

Neylan, T. C., M. Lenoci, K. W. Samuelson, T. J. Metzler, C. Henn-Haase, R. W. Hierholzer, S. E. Lindley, C. Otte, F. B. Schoenfeld, J. A. Yesavage, and C. R. Marmar. 2006. No improvement of posttraumatic stress disorder symptoms with guanfacine treatment. *American Journal of Psychiatry* 163(12):2186-2188.

NHMRC (National Health and Medical Research Council). 2007. *Australian guidelines for the treatment of adults with acute stress disorder and posttraumatic stress disorder*. Canberra, Australia: Australian Centre for Posttraumatic Mental Health.

Nixon, R. D. V., and D. M. Nearmy. 2011. Treatment of comorbid posttraumatic stress disorder and major depressive disorder: A pilot study. *Journal of Traumatic Stress* 24(4):451-455.

Othmer, S., and S. F. Othmer. 2009. Post traumatic stress disorder—the neurofeedback remedy. *Biofeedback* 37(1):24-31.

Otto, M. W., D. Hinton, N. B. Korbly, A. Chea, P. Ba, B. S. Gershuny, and M. H. Pollack. 2003. Treatment of pharmacotherapy-refractory posttraumatic stress disorder among Cambodian refugees: A pilot study of combination treatment with cognitive-behavior therapy vs sertraline alone. *Behaviour Research & Therapy* 41(11):1271-1276.

Ozer, E. J., S. R. Best, T. L. Lipsey, and D. S. Weiss. 2003. Predictors of posttraumatic stress disorder and symptoms in adults: A meta-analysis. *Psychological Bulletin* 129(1):52-73.

Padala, P. R., J. Madison, M. Monnahan, W. Marcil, P. Price, S. Ramaswamy, A. U. Din, D. R. Wilson, and F. Petty. 2006. Risperidone monotherapy for post-traumatic stress disorder related to sexual assault and domestic abuse in women. *International Clinical Psychopharmacology* 21(5):275-280.

Panahi, Y., B. R. Moghaddam, A. Sahebkar, M. A. Nazari, F. Beiraghdar, G. Karami, and A. R. Saadat. 2011. A randomized, double-blind, placebo-controlled trial on the efficacy and tolerability of sertraline in Iranian veterans with post-traumatic stress disorder. *Psychological Medicine* 41(10):2159-2166.

Paunovic, N., and L. G. Ost. 2001. Cognitive-behavior therapy vs exposure therapy in the treatment of PTSD in refugees. *Behaviour Research and Therapy* 39(10):1183-1197.

Peniston, E. O. 1998. The Peniston-Kulkosky brainwave neurofeedback therapeutic protocol: The future psychotherapy for alcoholism/PTSD/behavioral medicine. *The American Academy of Experts in Traumatic Stress*. http://www.aaets.org/article47.htm.

Peniston, E. O., and P. J. Kulkosky. 1991. Alpha-theta brainwave neuro-feedback therapy for Vietnam veterans with combat-related post-truamtic stress disorder. *Medical Psychotherapy: An International Journal* 4:47-60.

Peterson, A. L., C. A. Luethcke, E. V. Borah, A. M. Borah, and S. Young-McCaughan. 2011. Assessment and treatment of combat-related PTSD in returning war veterans. *Journal of Clinical Psychology in Medical Settings* 18:164-175.

Pfeiffer, P. N., D. Ganoczy, K. Zivin, and M. Valenstein. 2011. Benzodiazepines and adequacy of initial antidepressant treatment for depression. *Journal of Clinical Psychopharmacology* 31(3):360-364.

Pitman, R. K., K. M. Sanders, R. M. Zusman, A. R. Healy, F. Cheema, N. B. Lasko, L. Cahill, and S. P. Orr. 2002. Pilot study of secondary prevention of posttraumatic stress disorder with propranolol. *Biological Psychiatry* 51(2):189-192.

Pollack, M. H., E. A. Hoge, J. J. Worthington, S. J. Moshier, R. S. Wechsler, M. Brandes, and N. M. Simon. 2011. Eszopiclone for the treatment of posttraumatic stress disorder and associated insomnia: A randomized, double-blind, placebo-controlled trial. *Journal of Clinical Psychiatry* 72(7):892-897.

Power, K., T. McGoldrick, K. Brown, R. Buchanan, D. Sharp, V. Swanson, and A. Karatzias. 2002. A controlled comparison of eye movement desensitization and reprocessing versus exposure plus cognitive restructuring versus waiting list in the treatment of posttraumatic stress disorder. *Clinical Psychology & Psychotherapy* 9(5):299-318.

Powers, M. B., J. M. Halpern, M. P. Ferenschak, S. J. Gillihan, and E. B. Foa. 2010. A meta-analytic review of prolonged exposure for posttraumatic stress disorder. *Clinical Psychology Review* 30(6):635-641.

Pull, C. B. 2009. Current empirical status of acceptance and commitment therapy. *Current Opinion in Psychiatry* 22(1):55-60.

Raskind, M. A., E. R. Peskind, E. D. Kanter, E. C. Petrie, A. Radant, C. E. Thompson, D. J. Dobie, D. Hoff, R. J. Rein, K. Straits-Troster, R. G. Thomas, and M. M. McFall. 2003. Reduction of nightmares and other PTSD symptoms in combat veterans by prazosin: A placebo-controlled study. *American Journal of Psychiatry* 160(2):371-373.

Raskind, M. A., E. R. Peskind, D. J. Hoff, K. L. Hart, H. A. Holmes, D. Warren, J. Shofer, J. O'Connell, F. Taylor, C. Gross, K. Rohde, and M. E. McFall. 2007. A parallel group placebo controlled study of prazosin for trauma nightmares and sleep disturbance in combat veterans with post-traumatic stress disorder. *Biological Psychiatry* 61(8):928-934.

Reger, G. M., and G. A. Gahm. 2008. Virtual reality exposure therapy for active duty soldiers. *Journal of Clinical Psychology* 64(8):940-946.

Reger, G. M., G. A. Gahm, A. A. Rizzo, R. Swanson, and S. Duma. 2009. Soldier evaluation of the virtual reality Iraq. *Telemedicine Journal & E-Health* 15(1):101-104.

Reger, G. M., K. M. Holloway, C. Candy, B. O. Rothbaum, J. Difede, A. A. Rizzo, and G. A. Gahm. 2011. Effectiveness of virtual reality exposure therapy for active duty soldiers in a military mental health clinic. *Journal of Traumatic Stress*:1-4.

Reich, D. B., S. Winternitz, J. Hennen, T. Watts, and C. Stanculescu. 2004. A preliminary study of risperidone in the treatment of posttraumatic stress disorder related to childhood abuse in women. *Journal of Clinical Psychiatry* 65(12):1601-1606.

Reist, C., C. D. Kauffmann, R. J. Haier, C. Sangdahl, E. M. Demet, A. Chiczdemet, and J. N. Nelson. 1989. A controlled trial of desipramine in 18 men with posttraumatic stress disorder. *American Journal of Psychiatry* 146(4):513-516.

Resick, P. A., P. Nishith, T. L. Weaver, M. C. Astin, and C. A. Feuer. 2002. A comparison of cognitive-processing therapy with prolonged exposure and a waiting condition for the treatment of chronic posttraumatic stress disorder in female rape victims. *Journal of Consulting and Clinical Psychology* 70(4):867-879.

Resick, P. A., T. E. Galovski, M. O'Brien Uhlmansiek, C. D. Scher, G. A. Clum, and Y. Young-Xu. 2008. A randomized clinical trial to dismantle components of cognitive processing therapy for posttraumatic stress disorder in female victims of interpersonal violence. *Journal of Consulting and Clinical Psychology* 76(2):243-258.

Resick, P. A., L. F. Williams, M. K. Suvak, C. M. Monson, and J. L. Gradus. 2011. Long-term outcomes of cognitive-behavioral treatments for posttraumatic stress disorder among female rape survivors. *Journal of Consulting and Clinical Psychology*, Dec 19. [Epub ahead of print].

Ressler, K. J., B. O. Rothbaum, L. Tannenbaum, P. Anderson, K. Graap, E. Zimand, L. Hodges, and M. Davis. 2004. Cognitive enhancers as adjuncts to psychotherapy—use of D-cycloserine in phobic individuals to facilitate extinction of fear. *Archives of General Psychiatry* 61(11):1136-1144.

Ritchie, E. C. 2011. The therapeutic use of canines in medicine and psychiatry. Presentation at Saint Elizabeths Hospital/Department of Mental Health Continuing Medical Education Rounds. July 6.

Rizzo, A., T. D. Parsons, B. Lange, P. Kenny, J. G. Buckwalter, B. Rothbaum, J. Difede, J. Frazier, B. Newman, J. Williams, and G. Reger. 2011. Virtual reality goes to war: A brief review of the future of military behavioral healthcare. *Journal of Clinical Psychology in Medical Settings* 18(2):176-187.

Rodriguez-Romaguera, J., F. Sotres-Bayon, D. Mueller, and G. J. Quirk. 2009. Systemic propranolol acts centrally to reduce conditioned fear in rats without impairing extinction. *Biological Psychiatry* 65(10):887-892.

Rogers, S., S. M. Silver, J. Goss, J. Obenchain, A. Willis, and R. L. Whitney. 1999. A single session, group study of exposure and eye movement desensitization and reprocessing in treating posttraumatic stress disorder among Vietnam war veterans: Preliminary data. *Journal of Anxiety Disorders* 13(1-2):119-130.

Rosenberg, P. B., R. B. Mehndiratta, Y. P. Mehndiratta, A. Wamer, R. B. Rosse, and M. Balish. 2002. Repetitive transcranial magnetic stimulation treatment of comorbid posttraumatic stress disorder and major depression. *Journal of Neuropsychiatry and Clinical Neurosciences* 14(3):270-276.

Rosenthal, J. Z., S. Grosswald, R. Ross, and N. Rosenthal. 2011. Effects of transcendental meditation in veterans of Operation Enduring Freedom and Operation Iraqi Freedom with posttraumatic stress disorder: A pilot study. *Military Medicine* 176(6):626-630.

Rothbaum, B. O. 2008. Critical parameters for D-cycloserine enhancement of cognitive-behaviorial therapy for obsessive-compulsive disorder. *American Journal of Psychiatry* 165(3):293-296.

Rothbaum, B. O., and L. F. Hodges. 1999. The use of virtual reality exposure in the treatment of anxiety disorders. *Behavior Modification* 23(4):507-525.

Rothbaum, B. O., L. F. Hodges, D. Ready, K. Graap, and R. D. Alarcon. 2001. Virtual reality exposure therapy for Vietnam veterans with posttraumatic stress disorder. *Journal of Clinical Psychiatry* 62(8):617-622.

Rothbaum, B. O., M. C. Astin, and F. Marsteller. 2005. Prolonged exposure versus eye movement desensitization and reprocessing (EMDR) for PTSD rape victims. *Journal of Traumatic Stress* 18(6):607-616.

Rothbaum, B. O., S. P. Cahill, E. B. Foa, J. R. Davidson, J. Compton, K. M. Connor, M. C. Astin, and C. G. Hahn. 2006. Augmentation of sertraline with prolonged exposure in the treatment of posttraumatic stress disorder. *Journal of Traumatic Stress* 19(5):625-638.

Rothbaum, B. O., J. R. Davidson, D. J. Stein, R. Pedersen, J. Musgnung, X. W. Tian, S. Ahmed, and D. S. Baldwin. 2008a. A pooled analysis of gender and trauma-type effects on responsiveness to treatment of PTSD with venlafaxine extended release or placebo. *Journal of Clinical Psychiatry* 69(10):1529-1539.

Rothbaum, B. O., T. K. Killeen, J. R. T. Davidson, K. T. Brady, K. M. Connor, and M. H. Heekin. 2008b. Placebo-controlled trial of risperidone augmentation for selective serotonin reuptake inhibitor-resistant civilian posttraumatic stress disorder. *Journal of Clinical Psychiatry* 69(4):520-525.

Roy, M. J., J. Francis, J. Friedlander, L. Banks-Williams, R. G. Lande, P. Taylor, J. Blair, J. McLellan, W. Law, V. Tarpley, I. Patt, H. Yu, A. Mallinger, J. Difede, A. Rizzo, and B. Rothbaum. 2010. Improvement in cerebral function with treatment of posttraumatic stress disorder. *Annals of the New York Academy of Sciences* 1208:142-149.

Rudorfer, M. V., M. E. Henry, and H. A. Sackeim. 2003. Electroconvulsive therapy. In *Psychiatry*, edited by A. Tasman, J. Kay, and J. A. Lieberman, 2nd ed. Hoboken, NJ: John Wiley & Sons.

Sargant, W. W., E. Slater, and D. Kelly. 1972. *An introduction to physical methods of treatment in psychiatry*. 5th ed. New York: Science House.

Sarris, J., and D. J. Kavanagh. 2009. Kava and St. John's wort: Current evidence for use in mood and anxiety disorders. *Journal of Alternative & Complementary Medicine* 15(8):827-836.

Schneier, F. R., Y. Neria, M. Pavlicova, E. Hembree, E. J. Suh, L. Amsel, and R. D. Marshall. 2012. Combined prolonged exposure therapy and paroxetine for PTSD related to the World Trade Center attack: A randomized controlled trial. *American Journal of Psychiatry* 169(1):80-88.

Schnurr, P. P., M. J. Friedman, P. W. Lavori, and F. Y. Hsieh. 2001. Design of Department of Veterans Affairs cooperative study no. 420: Group treatment of posttraumatic stress disorder. *Controlled Clinical Trials* 22(1):74-88.

Schnurr, P. P., M. J. Friedman, D. W. Foy, M. T. Shea, F. Y. Hsieh, P. W. Lavori, S. M. Glynn, M. Wattenberg, and N. C. Bernardy. 2003. Randomized trial of trauma-focused group therapy for posttraumatic stress disorder—results from a Department of Veterans Affairs cooperative study. *Archives of General Psychiatry* 60(5):481-489.

Schnurr, P. P., M. J. Friedman, C. C. Engel, E. B. Foa, M. T. Shea, B. K. Chow, P. A. Resick, V. Thurston, S. M. Orsillo, R. Haug, C. Turner, and N. Bernardy. 2007. Cognitive behavioral therapy for posttraumatic stress disorder in women—a randomized controlled trial. *Journal of the American Medical Association* 297(8):820-830.

Seidler, G. H., and F. E. Wagner. 2006. Comparing the efficacy of EMDR and trauma-focused cognitive-behavioral therapy in the treatment of PTSD: A meta-analytic study. *Psychological Medicine* 36(11):1515-1522.

Shams, J., S. S. P Gudarzi, A.-R. Norouzi, B. Ghorbani, L. K. Habibi, and M.-T. Yasami. 2007. The efficacy and safety of add-on Ginko TD (*Ginkgo biloba*) treatment for PTSD: Results of a 12-week double-blind placebo-controlled study. *Iranian Journal of Psychiatry* 2:58-64.

Shapiro, D., I. A. Cook, D. M. Davydov, C. Ottaviani, A. F. Leuchter, and M. Abrams. 2007. Yoga as a complementary treatment of depression: Effects of traits and moods on treatment outcome. *Evidence-Based Complementary and Alternative Medicine* 4(4):493-502.

Shapiro, F. 1989a. Efficacy of the eye movement desensitization procedure in the treatment of traumatic memories. *Journal of Traumatic Stress* 2(2):199-223.

Shapiro, F. 1989b. Eye-movement desensitization—a new treatment for posttraumatic-stress-disorder. *Journal of Behavior Therapy and Experimental Psychiatry* 20(3):211-217.

Shapiro, S. 2001. Enhancing self-belief with EMDR: Developing a sense of mastery in the early phase of treatment. *American Journal of Psychotherapy* 55(4):531-542.

Sherman, M. D., F. Sautter, J. A. Lyons, G. M. Manguno-Mire, X. Han, D. Perry, and G. Sullivan. 2005. Mental health needs of cohabiting partners of Vietnam veterans with combat-related PTSD. *Psychiatric Services* 56(9):1150-1152.

Sherman, M. D., E. Fischer, U. B. Bowling, L. Dixon, L. Ridener, and D. Harrison. 2009. A new engagement strategy in a VA-based family psychoeducation program. *Psychiatric Services* 60(2):254-257.

Simon, N. M., K. M. Connor, A. J. Lang, S. Rauch, S. Krulewicz, R. T. LeBeau, J. R. Davidson, M. B. Stein, M. W. Otto, E. B. Foa, and M. H. Pollack. 2008. Paroxetine-CR augmentation for posttraumatic stress disorder refractory to prolonged exposure therapy. *Journal of Clinical Psychiatry* 69(3):400-405.

Simpson, T., D. Kaysen, S. Bowen, L. MacPherson, N. Chawla, A. Blume, G. Marlatt, and M. Larimer. 2007. PTSD symptoms, substance use, and vipassana mediation among incarcerated individuals. *Journal of Traumatic Stress* 20(3):239-249.

Smith, T. C., M. A. Ryan, B. Smith, R. J. Reed, J. R. Riddle, G. R. Gumbs, and G. C. Gray. 2007. Complementary and alternative medicine use among US Navy and Marine Corps personnel. *BMC Complementary and Alternative Medicine* 7:16.

Smucker, M. R., C. V. Dancu, E. B. Foa, and J. L. Niederee. 1995. Imagery rescripting: A new treatment for survivors of childhood sexual abuse suffering from post-traumatic stress. *Journal of Cognitive Psychotherapy: An International Quarterly* 9(1):3-17.

Southwick, S. M., C. A. Morgan, D. S. Charney, and J. R. High. 1999. Yohimbine use in a natural setting: Effects on posttraumatic stress disorder. *Biological Psychiatry* 46(3): 442-444.

Spates, C. R., E. Koch, K. Cusack, S. Pagoto, and S. Waller. 2009. Eye movement desensitization and reprocessing. In *Effective treatments for PTSD: Practice guidelines from the International Society for Traumatic Stress Studies*, edited by E. B. Foa, T. M. Keane, M. J. Friedman, and J. A. Cohen, 2nd ed. New York: Guilford Press.

Spiegel, D., C. Classen, E. Thurston, L. Butler. 2004. From child sexual abuse to adult sexual risk: Trauma, revictimization, and intervention. In *From child sexual abuse to adult sexual risk: Trauma, revictimization, and intervention*, edited by L. J. Koenig, 1st ed. Washington, DC: American Psychological Association.

Spiegel, H., and D. Spiegel. 1987. *Trance and treatment: Clinical uses of hypnosis*. Washington, DC: American Psychiatric Press

Stein, D. J., J. Davidson, S. Seedat, and K. Beebe. 2003. Paroxetine in the treatment of posttraumatic stress disorder: Pooled analysis of placebo-controlled studies. *Expert Opinion on Pharmacotherapy* 4(10):1829-1838.

Stein, D. J., J. C. Ipser, and S. Seedat. 2006. Pharmacotherapy for post traumatic stress disorder (PTSD). *Cochrane Database of Systematic Reviews* (1):CD002795.

Stein, M. B., N. A. Kline, and J. L. Matloff. 2002. Adjunctive olanzapine for SSRI-resistant combat-related PTSD: A double-blind, placebo-controlled study. *American Journal of Psychiatry* 159(10):1777-1779.

Stein, M. B., C. Kerridge, J. E. Dimsdale, and D. B. Hoyt. 2007. Pharmacotherapy to prevent PTSD: Results from a randomized controlled proof-of-concept trial in physically injured patients. *Journal of Traumatic Stress* 20(6):923-932.

Stewart, C. L., and T. A. Wrobel. 2009. Evaluation of the efficacy of the pharmacotherapy and psychotherapy in treatment of combat-related post-traumatic stress disorder: A meta-analytic review of outcome studies. *Military Medicine* 174(5):460-469.

Stowe, Z. N., and D. J. Newport. 2005. PTSD in pregnancy and the postpartum period. *Psychiatric Annals* 35(11):910-910.

Strauss, J., R. Coeytaux, J. McDuffie, and J. W. Williams. 2011. *Efficacy of complementary and alternative medicine therapies for posttraumatic stress disorder*. Washington, DC: Department of Veterans Affairs.

Such, E. A., B. E. Benson, D. A. Luckenbaugh, M. Geraci, R. M. Post, and U. McCann. 2009. Repetitive TMS combined with exposure therapy for PTSD: A preliminary study. *Journal of Anxiety Disorders* 23(1):54-59.

Tarrier, N., H. Pilgrim, C. Sommerfield, B. Faragher, M. Reynolds, E. Graham, and C. Barrowclough. 1999. A randomized trial of cognitive therapy and imaginal exposure in the treatment of chronic posttraumatic stress disorder. *Journal of Consulting & Clinical Psychology* 67(1):13-18.

Taylor, F. B., K. Lowe, C. Thompson, M. M. McFall, E. R. Peskind, E. D. Kanter, N. Allison, J. Williams, P. Martin, and M. A. Raskind. 2006. Daytime prazosin reduces psychological distress to trauma-specific cues in civilian trauma posttraumatic stress disorder. *Biological Psychiatry* 59(7):577-581.

Taylor, S., D. S. Thordarson, L. Maxfield, I. C. Fedoroff, K. Lovell, and J. Ogrodniczuk. 2003. Comparative efficacy, speed, and adverse effects of three PTSD treatments: Exposure therapy, EMDR, and relaxation training. *Journal of Consulting and Clinical Psychology* 71(2):330-338.

Telles, S., N. Singh, M. Joshi, and A. Balkrishna. 2010. Post traumatic stress symptoms and heart rate variability in Bihar flood survivors following yoga: A randomized controlled study. *BMC Psychiatry* 10:18.

Tucker, P., R. Zaninelli, R. Yehuda, L. Ruggiero, K. Dillingham, and C. D. Pitts. 2001. Paroxetine in the treatment of chronic posttraumatic stress disorder: Results of a placebo-controlled, flexible-dosage trial. *Journal of Clinical Psychiatry* 62(11):860-868.

Tucker, P., R. Potter-Kimball, D. B. Wyatt, D. E. Parker, C. Burgin, D. E. Jones, and B. K. Masters. 2003. Can physiologic assessment and side effects tease out differences in PTSD trials? A double-blind comparison of citalopram, sertraline, and placebo. *Psychopharmacology Bulletin* 37(3):135-149.

Tucker, P., R. P. Trautman, D. B. Wyatt, J. Thompson, S. C. Wu, J. A. Capece, and N. R. Rosenthal. 2007. Efficacy and safety of topiramate monotherapy in civilian posttraumatic stress disorder: A randomized, double-blind, placebo-controlled study. *Journal of Clinical Psychiatry* 68(2):201-206.

Twohig, M. P. 2009. Acceptance and commitment therapy for treatment-resistant posttraumatic stress disorder: A case study. *Cognitive and Behavioral Practice* 16(3):243-252.

Unutzer, J., W. Katon, C. M. Callahan, J. W. Williams, E. Hunkeler, L. Harpole, M. Hoffing, R. D. Della Penna, P. H. Noel, E. H. B. Lin, P. A. Arean, M. T. Hegel, L. Q. Tang, T. R. Belin, S. Oishi, C. Langston, and IMPACT Investigators. 2002. Collaborative care management of late-life depression in the primary care setting—a randomized controlled trial. *Journal of the American Medical Association* 288(22):2836-2845.

U.S. Army. 2012. Policy guidance on the assessment and treatment of post-traumatic stress disorder (PTSD). Memorandum for Commanders, MEDCOM regional medical commands. OTSG/MEDCOM Policy Memo 12-035. Fort Sam Houston, TX: U.S. Army Medical Comand. April 10.

VA and DoD (Department of Veterans Affairs and Department of Defense). 2004. *VA/DOD clinical practice guideline for the management of post-traumatic stress.* Washington, DC: VA and DoD.

VA and DoD. 2010. *VA/DOD clinical practice guideline for management of post-traumatic stress.* Washington, DC: VA and DoD.

Valenstein, M., K. K. Taylor, K. Austin, H. C. Kales, J. F. McCarthy, and F. C. Blow. 2004. Benzodiazepine use among depressed patients treated in mental health settings. *American Journal of Psychiatry* 161(4):654-661.

van Emmerik, A. A. P., J. H. Kamphuis, and P. M. G. Emmelkamp. 2008. Treating acute stress disorder and posttraumatic stress disorder with cognitive behavioral therapy or structured writing therapy: A randomized controlled trial. *Psychotherapy and Psychosomatics* 77(2):93-100.

Van Etten, M. L., and S. Taylor. 1998. Comparative efficacy of treatments for post-traumatic stress disorder: A meta-analysis. *Clinical Psychology & Psychotherapy* 5(3):126-144.

Van der Kolk, B. A., D. Dreyfuss, M. Michaels, D. Shera, R. Berkowitz, R. Fisler, and G. Saxe. 1994. Fluoxetine in posttraumatic-stress-disorder. *Journal of Clinical Psychiatry* 55(12):517-522.

Vaughan, K., M. S. Armstrong, R. Gold, N. O'Connor, W. Jenneke, and N. Tarrier. 1994. A trial of eye movement desensitization compared to image habituation training and applied muscle relaxation in post-traumatic stress disorder. *Journal of Behavior Therapy & Experimental Psychiatry* 25(4):283-291.

Velde, B. P., J. Cipriani, and G. Fisher. 2005. Resident and therapist views of animal-assisted therapy: Implications for occupational therapy practice. *Australian Occupational Therapy Journal* 52(1):43-50.

Von Korff, M. 2004. Commentary: Can care management enhance integration of primary and specialty care? *British Medical Journal* 329(7466):605-605.

Wagner, A. W., D. F. Zatzick, A. Ghesquiere, and G. J. Jurkovich. 2007. Behavioral activation as an early intervention for posttraumatic stress disorder and depression among physically injured trauma survivors. *Cognitive and Behavioral Practice* 14(4):341-349.

Walser, R. D., and D. Westrup. 2007. *Acceptance & commitment therapy for the treatment of post-traumatic stress disorder and trauma-related problems: A practitioner's guide to using mindfulness and acceptance strategies*. Oakland, CA: New Harbinger Publications.

Watts, B. V. 2007. Electroconvulsive therapy for comorbid major depressive disorder and posttraumatic stress disorder. *Journal of ECT* 23(2):93-95.

Wells, A., and S. Sembi. 2004a. Metacognitive therapy for PTSD: A core treatment manual. *Cognitive and Behavioral Practice* 11(4):365-377.

Wells, A., and S. Sembi. 2004b. Metacognitive therapy for PTSD: A preliminary investigation of a new brief treatment. *Journal of Behavior Therapy and Experimental Psychiatry* 35(4):307-318.

Wells, K. B., C. Sherbourne, M. Schoenbaum, N. Duan, L. Meredith, J. Unutzer, J. Miranda, M. F. Carney, and L. V. Rubenstein. 2000. Impact of disseminating quality improvement programs for depression in managed primary care—a randomized controlled trial. *Journal of the American Medical Association* 283(2):212-220.

World Federation of Societies of Biological Psychiatry, B. Bandelow, J. Zohar, E. Hollander, S. Kasper, H. J. Moller, G. Allgulander, J. Ayuso-Gutierrez, D. S. Baldwin, R. Bunevicius, G. Cassano, N. Fineberg, L. Gabriels, I. Hindmarch, H. Kaiya, D. F. Klein, M. Lader, Y. Lecrubier, J. P. Lepine, M. R. Liebowitz, J. J. Lopez-Ibor, D. Marazziti, E. C. Miguel, K. S. Oh, M. Preter, R. Rupprecht, M. Sato, V. Starcevic, D. J. Stein, M. van Ameringen, and J. Vega. 2008. World Federation of Societies of Biological Psychiatry (WFSBP) guidelines for the pharmacological treatment of anxiety, obsessive-compulsive and post-traumatic stress disorders—first revision. *World Journal of Biological Psychiatry* 9(4):248-312.

Zatzick, D. F., P. Roy-Byrne, J. Russo, F. P. Rivara, R. Droesch, A. Wagner, C. Dunn, G. J. Jurkovich, E. Uehara, and W. Katon. 2004. A randomized effectiveness trial of stepped collaborative care for acutely injured trauma survivors. *Archives of General Psychiatry* 61(May):498-506.

Zatzick, D., F. Rivara, G. Jurkovich, J. Russo, A. Wagner, J. Wang, C. Dunn, S. Lord, M. Petrie, S. O'Connor, and W. Katon. 2012. A randomized stepped care intervention trial targeting posttraumatic stress disorder for surgically hospitalized injury survivors. Accepted for publication. *Annals of Surgery* [Epub ahead of print].

Zhang, W., and J. R. Davidson. 2007. Post-traumatic stress disorder: An evaluation of existing pharmacotherapies and new strategies. *Expert Opinion on Pharmacotherapy* 8(12):1861-1870.

Zhang, Y., B. Feng, J.-P. Xie, F.-Z. Xu, and J. Chen. 2011. Clinical study on treatment of the earthquake-caused post-traumatic stress disorder by cognitive-behavior therapy and acupoint stimulation. *Journal of Traditional Chinese Medicine* 31(1):60-63.

Zlotnick, C., T. M. Shea, K. Rosen, E. Simpson, K. Mulrenin, A. Begin, and T. Pearlstein. 1997. An affect-management group for women with posttraumatic stress disorder and histories of childhood sexual abuse. *Journal of Traumatic Stress* 10(3):425-436.

8

Co-Occurring Psychiatric and Medical Conditions and Psychosocial Complexities

Many service members and veterans who have posttraumatic stress disorder (PTSD) have other conditions that require treatment and rehabilitation with treatment for PTSD—such psychiatric and medical conditions as depression, anxiety, substance abuse, chronic pain, and traumatic brain injury (TBI) and psychosocial conditions such as relationship problems, unemployment or underemployment, intimate partner violence (IPV), homelessness, and incarceration. This chapter focuses on co-occurring conditions that are most likely to interfere with effective PTSD-specific treatments (which themselves are discussed in Chapter 7) and whose treatment should be integrated into a comprehensive treatment program for PTSD. Three major categories of co-occurring conditions are considered: psychiatric (including depression and substance use disorders), medical (including chronic pain, TBI, and spinal cord injury), and psychosocial (including IPV, child maltreatment, homelessness, and incarceration). Discussion of each category includes a brief overview of the conditions and their co-occurrence with PTSD in military and veteran populations followed by a presentation of how to integrate their treatment into treatment for PTSD. The committee notes that evidence of the effectiveness of these approaches, as part of a broad overall rehabilitation program for service members or veterans who have PTSD, is sparse.

The committee recognizes that the prevalence of co-occurring psychiatric and medical conditions and psychosocial issues differs among the varied cohorts and subpopulations of service members and veterans (for example between women and men) and that the treatment needs of different groups will be different. For example, homelessness and vocational training are issues for veteran populations but not for active-duty service members. Among current service members, the needs of active-duty personnel differ from those of National Guard and reserve members and may vary according to service branch. Within veteran populations, the most important co-occurring medical and psychosocial treatment needs for patients who have PTSD may vary according to era and location of service. Dementia and other neurologic conditions that occur more frequently in aging populations, for example, constitute important comorbidity issues for veterans of World War II and Vietnam, but not for veterans of more recent conflicts.

CO-OCCURRING PSYCHIATRIC CONDITIONS AND PTSD

Comorbid conditions that include symptoms of depressive or anxiety disorders, substance use disorders, and high-risk behaviors appear to affect at least as many veterans returning from Operation Enduring Freedom (OEF) and Operation Iraqi Freedom (OIF) as PTSD alone (Hoge et al., 2004; Santiago et al., 2010). A large body of literature on trauma-exposed veteran and civilian populations supports the frequent co-occurrence of PTSD symptoms with depression (Erickson et al., 2001; Freuh et al., 2000; O'Donnell et al., 2004; Perlman et al., 2011; Shalev et al., 1998), traumatic grief (Prigerson, 2009; Shear, 2001, 2005), and alcohol use and drug use problems (Cerda et al., 2008; Cisler et al., 2011; Kulka, 1990; Zatzick and Galea, 2007) that may lead affected people to engage in high-risk behaviors that, in turn, are associated with exposure to additional traumatic events (Hearst et al., 1986; Kulka, 1990; Pat-Horenczyk et al., 2007). High rates of moral injury (defined as the perpetration of or failure to prevent atrocities or the witnessing of acts that transgress moral beliefs) (Litz et al., 2009) have been documented in active-duty military personnel deployed in the OEF and OIF theaters of war (MHAT IV, 2006).

The National Vietnam Veterans Readjustment Study, one of the first major epidemiologic investigations of Vietnam veterans, documented high rates of co-occurrence of PTSD and psychiatric disorders (Kulka, 1990). Three-fourths of male Vietnam veterans who had PTSD also had a lifetime diagnosis of alcohol abuse or dependence, 44% had a lifetime diagnosis of generalized anxiety disorder, and at least 20% had a lifetime diagnosis of depression or dysthymia. Of female Vietnam veterans who had PTSD, 44% had a lifetime diagnosis of depression and 23% had current depression. Research conducted in the 1980s also suggested that men who served in Vietnam were at increased risk for trauma, including fatal motor vehicle crashes and completed suicide (Hearst et al., 1986).

Stepped-care approaches begin with lower-intensity treatments, such as support groups, and phase in more intensive procedures, such as evidence-based interventions—such as cognitive behavioral therapy (CBT) and pharmacotherapy—for patients who have recalcitrant or recurrent symptoms of PTSD and related comorbidities (Engel and Katon, 1999). Collaborative stepped-care approaches and rehabilitative interventions that simultaneously target PTSD and comorbid conditions and psychosocial complexities have been proposed as an essential treatment delivery model for active-duty military and veteran populations (Engel and Katon, 1999; Engel et al., 2008; Gilbody et al., 2006; Zatzick et al., 2004, 2011, 2012). Collaborative stepped-care interventions are implemented by interdisciplinary teams of medical and mental health providers. Central to stepped-care approaches is regular assessment of PTSD symptoms and related comorbidities, coincident with evidence-based treatments. Collaborative stepped-care interventions that include care management and motivational interviewing can enhance a patient's initial engagement with treatment and diminish high-risk behaviors, such as binge drinking, and thereby optimize entry into and completion of evidence-based psychotherapy and pharmacotherapy for PTSD (Geiss Trusz et al., 2011; Zatzick et al., 2011). Those interventions can also incorporate emergency evaluations and treatments to target immediate and critical problems (such as suicide and interpersonal violence) directly.

Established treatments for PTSD, such as prolonged exposure (PE) therapy, can also address comorbid conditions, such as depression, anger, guilt, and general anxiety symptoms (Foa, 2011). Additional support for a stepped-care treatment approach comes from studies of veterans who have received multiple treatments that targeted their comorbidities before being randomized into efficacy trials of PTSD-targeted interventions. For example, a review of two major CBT efficacy trials found that many veterans in the studies received treatment for comorbid psychiatric and substance use conditions before their enrollment in the PTSD-specific treatment protocol, and following CBT treatment they had significant improvements in their PTSD and comorbid symptoms (Monson et al., 2006; Schnurr et al., 2007).

Combat experience is a known risk factor for both PTSD and substance use disorders (Jacobsen et al., 2001, 2008; Norman et al., 2010). In one study of OEF and OIF veterans who were treated in a Department of Veterans Affairs (VA) facility, 17% had co-occurring PTSD and a substance use disorder (Norman et al., 2010). One widely used treatment model is Seeking Safety, a manualized CBT program used to treat co-occurring PTSD and substance use disorder (Najavitz, 2009). A VA consensus conference noted that although there have been no randomized controlled trials (RCTs) of Seeking Safety, it may be an option for patients who are not ready for evidence-based treatment for PTSD (VA, 2010b). Central principles of the model include safety, both physically and psychologically in one's internal and external worlds; integrated treatment of PTSD and substance abuse; a focus on ideals and a search for meaning; and case management with an emphasis on cognitive, behavioral, and interpersonal domains (Najavitz, 2002). Several studies have evaluated the effectiveness of Seeking Safety in different populations and settings, including several veteran populations (Boden et al., 2012; Cook et al., 2006; Desai et al., 2008, 2009; Norman et al., 2010; Weaver et al., 2007; Weller, 2005); the results have been mixed.

In a recent RCT of 98 male veterans who had both substance use disorder and PTSD symptoms and who were recruited from an outpatient VA substance use disorders clinic, substituting Seeking Safety for part of the usual treatment was associated with better drug use outcomes than in the controls. However, alcohol use and PTSD severity decreased equally under both treatments (Boden et al., 2012). Findings of a pilot study of 14 male OEF and OIF veterans suggest that Seeking Safety may help to reduce alcohol use, depression, and PTSD in some participants at clinically significant levels. The investigators identified several features of the model that are especially helpful with combat veterans, including the case management component that helps persons to engage in other mental health and substance use disorder services. Veterans identified reintegration into civilian life and peer connections with other veterans as central to their recovery (Norman et al., 2010).

In another study, two nonequivalent cohorts of homeless female veterans who had psychiatric and substance abuse problems were recruited from VA homelessness programs. Seeking Safety appeared to have a moderately beneficial effect over 1 year on several clinical outcomes, including employment, social support, general symptoms of psychiatric distress, and symptoms of PTSD (Desai et al., 2008). In an uncontrolled pilot study of 18 male and female veterans in a VA setting, efficacy data on Seeking Safety indicated significant reduction in PTSD and substance use disorder symptoms, but in the absence of a randomized controlled condition it is unclear whether the reduction in symptoms was due to Safety Seeking or to other factors (Cook et al., 2006).

CO-OCCURING MEDICAL CONDITIONS AND PTSD

This section examines the treatment needs of people who have PTSD and co-occurring medical conditions. Chronic pain, TBI, amputation, spinal-cord injury, and severe burns—which may also result from the same trauma as that underlying PTSD—are each discussed. The section then examines the effect of PTSD on long-term health outcomes, including cardiovascular disease, inflammatory and autoimmune diseases, and diabetes mellitus.

Chronic Pain

Chronic pain is defined as pain that persists for at least 3 months after the resolution of a physical injury or disease process (Merskey and Bogduk, 1994). Such pain can affect social, occupational, and recreational function and can lead to problems of motivation, mood, social isolation, and estimates of self-worth.

The occurrence of physical injury that results in chronic pain is relatively common in the military, occurring from basic training to after discharge. Some 25% of male recruits and 50% of female recruits are predicted to experience at least one pain-related injury during basic combat training (McGeary et al., 2011). Chronic pain is the primary reason that OIF service members are evacuated from the theater of war (Harman et al., 2005), and combat-related orthopedic pain and musculoskeletal pain are the primary causes of disability (Masini et al., 2009). A review of medical records of OEF and OIF veterans who were seeking treatment at a VA polytrauma clinic found that 82% of them had documented chronic pain (Lew et al., 2009). Other studies of veterans have found that 50% of men and up to 78% of women report regular pain (Haskell et al., 2006; Kerns et al., 2003).

Chronic pain has adverse consequences on the cardiovascular, pulmonary, gastrointestinal, immunologic, and muscular systems. It also has been associated with increased anxiety, fear, anger, and depression and with a reduction in patient satisfaction and slower recovery from injury (Joshi and Ogunnaike, 2005). Starr et al. (2004) estimated the comorbidity of pain and PTSD to be greater than 50% for persons who sustained an orthopedic traumatic injury, and McGeary et al. (2011) report significantly higher rates of health care use by and poorer prognoses in patients who have comorbid PTSD and pain than those who have either diagnosis alone.

Treatment for Chronic Pain

Improvements in battlefield medicine practices and protective gear (body armor and helmet design) have led to increased survival of severely injured service members. Service members are also at risk for PTSD stemming from their physical injuries and the context in which they occurred. The symptoms that characterize chronic pain (for example, headache, irritability, sleep disturbance, and memory impairments) overlap with many symptoms of PTSD, and this complicates the diagnosis of, appropriate treatment for, and management of both conditions. The U.S. Army Surgeon General Pain Management Task Force Report (U.S. Army, 2010b) suggested the absence of pain-management practice guidelines in the theater of war has resulted in an "overreliance on opioid-based pain solutions, from point of injury throughout the care continuum."

Although a systematic literature review of treatments that targeted both chronic pain and PTSD symptoms found no combined treatment protocols, there is empirical evidence on the treatment of chronic pain in civilian and military populations with CBT and rehabilitation programs to restore function. Interdisciplinary chronic pain rehabilitation programs have empirical support for reducing pain and improving function in civilian populations (Gatchel et al., 2009; Gatchel and Okifuji, 2006; Guzman et al., 2001; Turk and Okifuji, 2002). Components of this approach typically include physical therapy, occupational therapy, CBT—including relaxation and biofeedback—and self-managed physical exercise. The U.S. Army Surgeon General Pain Management Task Force Report (U.S. Army, 2010b) made several recommendations for a comprehensive DoD and VA pain-management strategy that acknowledges the importance of treating pain. A number of studies have found CBT to be efficacious in reducing lower back pain (Hoffman et al., 2007), back and neck pain (Linton and Ryberg, 2001), osteoarthritis (Heinrich et al., 1985), and tension headache (Holroyd et al., 2001) and in improving function (Van Tulder et al., 2000). Key components of CBT pain programs include cognitive restructuring, relaxation training, time-based activity pacing, and graded homework assignments designed to target activity avoidance and improve engagement in an active lifestyle (Otis et al., 2011).

The functional-restoration approach is one example of an interdisciplinary program. Originally developed for use in sports medicine, this musculoskeletal pain management approach is individually tailored to the patient (on the basis of self-reported pain, medical history, structural measures, and functional-capacity measurements) with the goal of returning him or her to activity rather than focusing on pain symptoms (Mayer et al., 2003). Program components include objective and physical evaluation of physical and functional capacity, psychosocial assessment, identification of potential socioeconomic barriers to recovery, physician-directed treatment, and an interdisciplinary treatment-team approach. Evidence of the efficacy and robustness of functional-restoration approaches has been reported in several international populations (Gatchel and Okifuji, 2006).

The DoD Functional and Occupational Rehabilitation Treatment (FORT) program began in 2003 and uses a functional-restoration approach to decrease chronic musculoskeletal pain and increase functioning in service members (Gatchel et al., 2009). An RCT compared the FORT program with the usual treatment, standard anesthesia. The study used repeated measures in a treatment design that compared both groups immediately after and 6 and 12 months after treatment. The FORT participants had significantly better improvements in both psychosocial and physical outcomes immediately after treatment and at the 12-month follow-up than the treatment-as-usual group. The FORT group also had significant improvements in self-reported pain severity and intensity, perceived disability, pain-related concerns about physical activity and quality of life, sleep problems, emotional distress (depression and fear avoidance), functional lifting capacity (both floor-to-waist and waist-to-eye level), and lumbar active range of motion. At the 12-month follow-up, FORT participants were significantly less likely to seek high levels of treatment for pain, significantly less likely to rely on multiple pain medications, and twice as likely to remain on active duty. The DoD endorsed the functional-restoration approach in 2009 with a call for physical therapists to implement principles of sports medicine on the battlefield by 2013 (DoD, 2009).

An RCT is being conducted by the South Texas Research Organizational Network Guiding Studies on Trauma and Resilience (STRONG STAR) to evaluate the effectiveness of combined PE for PTSD and chronic pain treatment in active-duty orthopedic-trauma patients. The STRONG STAR RCT will compare outcomes in four study arms: a combined abbreviated PE and FORT-based pain approach, a PE group, a FORT group, and a treatment-as-usual group assessed immediately after treatment and at 6-month and 12-month follow-ups. This will be the first RCT to empirically test an integrated PTSD and pain treatment approach to improve functional outcomes in service members who have these co-occurring conditions (STRONG STAR, 2012).

Treatment for Co-Occurring Chronic Pain and PTSD

Besides the occurrence of physical combat wounds, extended time in service and multiple deployments have produced a population of active-duty service members who have had substantial wear and tear on their musculoskeletal systems. Because of concerns about stigma and appearing weak, service members often ignore or self-manage their pain until their condition impairs their ability to function and puts others at risk, at which time they are most likely to seek care (McGeary et al., 2011).

High levels of PTSD symptoms immediately after an injury have been shown to predict impairments in physical, role, and social functioning (Holbrook et al., 2005; O'Donnell et al., 2005; Ramchand et al., 2008; Zatzick et al., 2008a,b). Zatzick et al. (2008a) found that PTSD symptoms were independently associated with an inability to return to work 12 months after injury even after adjustment for all other relevant clinical, injury, and demographic characteristics. PTSD has also been shown to affect patient reports of physical symptoms and is a leading predictor of functional outcome after injury, including physical limitations and inability to return to work (Michaels et al., 1999). Co-occurring pain and PTSD from orthopedic trauma impede a patient's ability to benefit from pain treatment; such patients frequently have long periods of disability after trauma and poorer outcomes (McGeary et al., 2011). In a retrospective study of severely injured accident victims, Schnyder et al. (2001) found that PTSD predicted "perceived general health" more than injury severity or degree of physical functioning did. Thus, PTSD may lead to an increased focus on and perception of pain or an increased likelihood of reporting of pain symptoms. People who have PTSD also have a more negative perception of their general health, and this may also lead to complications in pain assessment and treatment. When chronic pain and PTSD are combined with a negative view of the future, there may be less participation in pain management programs that could lead to a reduction in symptoms.

Comorbid PTSD, depression, and chronic pain may interact to confound symptom presentation and treatment for each condition. PTSD and depression work together to exacerbate pain symptoms (Ahman and Stalnacke, 2008; Poundja et al., 2006; Roth et al., 2008). Several studies have found that pain and depression severity are strong predictors of each other and of functional status and quality of life (Bair, 2004; Kroenke et al., 2011; Lin et al., 2006). Treating depression with a selective serotonin reuptake inhibitor or other antidepressant or treating chronic pain with CBT has been shown to improve outcomes of both conditions (Bair, 2004; Institute for Clinical Systems Improvement, 2009; Kroenke et al., 2011). Concurrent treatment for pain and the psychiatric condition may result in greater improvement in both than sequential care. For example, when either pain or depression is initially treated with the goal of maximizing its treatment before addressing the comorbidity, neither is effectively treated, and treatment effect decreases as symptom severity of both the pain and the psychiatric condition increases (Kroenke et al., 2007, 2008, 2011; Lin et al., 2003, 2006). Therefore, combining pharmacologic and psychologic treatments for PTSD, depression, and chronic pain is likely to result in improved outcomes.

Traumatic Brain Injury

TBI is defined by the DoD and the VA (DCoE and DVBIC, 2009) as a traumatically induced structural injury and/or physiological disruption of brain function as a result of external force that is indicated by new onset or worsening of at least one of the following clinical signs, immediately following the event:

- Any period of loss of or a decreased level of consciousness;
- Any loss of memory for events immediately before or after the injury;

- Any alteration in mental state at the time of the injury (confusion, disorientation, slowed thinking, etc.);
- Neurological deficits (weakness, loss of balance, change in vision, praxis, paresis/plegia, sensory loss, aphasia, etc.) that may or may not be transient; and
- Intracranial lesion.

From 2000 through the end of 2011, a total of 229,106 service members in all services suffered TBI, of whom 77% experienced mild TBI (mTBI), as shown in Table 8-1 (DVBIC, 2011). On the basis of data collected from the postdeployment health questionnaires, 12% of returning service members had experienced mTBI while deployed (Schneiderman et al., 2008); when a structured interview was used, the prevalence of mTBI was almost twice as high (23%) as the questionnaire rate (Terrio et al., 2009).

TBI may be caused by a bump, blow, or jolt to the head; by acceleration or deceleration force without impact; or by penetration to the head that disrupts the normal function of the brain (DVBIC, 2011). The primary cause of TBI in OEF and OIF service members and veterans is an explosion or blast injury (Owens et al., 2008); the majority are closed head injuries that result from improvised explosive devices (IEDs) (Galarneau et al., 2008). Falls, motor vehicle incidents, and assault also cause TBIs in this population. However, blast-related TBI has been a focus of research because of its frequency and the difficulties that it presents for diagnosis. For example, concussive injuries associated with strong blasts may not be identified immediately if they occurred at the same time as more life-threatening injuries that dominate medical treatment. Additionally, mTBI resulting from a blast may produce no outward sign of injury and leave service members reluctant to report acute symptoms because they do not want to be medically evacuated and separated from their units. Thus, mTBI may not be identified as

TABLE 8-1 Incidence of TBI by Severity in All Armed Forces (Cumulative, 2000–2011)

TBI Severity	Number
Penetrating	3,738
Severe	2,360
Moderate	38,235
Mild	175,674
Not classifiable	9,099
Total	229,106

SOURCE: DVBIC, 2011.

a concern until a service member returns home from deployment (DVBIC, 2011).

The higher-level cognitive domains typically affected by TBI include attention, speed of processing, working memory, visuospatial ability and praxis, language and communication, and executive function. In the case of mTBI, postconcussion syndrome is considered to have occurred when three or more concussion symptoms persist for 3 months or more after injury (APA, 2000). Symptoms of concussion include fatigue, disordered sleep, headache, vertigo or dizziness, irritability or aggression with little or no provocation, anxiety, depression or affective liability, changes in personality, and apathy or lack of spontaneity. Postconcussion syndrome has been reported to occur in 10–20% of TBI cases (e.g., Ruff, 2005; Wood, 2004) and as many as 44% of hospitalized mTBI cases (Dikmen et al., 2010). In a U.S. Army brigade sample of clinically confirmed mTBI, memory deficits (16%), headache (20%), and irritability (21%) were reported to be the most frequent symptoms of postconcussion syndrome (Terrio et al., 2009). Belanger et al. (2005) failed to show a difference in neuropsychologic performance between blast and non-blast TBI, although anecdotal reports suggest otherwise (no data were available to confirm this observation). Many authors cite the need for more research to determine the effect of multiple trauma because they suspect the brain may adapt to the first concussion quickly but be more susceptible to injury with additional trauma owing to residual effects of the first one (Bigler, 2008; Moser et al., 2005; Omalu et al., 2005; Wall, 2006).

Co-Occurrence of TBI and PTSD

Symptoms of PTSD and mTBI may have considerable overlap, and this presents a diagnostic challenge. Studies indicate that the co-occurrence of TBI, pain, and psychosocial health problems is more common than is their isolated occurrence in OEF and OIF service members and veterans. The presence of PTSD after mTBI may prolong the duration of and potentially exacerbate the mTBI symptoms (Brenner et al., 2010). A recent systematic review found the frequency of comorbid probable PTSD in people who had probable mTBI was 33–39% (Carlson et al., 2010). Sayer et al. (2009) found there was a high comorbidity of pain, PTSD, and mTBI in patients who were treated at VA level-1 polytrauma rehabilitation centers (treatment facilities for the most-impaired veterans). Of 188 combat-injured service members, 93% had incurred combat-related TBI, 81% reported a pain problem, and 53% received some type of mental health service. A similar study of 50 OEF and OIF veterans who were treated at a VA level-1 polytrauma rehabilitation center found that 80% reportedly incurred combat-related TBI (58% were penetrating, 22% were closed), 96% reported at least one pain problem, and 44% reported experiencing PTSD (Clark et al., 2007). Of 62 patients at a level-2 polytrauma network site, Lew et al. (2007) found that 97% reported three or more postconcussive symptoms (for example, headache, dizziness, and fatigue), 97% reported chronic pain, and 71% met the criteria for PTSD. In a comprehensive review of medical records of 340 OEF and OIF veterans seen at a level-2 polytrauma network site, Lew et al. (2009) found that 82% had more than one diagnosis and 42% had three co-occurring diagnoses, including pain, PTSD, and post-concussion syndrome. Veterans who had positive TBI screens were also more likely to have a diagnosis of PTSD, depression, and substance abuse disorder; these three conditions were present in isolation in only 5%, 10%, and 3% of veterans, respectively—significantly lower frequencies than those at which they were present in combination (Lew, 2009). In another study by Ruff et al. (2008), approximately 66% of veterans who presented with headache and TBI had cognitive deficits on examination, more severe and more frequent headaches, more reports of pain, higher rates of PTSD, and impaired sleep with nightmares than veterans with mTBI who did not have a neurologic impairment.

A large study of approximately 3,000 hospitalized patients found that those who had mild, moderate, or severe TBI and PTSD had significantly worse physical, role, and social functioning than patients who had TBI of any severity without PTSD. Regardless of TBI severity, patients who had PTSD had greater impairments in self-reported cognitive functioning—including reasoning, memory, problem solving, concentration, and thinking—than those who did not have PTSD. Patients who had severe TBI had the highest cognitive impairments and had the least improvement during the 12-month follow-up. Increasing severity of TBI (moderate and severe) was associated with lower rates of PTSD symptoms in this population than mTBI; this supports the theory that a more severe head injury may disrupt memory consolidation and associated PTSD symptoms (Zatzick et al., 2010).

Depression is frequently reported in people who have chronic postconcussion syndrome (Hesdorffer et al., 2009). People who have mTBI and experience depression after the injury report more symptoms and more severe symptoms than those who have mTBI without depression (Lange et al., 2010). People who have mTBI report more problems with cognitive function if they have comorbid depression, anxiety, or PTSD than if they do not have these conditions (Spencer et al., 2010). Depression after mTBI has been associated with older age at time of injury and higher levels of depressive symptoms in the week after injury (Bay, 2009).

When the Minneapolis VA Evidence Synthesis Program reviewed the literature on patient care for TBI and PTSD from 1980 to April 2009 (VA, 2009), they had two key findings: the reported prevalence of comorbid

TBI and PTSD varied widely among study populations, none of which was a large, representative population; and no published studies reviewed the accuracy of diagnostic tests that were used for assessing co-occurring mTBI and PTSD. Those findings suggest that the frequent, albeit variable, co-occurrence of TBI, PTSD, and other health conditions presents serious challenges for optimizing treatment-planning and outcomes. PTSD may also exacerbate other conditions that are often reported after deployment, including pain and headache, because of its effects on sleep and the perception of pain. There is some question as to whether the neuropathology of PTSD associated with TBI differs from that of PTSD arising from trauma that is not due to direct physical or neurologic injury to the brain (Stein and McAllister, 2009; see also Chapter 3).

Treatment for Co-Occurring TBI and PTSD

Few empirical studies have examined treatment protocols that specifically targeted co-occurring TBI and PTSD symptoms in civilian populations (Bryant et al., 2003; McAllister, 2009; McMillan et al., 2003). In recognition of this, the VA Consensus Conference report (2010) stated that, "there was complete consensus that the current VA/DoD clinical practice guidelines for PTSD, mTBI, and pain should be followed at this time, until new research suggests other approaches or demonstrates that current clinical practice guidelines are ineffective or inappropriate for this complex population."

Many approaches to the rehabilitation of the neurocognitive, vocational, and psychosocial sequelae of TBI have been developed and evaluated over the last 30 years. Cognitive neurorehabilitation has been defined by Robertson and Fitzpatrick (2008) as a "structured, planned experience derived from an understanding of brain function which ameliorates dysfunctional cognitive and brain processes caused by disease or injury and improves everyday life function." The efforts are as varied as the types of impairments they try to address.

The American Congress of Rehabilitation Medicine Brain Injury Interdisciplinary Special Interest Group Cognitive Rehabilitation Task Force has published three systematic reviews of the efficacy of neurocognitive rehabilitation after TBI or stroke (Cicerone et al., 2000, 2005, 2011). The most recent presented a set of practice standards, guidelines, and options based on the array of evidence supporting various cognitive rehabilitation strategies. This provided clear standards for implementation of cognitive rehabilitation therapy (CRT) primarily on the basis of civilian TBI literature on the remediation of neurocognitive impairments (attention, visuospatial, and praxic deficits and impairments in language and communication, memory, and executive function).

Two efforts have served as the basis of the most up-to-date and specific analysis of the treatment literature and of practice recommendations for the remediation of TBI-related impairments in neurocognitive, emotional, and psychosocial functioning and for addressing the future of assessment of and intervention in co-occurring TBI and PTSD: the 2010 VA Consensus Conference and the Institute of Medicine (IOM) consensus report on CRT after TBI. The VA Consensus Conference (VA, 2010a) provided a series of recommendations that address comorbid TBI and PTSD in veterans, including the following:

- Identify best practices for co-occurring TBI, PTSD, and pain through further research.
- Enhance collaborative-care coordination among disciplines.
- Determine special and unique issues for PTSD, mTBI, and pain patients in rural health settings.
- Improve collection and monitoring of treatment outcomes of patients who have these comorbidities to examine variables relevant to the wide variety of treatment approaches that are being implemented.
- Include family members in the treatment planning and process.
- Provide support to family members when possible.
- Increase opportunities for educating clinical care providers regarding outcome measurement.

Clear action plans for research priorities, with timelines, for treating persons who have PTSD, mTBI, and pain were also recommended (VA, 2010a).

The IOM (2011) report on the use of CRT for TBI reviewed 90 TBI studies. The report described CRT as, "a collection of treatments, generally tailored to an individual depending on the pattern of the impairments and activity limitations, related disorders (e.g., preexisting conditions or comorbidities), and the presence of a family or social support system" and acknowledged that although there is some benefit of some forms of CRT for TBI, the evidence of its therapeutic value is variable and insufficient overall to provide definitive guidance for clinical best practices. The report also acknowledged the many current limitations in the literature, including lack of operational definitions of different forms of CRT, small sample sizes, and the many premorbid conditions, comorbidities, and environmental factors that may affect the outcome of CRT in heterogeneous populations. Because of the lack of a heterogeneous definition and varied study designs, a substantial effort is needed to address TBI and co-occurring conditions, such as PTSD.

The *Co-occurring Conditions Toolkit: Mild Traumatic Brain Injury and Psychological Health* (DCoE, 2011) evolved from a 2009 VA conference to develop consensus recommendations for the treatment of veterans who have comorbid concussion, PTSD, and pain. At the conference, subject-matter experts in the VA and the DoD determined that current VA/DoD clinical practice guidelines aimed at patients who presented with a single condition would be applicable to patients who had comorbid conditions until there was evidence that the guidelines were contraindicated. The toolkit was designed to assist primary care providers in evaluating and managing patients who present with multiple conditions by synthesizing information from the existing guidelines. The primary focus of the toolkit is on improving the evaluation and specification of conditions that may result from conflicting sets of presenting symptoms rather than on diagnosing co-morbid conditions. An electronic version of the toolkit was recently created for smartphones and tablet devices by the National Center for Telehealth and Technology. The application contains the entire contents of the hard-copy form of the toolkit and provides digital interactive decision trees to aid in the identification of appropriate interventions and timing of services for patients who have co-occurring conditions, including PTSD, depression, chronic opioid therapy, and substance use disorders (DoD, 2012).

Amputation, Spinal Cord Injury, and Burns

IEDs and other blasts have caused many of the physical injuries sustained in OEF and OIF. Adoption of body armor and armored vehicles has improved battlefield injury survival rates; however, the enhanced protection from injuries to vital organs has meant that a number of service members have survived catastrophic spinal cord injury, amputation, and burns (in addition to TBI). Compared with the incidence of TBI, the number of service members who have suffered such polytrauma is relatively small. For example, as of September 2010, there have been 1,222 major limb amputations and 399 minor (finger, toe, hand, and foot) amputations in OEF and OIF service members (Fischer, 2010). As of September 2007, spinal cord injury was reported in approximately 100 active-duty service members, often as a result of blast injuries that damaged the more exposed cervical spinal region and typically led to quadriplegia (Weaver et al., 2009).

Polytrauma survivors who have suffered complex combinations of injuries and are at risk for developing PTSD will require substantial, and in many cases long-term, care and rehabilitation. In a recent study of 382 military amputees, Melcer et al. (2010) reported that two-thirds had at least one mental health diagnosis, the most prevalent of which was PTSD, followed by acute stress reaction and depressive disorder. Virtually all the injuries (91.4%) were caused by traumatic exposures to explosions, including those of IEDs, rocket-propelled grenades, mortars, and landmines. In an analysis of 221 amputee veterans (92.3% served in OEF and OIF) discharged between July 1, 2005, and September 30, 2006, 61.5% had been diagnosed with PTSD in the VA compared with 11.7% of all nonamputee veterans discharged from the military during this same time period (n = 490,936) (VA, 2012a).

Gaylord et al. (2009) followed 372 service members whose burns were treated at an Army burn center during the period October 2003–May 2008 and found 25% of them screened positive for PTSD. Those findings are within the range of previous estimates of the 12-month prevalence of PTSD in civilian burn patients, which have been estimated to range from 9% to 45% (Dyster-Aas et al., 2008; McKibben et al., 2008).

In a 2001 review of spinal cord injury and co-occurring mental disorders, Kennedy and Duff (2001) reported the prevalence of PTSD after spinal cord injury to be 16% in veterans who had suffered combat trauma and 10–40% in the general population (Radnitz et al., 1998a,b). In civilian victims of fire and motor vehicle incidents, depression is the most common comorbid disorder for those diagnosed with PTSD (Maes et al., 2000). As in the case of TBI, no empirical studies have examined treatment protocols specifically targeted at PTSD after multiple, complex traumatic injuries.

Other Medical Conditions and PTSD

Conditions other than those related to the trauma co-occur with PTSD in military and veteran populations and have implications for treatment of both PTSD and the comorbid condition. For example, many studies have shown PTSD to be associated with increased risk of cardiovascular disease (Boscarino, 2008a; Cohen et al., 2009a; Kubzansky et al., 2007), specifically, coronary heart disease, which may be an effect of PTSD on hypertension, hyperlipidemia, and obesity (Coughlin, 2011). Cohen et al. (2010) examined the effect of mental health diagnoses on cardiovascular risk factors—including hypertension, dyslipidemia, and diabetes—in a sample of approximately 303,000 OEF and OIF veterans who received care at VA facilities from 2001 through 2008. Veterans were categorized as having no mental health diagnoses, having mental health diagnoses but not PTSD, or having PTSD with or without comorbid mental health diagnoses. When the group that had no mental health diagnoses was used as the reference and after adjustment for demographic and military factors and for number of visits to primary care subspecialties, both men and women in the PTSD group and the group that had mental health diagnoses but not PTSD had significantly higher rates of hypertension and dyslipidemia.

Three prospective studies indicate that PTSD may be involved in the etiology of coronary heart disease. In the first, of 1,002 veterans enrolled in the Normative Aging Study, the authors found that after controlling for depressive symptoms and other factors, the adjusted relative risk of combined nonfatal myocardial infarction and fatal coronary heart disease increased significantly for each standard deviation increase in score on the Mississippi Scale for Combat-Related PTSD. That a similar significant association was found when angina was included constituted evidence that higher levels of PTSD symptoms may increase the risk of incident coronary heart disease in older male veterans (Kubzansky et al., 2007). In a related study of Vietnam Army veterans, Boscarino (2008a) found that after adjustment for coronary risk factors and depression, a diagnosis of PTSD more than doubled the risk of death from early-age heart disease. The third prospective study, which sampled 1,059 civilian women, found that after adjustment for coronary risk factors and depression, participants who had five or more PTSD symptoms were at significantly higher risk of incident coronary heart disease than participants who had no PTSD symptoms (Kubzansky et al., 2009). PTSD is also associated with decreased adherence to treatment regimens for myocardial infarction (Shemesh et al., 2004).

Metabolic syndrome is defined as a cluster of several risk factors—such as hypertension, obesity, diabetes, and hyperlipidemia—that when they occur together increase the risk of cardiovascular diseases (including coronary heart disease, coronary artery disease, and stroke). Psychologic factors have been associated with the individual components of metabolic syndrome and with metabolic syndrome as a whole (Vaccarino et al., 2008). Cohen et al. (2009a) found that higher levels of depression, anger expression, hostility, and pessimism, assessed with validated measures, were significantly associated with increased prevalence of metabolic syndrome. However, the association was largely explained by income and lifestyle mediators (smoking, body mass index, regular alcohol use, physical activity).

In addition to the significant association between PTSD and cardiac disease, PTSD is associated with lower health-related quality of life. In a sample of 1,022 men and women who had coronary heart disease (about 40% of whom were veterans), after adjustment for cardiovascular risk factors, including demographic factors and smoking status, objective measures of cardiac function (such as exercise capacity and ejection fraction) and comorbid depression, PTSD was independently associated with greater symptom burden, greater physical limitation, and worse quality of life (Cohen et al., 2009b).

In addition to its association with heart disease, PTSD has been associated with inflammatory and autoimmune diseases (Boscarino, 2008b; O'Toole and Catts, 2008), proinflammatory and anti-inflammatory activity (von Känel et al., 2007), endothelial dysfunction (von Känel et al., 2008), and diabetes mellitus (Boyko et al., 2010; Qureshi et al., 2009). The association between PTSD and diabetes has been mixed. Qureshi et al. (2009) reviewed four studies that examined the relationship between physical disease and PTSD. Two of the studies of the general population (Lauterbach et al., 2005; Weisberg et al., 2002) found positive associations, and two (Boscarino, 2004; Norman et al., 2006), including one that used a sample of 2,490 male Vietnam veterans, were negative. Using a large sample from the Millennium Cohort Study, Boyko et al. (2010) found that after adjustment for several factors—including demographic factors, military service characteristics, physical health factors, and mental health conditions—baseline PTSD was the only factor significantly associated with increased risk of diabetes. Cohen et al. (2009a) found that after adjustment for demographic factors and number of deployments, a PTSD diagnosis (and mental health diagnoses but not PTSD) was significantly associated with diabetes in both men and women; however, after adjustment for number of primary care visits and number of subspecialty visits, PTSD was not statistically associated with diabetes in men.

There is also evidence that PTSD is associated with an increased susceptibility to future health conditions (such as dementia) and with an increased use of health care services; the latter finding suggests that the successful early treatment of PTSD may contribute to future health care savings (Boscarino, 2004, 2008a,b; Cohen et al., 2010; Spiro, 1994; Yaffe et al., 2010).

CO-OCCURRING PSYCHOSOCIAL PROBLEMS AND PTSD

Recently, more recognition that some people who have PTSD also have severe psychologic symptoms; experience difficulties with their partnerships and families, social environments, and work settings; and make more use of community and psychiatric services has resulted in improved treatment for PTSD. Psychosocial rehabilitation typically involves family psychoeducation and supported employment, education, and housing. Some clinicians may serve as case managers for their patients; in other cases, patients work with peer counselors. The 2010 VA/DoD guideline recommends psychosocial rehabilitation and expanding services offered by inpatient and outpatient programs in primary care settings, outpatient clinics, Vet Centers, and home-based care programs, including partnerships with agencies and providers in the communities (VA and DoD, 2010).

Empirically validated data support an integrated and collaborative treatment plan for PTSD (VA and DoD, 2010). Although currently underused, this approach combines trauma-focused therapies with psychosocial rehabilitation. Once a patient and a clinician identify the patient's PTSD-related problems, they must determine whether the issues are associated with core symptoms of PTSD or with some other problem and ensure that any interventions are provided in the context of integrative treatment for PTSD. The timing and pacing of interventions are critical because safety, self-care, and stabilization must be ensured before any of the treatment approaches are introduced to a client and his or her family.

Most research findings emphasize that positive social support is a central moderating influence in mitigating the adverse effects of trauma (IOM, 2008). Social support also facilitates effective treatment, healing, and recovery for service members, veterans, and their families. Consequently, health care providers should be attuned to a patient's psychosocial issues, and these issues should be central to all phases of a multimodal, integrative, comprehensive treatment and rehabilitation approach, including assessment, engagement, and planning of interventions (VA and DoD, 2010).

Relationship Problems

Most service members, veterans, and their families handle deployment and combat stressors without developing mental health problems. However, trauma can disrupt social connections, and deployment-related separations and reunions can exacerbate already stressful situations. Many service members confront substantial problems with relationships throughout the deployment cycle, including relationships with partners, family members, friends, extended family members, and coworkers (Davidson et al., 1989).

Although the committee did not find any studies that specifically associate divorce with the presence of PTSD in one or both partners, some general divorce statistics are applicable. Recent research consistently shows a higher prevalence of marital conflict and higher rates of divorce in OEF and OIF veteran couples than in civilian couples (Finley et al., 2010; Foran et al., 2011). That finding is similar to the significantly higher divorce rate in Vietnam veterans than in the general population; rates of divorce are even higher in Vietnam veterans who have PTSD (Kulka, 1990). An estimated 38% of Vietnam veterans' marriages failed within 6 months of veterans' return from deployment (PCMH, 1978). In addition to divorce, increasing rates of intimate partner violence (IPV) and child maltreatment by OEF and OIF couples have been noted (IOM, 2010; Rentz et al., 2007; Tanielian and Jaycox, 2008). This section discusses those and other psychosocial problems and clinical and program interventions to address them.

Multiple types of acts and degrees of violence fall under the umbrella definition of IPV. Milder, but no less serious, acts include pushing and slapping; more severe forms of IPV include punching, strangling, and burning. The U.S. military has recently adopted the definition of clinically significant IPV—physical aggression by a partner that results in injury, significant potential for injury, or significant fear—as the standard definition of abuse to be used as a threshold for whether IPV allegations should be labeled as abusive, and thereby result in more severe consequences (Slep et al., 2011). Recent research findings indicate high rates of IPV by returning OEF and

OIF service members and veterans (IOM, 2010; Jakupcak et al., 2007; Wadsworth and Riggs, 2010). A study of the prevalence of IPV, clinically significant IPV, and clinically significant emotional abuse found widespread partner maltreatment in military samples. Lower rank was a risk factor for perpetration and victimization. Men were more likely than women to perpetrate clinically significant IPV (Foran et al., 2011). Veterans who have PTSD have consistently had a higher incidence of IPV and significantly higher rates of aggression and violence than veterans who do not have PTSD (Beckham et al., 1997; Byrne and Riggs, 1996; Freeman and Roca, 2001; Jordan et al., 1992; Kulka, 1990; Taft et al., 1999; Teten et al., 2010; Tinney and West, 2011).

Teten et al. (2010) grouped OEF and OIF veterans according to their results on the PTSD Checklist–Military version (PTSD, subthreshold, and no PTSD) and compared the groups on self-report measures of hostility, aggression, and trait anger. Veterans in the PTSD group reported significantly greater anger and hostility than those in the subthreshold PTSD group, and those who did not have PTSD reported the least anger and hostility. There were no significant differences between the subthreshold PTSD and PTSD groups with respect to aggression, but both groups were significantly more likely to have endorsed aggression than the non-PTSD group. Those results suggest that it may be beneficial for clinicians to screen for anger and aggression in veterans who exhibit symptoms of PTSD in order to incorporate early treatment interventions that address affect dysregulation and problems with anger management. Jakupcak et al. (2007) examined partner aggression in male OIF and OEF veterans and compared their aggressiveness with that reported by Vietnam veterans who had PTSD. When age was controlled for, odds ratios showed that male OEF and OIF veterans who had PTSD were 1.9–3.1 times more likely to perpetrate aggression toward their female partners and 1.6–6.0 times more likely to report experiencing female-perpetrated aggression than OEF and OIF veterans who did not have PTSD and Vietnam veterans who had PTSD.

Typically, deployment and reintegration stressors weigh heavily on service members or veterans and their partners as they navigate complicated adjustments and transitions back into the community. Coping with war-theater combat and deployment stressors is moderated by the resilience and problem-solving capacities of service members, veterans, and their partners. In many cases, couples renew their connections after deployment without engaging in acute interpersonal conflict, but some service members and veterans who have PTSD, depression, TBI, or substance use disorders may find themselves more vulnerable to behaving in abusive and violent ways (Martin et al., 2010; Teten et al., 2010).

Several hypotheses have been offered to explain the heightened volatility. The hyperarousal cluster (Criterion D) of PTSD symptoms translates into affect dysregulation, alternating numbness and hyperarousal, emotional lability, and intermittent rage outbursts. The physiologic traumatic stress response can be triggered by stimuli that are associated with the original traumatic event. The biologic determinants intersect with a full range of intense emotions to create an incendiary milieu in the home (Finley et al., 2010). Such emotions may include estrangement; feelings of abandonment, loss, and rejection; isolation; and powerlessness related to a loss of military identity or a gap in resuming family and work roles on homecoming. In a study of returning OEF and OIF service members, the intensity of combat experience and exposure to violent human trauma were predictive of verbal and physical aggression toward others 3 months after deployment (Killgore et al., 2008).

A small study that examined IPV in a sample of mainly OEF and OIF veterans (84% who had PTSD) and their spouses found three general patterns of PTSD-related partner violence: violence committed in anger, dissociative violence, and parasomniac/hypnopompic violence (violence occurring during sleep or just before waking). The form of violence may be related to the specific PTSD symptom clusters affecting the veteran. Recognition of the form partner violence may take, when it may occur, and how both the veteran and his or her partner may perceive and respond to it has important implications for informing and developing appropriate plans for coping and safety-seeking (Finley et al., 2010). A recent study investigated the association between committing IPV and PTSD in a clinical sample of 302 men who sustained intimate terrorism—a form of IPV that involves intense violence—and a community sample of 520 men. Men who sustained intimate terrorism were at a much higher risk for exceeding the clinical cutoff on the PTSD measure than men who sustained common couple violence or no violence. The authors suggest that treatment approaches might also differ according to the degree of violence suffered (Hines and Douglas, 2011).

To facilitate a smooth transition after deployment, the DoD and the VA each use many treatment programs, but there is a lack of empirical evidence to support their efficacy. In the DoD, family advocacy programs are supported by each service branch. After a partner, family member, or clinician reports an incident of IPV to a superior officer, the command activates a referral for an assessment with a family advocacy program. If a victim reports to a victim advocate or health care provider, the victim can request a restricted report, in which case the command is not notified and a full assessment is not performed. If the provider feels that some aspects of the case are too risky to warrant a restricted report, he or she may refuse to issue a restricted report and may inform command while starting the assessment process.

Treatment programs typically involve individual and group therapy for the offender and individual support and therapy for the victimized partner. When safety has been achieved for both partners, couples therapy is often indicated to renew connections, foster sound problem solving and communication skills, and discuss symptoms and phenomena associated with PTSD (Robichaux and McCarroll, 2011). Anger-management groups constitute another common treatment option for offenders. For example, the VA Medical Center in Boston sponsors a 12-session program for men to help with anger management and conflict resolution in intimate relationships. The program has not been evaluated, but evaluation data are being collected (VA, 2012b).

A number of prevention and treatment programs that address IPV in the civilian and military sectors are being evaluated. For example, Families OverComing Under Stress (FOCUS), is a family-centered and evidence-based resilience training program adapted for use by the U.S. Marine Corps at Camp Pendleton, California (the largest Marine base on the West Coast), in 2006. In 2008, the Navy Bureau of Medicine and Surgery collaborated with the University of California, Los Angeles, in launching a large demonstration project with Navy and Marine Corps families. In 2009, FOCUS services were made available to Army and Air Force families at selected installations throughout the United States. The preventive interventions in the program use psychoeducation, emotional regulation skills, problem solving skills, communication skills, and management of traumatic stress reactions (Lester et al., 2011).

A recent RCT conducted by Iverson et al. (2011) explored the efficacy of CBT for reducing the risk of IPV in 150 civilian women who experienced interpersonal trauma and who had PTSD. After controlling for recent IPV, reduced symptoms of PTSD and depression were associated with a decreased likelihood of IPV victimization within 6 months; this highlights the importance of treating the co-occurring conditions of PTSD and depression in survivors of IPV as one method of reducing the risk of IPV. However, the study included only civilians, and it should be replicated in a military population to assess the generalizability of the findings.

Tinney and West (2011) emphasize the importance of ensuring the safety of the victims, the veterans, and all family members, and they recommend a coordinated, integrated multimodal community response to IPV and family violence. They describe an integrated best-practice model called the Praxis International "Saint Paul Blueprint for Safety" to respond to IPV in families affected by military service. The model involves a nexus of agencies that address domestic violence to maximize safety while holding offenders accountable and facilitating change (Praxis International, 2010). The program is a prototype that can be used by any community to link its criminal justice agencies in a coherent, research-informed domestic violence model. Although it has not been evaluated for IPV in military couples, the program developers report positive outcomes in addressing IPV crimes.

Effects of Parental Deployment and PTSD on Children

Slightly more than 2 million children have been affected by parental deployment to OEF and OIF, including 40% younger than 5 years old (Boston University School of Social Work, 2012). Although many military families harness their resilience and handle deployments well, some have difficulties with reconnecting and parenting, especially when a returning service member has PTSD (Chandra et al., 2010; Davidson et al., 1989; MacDermid et al., 2005; MHAT 7, 2011). Very young children are particularly vulnerable to deployment separations as a result of normative developmental challenges, including their emotional and cognitive immaturity and their reliance on parents for healthy development (Cozza and Lieberman, 2007; Paris et al., 2010). The relationship between parental functioning and the adaptation of children in the context of trauma and separation is well established. For example, studies of the effects of PTSD in Vietnam War veterans on family and marital functioning, including effects on children, found reduced family cohesion and less effective coping by both partners (Galovski and Lyons, 2004) and problematic parenting styles of over control, overprotection, disengagement, or enmeshment (extreme or inappropriate closeness) with children (Rosenheck and Nathan, 1985). Researchers have established the relationship between specific symptom clusters associated with PTSD (for example, intrusion, avoidance and numbing, and hyperarousal) and the quality of parent–child relationships. In particular, the emotional numbing associated with PTSD interferes with a parent's capacity to engage with and sustain interactions with his or her children (Ruscio et al., 2002).

Child maltreatment typically refers to physical, sexual, or emotional abuse inflicted by adults or adolescents toward children or neglect of basic needs of safety, shelter, nutrition, and education. A historical perspective provides a window into shifting rates of child maltreatment from 1990, before the 1990–1991 Gulf War to the present. In 1990, the child maltreatment rate was 6.9 per 1,000 children based on data from the Army Central Registry (Robichaux and McCarroll, 2011). In general, the rates of child maltreatment in military families decreased through the 1990s, increased to 5.2 per 1,000 children in 2000 and 6.2 per 1,000 children in 2004, and decreased to 5.0 per 1,000 children in 2007, the latest year for which data are available (Robichaux and McCarroll, 2011).

Child neglect as a form of maltreatment appears to be correlated with deployment. Cases of neglect of children in military families decreased from a high of 3.6 per 1,000 children in 1991 (during the 1990–1991 Gulf War) to a low of 2.7 per 1,000 in 2000 (before the start of OEF and OIF)—an overall decline of 25%. Child neglect rates rose to 4.5 per 1,000 in 2004, fell to 3.3 per 1,000 in 2006 and rose to 3.7 per 1,000 in 2007 (the latest data available). Neglect rates were highest in the youngest children. Clinical depression of the nondeployed spouse may contribute substantially to the observed increase in child neglect rates during combat deployments. PTSD has not been designated as a co-occurring condition but may exist in some of the nondeployed partners; however, the rate of PTSD in this group is unknown. The rates of physical child abuse decreased from 3.1 per 1,000 children in 1990 to 1.0 per 1,000 in 2007 (Robichaux and McCarroll, 2011).

Although it has not been PTSD specific, research points to a probable positive association between increased length of deployment and risk of child maltreatment, especially child neglect (Gibbs et al., 2007; McCarroll et al., 2008; Rentz et al., 2007). Most prevention and treatment approaches for reducing violence related to child maltreatment have not been systematically evaluated. One RCT found child–parent psychotherapy to be more efficacious than case management plus treatment-as-usual for preschool children exposed to IPV. Children in the child–parent psychotherapy group had decreased total behavior problems and PTSD symptoms, and their mothers (most of whom had PTSD) had significantly fewer PTSD avoidance symptoms at the end of treatment than did the control mothers (Lieberman et al., 2005). Two other programs, a Nurse–Family Partnership home-visiting program and the Positive Parenting Program (Triple P) have been shown to reduce child maltreatment. Other prevention and treatment programs are focused on supporting children and families of combat-injured service members and seek to enhance family cohesion, communication, secure attachments, education, and, when necessary, capacities for bereavement. All those programs have been found to serve as protective factors in reducing the risk of child maltreatment, including abuse and neglect (Cozza et al., 2011).

Strong Families Strong Forces is a three-phase project funded through a DoD grant and administered by a team of researchers in the Boston University School for Social Work (2012) to help veterans of OEF and OIF to reintegrate into their families after deployment. Phases 1 and 2 of the 4-year research program served to develop and test a home-based intervention to mitigate the stresses of the deployment life cycle on families, particularly those with children 1–5 years old, including the effects of a parent's PTSD on young children. Preliminary results found strains related to deployment separation, parenting, role adjustments, and mental health concerns, including PTSD. An eight-module home-based therapeutic program was developed to address the emotional cycle of deployment and reintegration and to provide guidance on more effective parenting and reestablishing relationships with children. The research team is in phase 3 of the project and is using an RCT to compare the efficacy of this treatment with the efficacy of usual treatment of a control group that takes place 1 month after the treatment group completes the program (Paris et al., 2011).

Suicide

At the start of OEF, the rate of suicide in the U.S. Army (10 suicides per 100,000 soldiers per year) was about half the civilian suicide rate of 18 per 100,000 (adjusted for age and sex). However, in 2003–2010, coinciding with the conflicts in Afghanistan and Iraq, the suicide rate in active-duty soldiers nearly doubled to about 22 suicides per 100,000 soldiers per year (CDC and NCHS, 2009; Ritchie, 2012). Although the suicide rate has leveled off in active-duty soldiers, it has continued to rise in National Guard soldiers (Ritchie, 2012). In response, the Army and the DoD have created task forces to understand the risk factors for suicide, especially factors peculiar to the military. The task forces' recommendations include standardized treatment protocols for at-risk military personnel and expanded primary health screenings that include mental health assessments (U.S. Army, 2010a).

As is the case with civilian suicides, many military suicides involve relationship problems with intimate partners, parents, or fellow unit members (CDC, 2012). Approximately two-thirds of military suicides appeared to be triggered by a relationship breakup. Like most civilian suicides, most military suicides are males, who tend to be more impulsive and use more violent methods of suicide (Styka et al., 2010). Black et al. (2011) found that the accumulation of multiple stressors—including relationship problems, job difficulties, and physical problems that many soldiers experience during their active-duty careers—is associated with completing suicide. In 2009, 9% of soldiers who committed suicide had received a diagnosis of PTSD (U.S. Army, 2010a). The National Comorbidity Survey found that PTSD (but not other anxiety disorders) was significantly associated with both suicidal ideation and attempts (Sareen et al., 2005). Therefore, monitoring for suicidal ideation and providing appropriate preventive interventions for persons being treated for PTSD in any sector is imperative. There are often concerns that some treatments for PTSD, such as prolonged exposure, may increase the risk for suicide or psychiatric hospitalization. However, these concerns do not appear to be supported by the scientific literature. For example, in a RCT of female veterans who had PTSD, Schnurr et al. (2007) compared PE (n = 141) with present-centered therapy (n = 143). Women who received PE experienced a significantly greater reduction of PTSD symptoms and were significantly less likely to meet PTSD diagnostic criteria than women who received present-centered therapy. Furthermore, there were more suicide attempts (3 vs. 1) and more than twice as many psychiatric hospitalizations (9 vs. 4) for the women who received the present-centered therapy compared with those who received PE. Those results suggest that rather than increasing risk, effective treatments for PTSD may reduce the risk for suicide and psychiatric hospitalization in those who have PTSD.

Unemployment and Vocational Rehabilitation

Rates of unemployment are high in OEF and OIF veterans. The Bureau of Labor Statistics reported that during 2011 the overall unemployment rate in veterans who had served in the military since 2001 was 12.1%. The rate was especially high (29.1%) in younger male veterans (18–24 years old) and was also higher in members of the National Guard and reserves (9.1%) and in veterans who had served in a combat zone since 2001 (11.6%). Veterans who had more education had an increased likelihood of employment (DoL, 2010).

Using data from the National Survey of the Vietnam Generation, Savoca and Rosenheck (2000) found that a lifetime diagnosis of PTSD was associated with an almost 50% lower likelihood of current employment. Similar findings have been reported by other large-scale studies of Vietnam veterans (McCarren et al., 1995; Zatzick et al., 1997). More recently, Smith et al. (2005) found that the severity of PTSD symptoms correlated with work performance. Of Vietnam veterans who were in treatment for PTSD in the VA, those with more severe symptoms were more likely to be working only part-time or not at all. The high rates of general unemployment, particularly in those who experienced combat, and earlier employment findings on Vietnam veterans who have PTSD underscore the importance of addressing vocational issues for veterans who have PTSD.

Veterans who have been adjudicated to have PTSD that is at least 20% disabling and related to their time in service are offered a comprehensive array of vocational services by the VA Vocational Rehabilitation and Employment Program, including funds for schooling or training, comprehensive vocational evaluation, work-readiness services, and case management and vocational-placement services. The program reimburses employers for initial on-the-job training and provides other incentives to hire veterans who have service-connected PTSD. A comprehensive rehabilitation plan is developed in collaboration with the veteran. The VA also provides vocational services through its compensated work therapy (CWT) program, which includes preemployment programs to prepare veterans for seeking work, sheltered workshops managed by VA staff, transitional housing while veterans begin work and become financially established in the community, and a robust supportive employment program that consists of competitive employment with integrated therapeutic supports. The focus of supportive employment is on assisting veterans who have mental illnesses in gaining access to meaningful employment.

In a study conducted more than 10 years ago, veterans who had PTSD were 19% less likely to be employed after discharge from the CWT program than veterans who had substance abuse disorders or who were homeless but did not have PTSD (Crowther, 2010). However, a recent RCT found that an evidence-based intervention for vocational rehabilitation was successful in veterans who had PTSD. This study randomized 85 veterans who had PTSD into a supportive employment program—Individual Placement and Support—or standard vocational rehabilitation and followed them for 12 months after enrollment. The manualized Individual Placement and Support program had previously been shown to be effective in improving employment outcomes in seriously mentally ill patients. Veterans enrolled in the Individual Placement and Support intervention were much more likely to obtain competitive employment in the community than those who did not receive the intervention (76% vs. 28%), worked more of the eligible weeks (42% vs. 16%), and had significantly more earnings during the follow-up period ($9,264 vs. $2,601). The study did not specify the era of service of the participants, who had a mean age of 40 years and were enrolled in the study during 2006–2010. Patients had high rates of co-occurring other psychiatric conditions, including alcohol dependence (42%), alcohol abuse (21%), drug dependence (37%), drug abuse (18%), and major depression (89%) (Davis et al., 2011).

High-Risk Behaviors

Service members returning from combat deployment are prone to high-risk behaviors that may endanger themselves and others. The most common high-risk behaviors include hazardous use of alcohol, aggressive or dangerous driving, and excessive gambling. Those behaviors can cause substantial adjustment problems for service members and veterans and may contribute to and compound other problems, including PTSD. Recent evidence suggests that high-risk behaviors are associated with the intensity of combat experienced during deployment. Deployed service members have a greater probability of morbidity and mortality from motor vehicle incidents and other unintentional sources of injury than nondeployed service members. A few studies of earlier conflicts suggest this vulnerability decreases over time, but there are few data on a similar decline in risk for service members returning from Iraq and Afghanistan, especially those who had repeated deployments and are at higher risk of PTSD (Killgore et al., 2008). Addressing these behaviors should be considered part of overall PTSD treatment and rehabilitation in such populations.

High-risk behaviors are seldom noted in clinical records of service members or veterans who are seeking mental health treatment in military or VA settings. Moreover, many clinicians do not perceive themselves as adequately trained to treat high-risk behaviors (Drebing et al., 2001; Weis and Manos, 2007). Short, validated screening and assessment tools exist for the most studied behaviors, such as the three-item AUDIT-C (Kriston et al., 2008) for hazardous use of alcohol; problem gambling (Westermeyer et al., 2005); and aggressive and unsafe driving (Killgore et al., 2008). Screening for those behaviors in high-risk populations, such as veterans who have had multiple deployments, may be an important first step in initiating treatment for these and related psychiatric comorbidities.

Alcohol Use

Separate from the psychiatric condition of alcohol abuse discussed earlier in this chapter, the hazardous or harmful use of alcohol is a major public health problem, accounting for as much disability and mortality as tobacco use and hypertension (Room et al., 2005). Alcohol-related incidents have increased since the beginning of OEF and OIF (DoD, 2007). A recent analysis from the Millennium Cohort Study of 48,481 active-duty, reserve, and National Guard service members found that rates of the following alcohol consumption behaviors were particularly high in reserve and National Guard members (Jacobson et al., 2008): heavy weekly drinking—men who consumed greater than 14 alcoholic drinks per week or women who consumed greater than 7—(9%), binge drinking—consuming 5 or more alcoholic drinks (4 or more for women) on at least one day per week or on a single occasion—(53%), and alcohol-related problems—positive response to one of several scenarios including consuming alcohol against physician orders; drinking, intoxicated, or hung over from alcohol while working, going to school, or taking care of children; and driving a vehicle after consuming several drinks—(15%). Similarly, a recent study of 1,508 OEF and OIF veterans who were using VA medical, surgical, or mental health services found that 40% screened positive for hazardous alcohol use (Calhoun et al., 2008). A recent survey of 596 OEF and OIF veterans from all services and components found 39% screened positive for probable alcohol abuse. Although OEF and OIF veterans did not differ significantly with regard to PTSD symptoms, OIF veterans reported significantly more depression, alcohol use, and substance use than OEF veterans (Eisen et al., 2012).

A recent study surveyed 1,252 OIF combat soldiers immediately after and 3 months after deployment to assess the relationship between combat experiences, selected high-risk behaviors, alcohol use, and aggression. Greater exposure to violent combat, human trauma, and killing another person were predictive of risk-taking behaviors, including more frequent alcohol use and consuming alcohol in increased quantities (Killgore et al., 2008). Similarly, in a study of 1,120 OIF infantry soldiers, 25% screened positive for alcohol misuse, and those reporting higher rates of exposure to threats of death and injury were significantly more likely to screen positive for alcohol misuse (Wilk et al., 2010). Moreover, PTSD has repeatedly been correlated with abuse of alcohol in veteran and active-duty populations. For example, alcohol misuse was recently shown to be related to PTSD symptoms in OEF and OIF veterans (Jakupcak, 2010). In response, the military has developed and piloted programs to identify and reduce alcohol misuse in active-duty service members. Williams et al. (2009) reported the results of the modification of two Internet-based alcohol interventions delivered to active-duty military personnel: 2,171 received the intervention and 919 served as controls. The modified drinker-checkup program (Hester et al., 2005) was effective in reducing alcohol misuse. Similarly, an Internet-based intervention for marines was found to be generally acceptable to many potential participants (Simon-Arndt et al., 2006). In a study of 963 Army National Guard members recently returned from deployment, of the 113 (11.7%) who reported an alcohol abuse disorder that first occurred during or following deployment, 35 reported coincident depression, 23 reported coincident PTSD, and 15 reported both depression and PTSD. After adjustment for several potentially confounding factors, peri- and postdeployment PTSD was found to be significantly associated with alcohol abuse disorders. The authors concluded that coincident PTSD and depression were predictive of developing peri- and postdeployment alcohol abuse, and therefore, deployment-related exposures may increase the risk of alcohol-related problems and disorders (Marshall et al., 2012). Although it did not examine temporality of diagnoses, a large study of 18,305 active-duty and National Guard soldiers found that at 3 months and 12 months following deployment to Iraq, about half of the soldiers who screened positive, using the strictest definition developed for the study, for PTSD or depression also screened positive for alcohol misuse or aggressive behaviors (Thomas et al., 2010).

During its site visit to Fort Hood, Texas, the committee heard about the intensive outpatient program in which PTSD treatment is embedded in alcohol- and substance-abuse treatment. Practitioners and patients both reported that the program is less stigmatizing than PTSD-specific programs.

Unsafe and Aggressive Driving

Aggressive and unsafe driving can be problematic for active-duty service members (Killgore et al., 2008). Although most research focuses on veterans from earlier eras, the likelihood of high-risk behavior is expected to be high in OEF and OIF veterans because this population is younger and unsafe driving correlates highly with age. For example, UK military personnel who had been deployed to Iraq had higher rates of dangerous driving than older veterans. OEF and OIF service members who drove in combat areas were often attacked and had learned to adapt more aggressive driving techniques and to not use seat belts so they could leave their vehicles quickly (Kuhn et al., 2010). A recent study explored unsafe driving in 474 male U.S. veterans who were receiving treatment for PTSD. Approximately two-thirds of them reported lifetime aggressive driving, and one-third reported current aggressive driving. Severity of PTSD was associated with aggressive driving but not with other forms of unsafe driving, such as lack of seatbelt use. OEF and OIF veterans had higher rates of aggressive driving and other forms of unsafe driving than Vietnam and 1990–1991 Gulf War veterans even after controlling for age, other demographics, and severity of PTSD (Kuhn et al., 2010).

Gambling

Problem gambling has been associated with anxiety disorders in large epidemiologic studies of civilians (Kessler et al., 2008), and several studies have corroborated the significant association between PTSD and problem gambling in veteran populations. Lifetime PTSD was related to current pathologic gambling in Vietnam twin-study veterans, and active PTSD symptoms predicted gambling problems in older veterans (Levens et al., 2005; Scherrer et al., 2007). In a national survey of more than 8,000 male Vietnam-era veterans, 10% had a lifetime diagnosis of PTSD and 2.3% had pathologic gambling, but the overlap between the two conditions was not given (Eisen et al., 2004). In a study of pathologic gambling in American Indian and Hispanic veterans of all eras combined, a diagnosis of current PTSD was significantly associated with lifetime pathologic gambling (Westermeyer et al., 2005).

In a sample of 111 male and female veterans who were admitted to a VA gambling treatment program, 64% reported a history of emotional trauma, 41% reported physical trauma, and 24% reported sexual trauma, primarily in childhood (Kausch et al., 2006). A group of 149 treatment-seeking problem gamblers were assessed for PTSD symptoms; 34% reported a high frequency of PTSD symptoms and were found to have greater lifetime gambling severity, psychiatric symptom severity, and impulsivity than those who had a low frequency of PTSD symptoms (Ledgerwood and Petry, 2006). Conversely, a study of 153 Australian veterans who were in treatment for PTSD found that although 28% screened positive for problem gambling, no significant relationship was found between problem gambling and PTSD (Biddle et al., 2005).

Incarceration

As noted earlier in this chapter, PTSD is commonly associated with substance abuse, unregulated anger, aggressive behavior, and hazardous use of alcohol, all of which are themselves associated with legal problems and incarceration. Few studies have examined the association between PTSD and incarceration.

Saxon et al. (2001) studied 129 jailed veterans, 87% of whom reported a history of trauma and 39% of whom screened positive for PTSD. Those who screened positive for PTSD reported more trauma, more serious legal problems, higher lifetime alcohol and drug use, and more mental health and general health problems. In those who screened positive for PTSD, the most common trauma was witnessing the death or serious injury of someone; 28% had been in combat. Those findings in veterans are consistent with findings of other studies of incarcerated adults in the general population. Black et al. (2005) studied 4,886 subjects randomly drawn from four groups: active-duty and National Guard and reserve veterans of the 1990–1991 Gulf War and active-duty and National Guard and reserve veterans from other periods. Overall, 23% had been incarcerated at some time in their lives. Veterans of the 1990–1991 Gulf War who had been incarcerated were three times more likely to report PTSD symptoms and depression and twice as likely to report alcohol abuse and anxiety. Gulf War veterans who had participated in combat had a higher rate of incarceration than those who had not. The findings from those two studies suggest that outreach to veterans who have PTSD and who are incarcerated or have been recently released may help them to access comprehensive treatment and rehabilitation options to improve functioning and reduce the risk of recidivism and future legal problems.

Homelessness

Homelessness is an impediment to the rehabilitation and recovery of veterans who have PTSD. Although estimates of homelessness of veterans vary, the federal government estimates that 75,609 veterans were homeless on a single night in January 2009, and that at least 136,334 were homeless at some time from October 2008 to September 2009 (HUD and VA, 2010). Veterans are twice as likely to be homeless as other adults, and minority-group veterans are 2–3 times more likely to be homeless than non-Hispanic white veterans. Disability is a major factor in homelessness of veterans: 52% of the homeless are estimated to have a disability, most often a mental disorder or substance abuse. A 2011 report found that homelessness of veterans had declined by 11% since January 2009. That may, in part, be a result of the national initiative by the VA and the U.S.

Department of Housing and Urban Development to reduce homelessness of veterans (VA, 2012c).

The VA provided specialized homelessness services to 92,625 veterans during 2009, including case-management services at every medical center, a national 24-hour help line, programs for incarcerated veterans and mentally ill veterans in the justice system, Stand Downs (health outreach efforts in conjunction with communities), supportive housing services, community partnerships, and more intensive residential services. In 2011, the VA announced grants to 85 community organizations in 40 states to establish a new homeless-prevention program for veterans and their families (VA, 2012bc).

VA homelessness programs predominantly serve veterans who have mental disorders and substance abuse. These programs have demonstrated through program evaluations that they are effective in reducing homelessness. A recent uncontrolled study of three residential care programs, the most intensive interventions, indicated that of 1,003 participating veterans, all but 11% had a serious mental health or substance abuse disorder. Although 47% had a substance abuse disorder, only 9% had PTSD and 37% had a dual diagnosis of substance abuse and a psychiatric diagnosis. A comorbid psychiatric disorder and substance abuse disorder was predictive of poorer mental health functioning and quality of life outcomes, but does not appear to adversely affect the ability to gain independent housing through these programs. At 12-month follow-up, 78% were no longer homeless, a result comparable to other reports of VA residential homelessness care (McGuire et al., 2011).

Other factors associated with homelessness are experiencing sexual assault while serving in the military and being a member of the National Guard or reserves. With the increasing number of women in the military, sexual assault during military service is an increasingly important trauma-associated risk factor for homelessness evidenced by one study that compared housed and homeless female veterans in Los Angeles and found that sexual assault during military service was associated with increased rates of homelessness (Washington et al., 2010).

SUMMARY

Many service members returning from deployments in Iraq and Afghanistan suffer a constellation of signature injuries that include PTSD, depression, substance abuse, TBI, and IPV. Given the complexity of those mental health and psychosocial problems, treatment approaches need to provide complex solutions. The committee finds that treatment for co-occurring conditions and functional impairments is critical for the success of treatment of all service members and veterans who have PTSD. As informed by the review of the empiric literature on the treatment of PTSD and related physical, mental, and psychosocial comorbidities presented in the chapter, a collaborative care model should be introduced before or concurrently with evidence-based PTSD treatment models.

REFERENCES

Ahman, S., and B. M. Stalnacke. 2008. Post-traumatic stress, depression, and anxiety in patients with injury-related chronic pain: A pilot study. *Journal of Neuropsychiatric Disease and Treatment* 4(6):1245-1249.

APA (American Psychiatric Association). 2000. *Diagnostic and statistical manual of mental health disorders: Fourth edition: Text revision.* Washington, DC: American Psychiatric Association.

Bair, M. J. 2004. Impact of pain on depression treatment response in primary care. *Psychosomatic Medicine* 66(1):17-22.

Bay, E. 2009. Current treatment options for depression after mild traumatic brain injury. *Current Treatment Options in Neurology* 11(5):377-382.

Beckham, J. C., M. E. Feldman, A. C. Kirby, M. A. Hertzberg, and S. D. Moore. 1997. Interpersonal violence and its correlates in Vietnam veterans with chronic posttraumatic stress disorder. *Journal of Clinical Psychology* 53(8):859-869.

Belanger, H. G., G. Curtiss, J. A. Demery, B. K. Lebowitz, and R. D. Vanderploeg. 2005. Factors moderating neuropsychological outcomes following mild traumatic brain injury: A meta-analysis. *Journal of the International Neuropsychological Society* 11(3):215-227.

Biddle, D., G. Hawthorne, D. Forbes, and G. Coman. 2005. Problem gambling in Australian PTSD treatment-seeking veterans. *Journal of Traumatic Stress* 18(6):759-767.

Bigler, E. D. 2008. Neuropsychology and clinical neuroscience of persistent post-concussive syndrome. *Journal of the International Neuropsychological Society* 14(1):1-22.

Black, D. W., C. P. Carney, P. M. Peloso, R. F. Woolson, E. Letuchy, and B. N. Doebbeling. 2005. Incarceration and veterans of the first Gulf War. *Military Medicine* 170(7):612-618.

Black, S. A., M. S. Gallaway, M. R. Bell, and E. C. Ritchie. 2011. Prevalence and risk factors associated with suicides of Army soldiers. *Military Psychology* 23(4):433-451.

Boden, M. T., R. Kimerling, J. Jacobs-Lentz, D. Bowman, C. Weaver, D. Carney, R. Walser, and J. A. Trafton. 2012. Seeking safety treatment for male veterans with a substance use disorder and post-traumatic stress disorder symptomatology. *Addiction* 107(3):578-586.

Boscarino, J. A. 2004. Posttraumatic stress disorder and physical illness: Results from clinical and epidemiological studies. *Annals of the New York Academy of Sciences* 1032:141-153.

Boscarino, J. A. 2008a. A prospective study of PTSD and early-age heart disease mortality among Vietnam veterans: Implications for surveillance and prevention. *Psychosomatic Medicine* 70(6):668-676.

Boscarino, J. A. 2008b. Psychobiologic predictors of disease mortality after psychological trauma: Implications for research and clinical surveillance. *Journal of Nervous and Mental Disease* 196(2):100-107.

Boston University School of Social Work. 2012. *Strong families strong forces.* http://www.bu.edu/sfsf/ (accessed February 1, 2012).

Boyko, E. J., I. G. Jacobson, B. Smith, M. A. Ryan, T. I. Hooper, P. J. Amoroso, G. D. Gackstetter, E. Barrett-Connor, and T. C. Smith. 2010. Risk of diabetes in U.S. military service members in relation to combat deployment and mental health. *Diabetes Care* 33(8):1771-1777.

Brenner, L. A., B. J. Ivins, K. Schwab, D. Warden, L. A. Nelson, M. Jaffee, and H. Terrio. 2010. Traumatic brain injury, posttraumatic stress disorder, and postconcussive symptom reporting among troops returning from Iraq. *Journal of Head Trauma Rehabilitation* 25(5):307-312.

Bryant, R. A., M. Moulds, R. Guthrie, and R. D. Nixon. 2003. Treating acute stress disorder following mild traumatic brain injury. *American Journal of Psychiatry* 160(3):585-587.

Byrne, C. A., and D. S. Riggs. 1996. The cycle of trauma; Relationship aggression in male Vietnam veterans with symptoms of posttraumatic stress disorder. *Violence & Victims* 11(3):213-225.

Calhoun, P. S., J. R. Elter, E. R. Jones, H. Kudler, and K. Straits-Troster. 2008. Hazardous alcohol use and receipt of risk-reduction counseling among U.S. veterans of the wars in Iraq and Afghanistan. *Journal of Clinical Psychiatry* 69(11):1686-1693.

Carlson, K. F., D. Nelson, R. J. Orazem, S. Nugent, D. X. Cifu, and N. A. Sayer. 2010. Psychiatric diagnoses among Iraq and Afghanistan war veterans screened for deployment-related traumatic brain injury. *Journal of Traumatic Stress* 23(1):17-24.

CDC (Centers for Disease Control and Prevention). 2012. *National violent death reporting system*. http://wisqars.cdc.gov:8080/nvdrs/nvdrsDisplay.jsp (accessed February 29, 2012).

CDC and NCHS (National Center for Health Statistics). 2009. *Suicide rates in the Army and civilian population 1990-2009*. U.S. Army Public Health Command (Provisional) Behavioral and Social Health Outcomes Program.

Cerda, M., D. Vlahov, M. Tracy, and S. Galea. 2008. Alcohol use trajectories among adults in an urban area after a disaster: Evidence from a population-based cohort study. *Addiction* 103(8):1296-1307.

Chandra, A., S. Lara-Cinisomo, L. H. Jaycox, T. Tanielian, R. M. Burns, T. Ruder, and B. Han. 2010. Children on the homefront: The experience of children from military families. *Pediatrics* 125(1):16-25.

Cicerone, K. D., C. Dahlberg, K. Kalmar, D. M. Langenbahn, J. F. Malec, T. F. Bergquist, T. Felicetti, J. T. Giacino, J. P. Harley, D. E. Harrington, J. Herzog, S. Kneipp, L. Laatsch, and P. A. Morse. 2000. Evidence based cognitive rehabilitation: Recommendations for clinical practice. *Archives of Physical Medicine and Rehabilitation* 81(12):1596-1615.

Cicerone, K. D., C. Dahlberg, J. F. Malec, D. M. Langenbahn, T. Felicetti, S. Kneipp, W. Ellmo, K. Kalmar, J. T. Giacino, J. P. Harley, L. Laatsch, P. A. Morse, and J. Catanese. 2005. Evidence-based cognitive rehabilitation: Updated review of the literature from 1998 through 2002. *Archives of Physical Medicine and Rehabilitation* 86(8):1681-1692.

Cicerone, K. D., D. M. Langenbahn, C. Braden, J. F. Malec, K. Kalmar, M. Fraas, T. Felicetti, L. Laatsch, J. P. Harley, T. Bergquist, J. Azulay, J. Cantor, and T. Ashman. 2011. Evidence-based cognitive rehabilitation: Updated review of the literature from 2003 through 2008. *Archives of Physical Medicine and Rehabilitation* 92(4):519-530.

Cisler, J. M., A. B. Amstadter, A. M. Begle, H. S. Resnick, C. K. Danielson, B. E. Saunders, and D. G. Kilpatrick. 2011. PTSD symptoms, potentially traumatic event exposure, and binge drinking: A prospective study with a national sample of adolescents. *Journal of Anxiety Disorders* 25(7):978-987.

Clark, M. E., M. J. Bair, C. C. Buckenmaier, R. J. Gironda, and R. L. Walker. 2007. Pain and combat injuries in soldiers returning from Operations Enduring Freedom and Iraqi Freedom: Implications for research and practice. *Journal of Rehabilitation Research and Development* 44(2):179-193.

Cohen, B. E., C. Marmar, L. Ren, D. Bertenthal, and K. H. Seal. 2009a. Association of cardiovascular risk factors with mental health diagnoses in Iraq and Afghanistan war veterans using VA health care. *Journal of the American Medical Association* 302(5):489-492.

Cohen, B. E., C. R. Marmar, T. C. Neylan, N. B. Schiller, S. Ali, and M. A. Whooley. 2009b. Posttraumatic stress disorder and health-related quality of life in patients with coronary heart disease: Findings from the heart and soul study. *Archives of General Psychiatry* 66(11):1214-1220.

Cohen, B. E., P. Panguluri, B. Na, and M. A. Whooley. 2010. Psychological risk factors and the metabolic syndrome in patients with coronary heart disease: Findings from the heart and soul study. *Psychiatry Research* 175(1-2):133-137.

Cook, J. M., R. D. Walser, V. Kane, J. I. Ruzek, and G. Woody. 2006. Dissemination and feasibility of a cognitive-behavioral treatment for substance use disorders and posttraumatic stress disorder in the veterans administration. *Journal of Psychoactive Drugs* 38(1):89-92.

Coughlin, S. S. 2011. Post-traumatic stress disorder and cardiovascular disease. *Open Cardiovascular Medical Journal* 5:164-170.

Cozza, S. J., and A. F. Lieberman. 2007. The young military child: Our modern Telemachus. *Zero to Three* 27(6):6.

Cozza, S. J., R. S. Chun, and C. Miller. 2011. The children and families of combat-injured service members. In *Combat and operational behavioral health*, edited by E. C. Ritchie. Ft. Detrick, MD: Borden Institute. Pp. 503-534.

Crowther, R., M. Marshall, G. R. Bond, and P. Huxley. 2010. Vocational rehabilitation for people with severe mental illness (review). *Cochrane Database of Systematic Reviews* 2001(2). DOI: 10.1002/14651858.CD003080.

Davidson, J., R. Smith, and H. Kudler. 1989. Familial psychiatric illness in chronic posttraumatic stress disorder. *Comprehensive Psychiatry* 30(4):339-345.

Davis, L. L., A. Leon, R. Toscano, C. Drebing, L. C. Ward, P. E. Parker, T. M. Kashner, and R. E. Drake. 2011. A randomized controlled trial of supported employment among veterans with posttraumatic stress disorder. *Psychiatric Services in Advance* 1-7.

DCoE (Defense Centers of Excellence for Psychological Health and Traumatic Brain Injury). 2011. *Co-occurring conditions toolkit: Mild traumatic brain injury and psychological health*. Washington, DC: Department of Defense.

DCoE and DVBIC (Defense and Veterans Brain Injury Center). 2009. *Mild traumatic brain injury pocket guide (CONUS)*. http://www.dcoe.health.mil/Content/Navigation/Documents/Mild%20Traumatic%20Brain%20Injury%20Pocket%20Guide.pdf (accessed January 30, 2012).

Desai, R. A., I. Harpaz-Rotem, L. M. Najavits, and R. A. Rosenheck. 2008. Impact of the seeking safety program on clinical outcomes among homeless female veterans with psychiatric disorders. *Psychiatric Services* 59(9):996-1003.

Desai, R. A., I. Harpaz-Rotem, L. M. Najavits, and R. A. Rosenheck. 2009. Seeking safety therapy: Clarification of results. *Psychiatric Services* 60(1):125.

Dikmen, S., J. Machamer, J. R. Fann, and N. R. Temkin. 2010. Rates of symptom reporting following traumatic brain injury. *Journal of the International Neuropsychological Society* 16(03):401.

DoD (Department of Defense). 2007. *An achievable vision: Report of the Department of Defense Task Force on Mental Health*. Falls Church, VA: Defense Health Board.

DoD. 2009. *Brigade combat team physical therapy guide*. Washington, DC: Department of Defense Office of the Surgeon General.

DoD. 2012. *Co-occurring conditions toolkit (CCT)*. http://t2health.org/apps/cct (accessed January 30, 2012).

DoL (Department of Labor). 2012. *Employment situation of veterans—2011*. USDL-12-0493. http://www.bls.gov/news.release/pdf/vet.pdf (accessed April 2, 2012).

Drebing, C. E., A. Mello, W. Penk, C. Krebs, E. A. Van Ormer, R. L. Peterson, and E. J. Federman. 2001. Clinical care of gambling disorders: Training, experience, and competence among VHA psychologists. *Journal of Gambling Studies* 17(2):117-136.

DVBIC (Defense and Veterans Brain Injury Center). 2011. TBI *numbers by severity*. http://www.dvbic.org/TBI---The-Military/TBI-Facts.aspx (accessed January 8, 2012).

Dyster-Aas, J., M. Willebrand, B. Wikehult, B. Gerdin, and L. Ekselius. 2008. Major depression and posttraumatic stress disorder symptoms following severe burn injury in relation to lifetime psychiatric morbidity. *Journal of Trauma-Injury Infection & Critical Care* 64(5):1349-1356.

Eisen, S. A., K. H. Griffith, H. Xian, J. F. Scherrer, I. D. Fischer, S. Chantarujikapong, J. Hunter, W. R. True, M. J. Lyons, and M. T. Tsuang. 2004. Lifetime and 12-month prevalence of psychiatric disorders in 8,169 male Vietnam war era veterans. *Military Medicine* 169(11):896-902.

Eisen, S. A., M. R. Shultz, D. Vogt, M. E. Glickman, R. Elwy, M. L. Drainoni, P. E. Osei-Bonsu, and J. Martin. 2012. Mental and physical health status and alcohol and drug use following return from deployment to Iraq or Afghanistan. *American Journal of Public Health* 102(S1):S66-S73.

Engel, C. C., and W. J. Katon. 1999. Population and need based prevention of unexplained physical symptoms in the community. In *Strategies to protect the health of deployed U.S. forces: Medical surveillance, record keeping, and risk reduction*, edited by Institute of Medicine. Washington, DC: National Academy Press. Pp. 173-212.

Engel, C. C., T. Oxman, C. Yamamoto, D. Gould, S. Barry, P. Stewart, K. Kroenke, J. W. Williams, Jr., and A. J. Dietrich. 2008. RESPECT-MIL: Feasibility of a systems-level collaborative care approach to depression and post-traumatic stress disorder in military primary care. *Military Medicine* 173(10):935-940.

Erickson, D. J., J. Wolfe, D. W. King, L. A. King, and E. J. Sharkansky. 2001. Posttraumatic stress disorder and depression symptomatology in a sample of Gulf War veterans: A prospective analysis. *Journal of Consulting & Clinical Psychology* 69(1):41-49.

Finley, E. P., M. Baker, M. J. Pugh, and A. L. Peterson. 2010. Patterns and perceptions of intimate partner violence committed by returning veterans with post-traumatic stress disorder. *Journal of Family Violence* 25:737–743.

Fischer, H. 2010. *U.S. military casualty statistics: Operation New Dawn, Operation Iraqi Freedom, and Operation Enduring Freedom*. Washington, DC: Congressional Research Service.

Foa, E. B. 2011. Prolonged exposure therapy: Past, present, and future. *Depression & Anxiety* 28(12):1043-1047.

Foran, H. M., A. M. S. Slep, and R. E. Heyman. 2011. Prevalences of intimate partner violence in a representative U.S. Air Force sample. *Journal of Consulting and Clinical Psychology* 79(3):391-397.

Freeman, T. W., and V. Roca. 2001. Gun use, attitudes toward violence, and aggression among combat veterans with chronic posttraumatic stress disorder. *Journal of Nervous and Mental Disease* 189(5):317-320.

Frueh, B. C., P. B. Gold, M. Dammeyer, K. L. Pellegrin, M. B. Hamner, M. R. Johnson, S. P. Cahill, and G. W. Arana. 2000. Differentiation of depression and PTSD symptoms in combat veterans. *Depression and Anxiety* 11(4):175-179.

Galarneau, M. R., S. I. Woodruff, J. L. Dye, C. R. Mohrle, and A. L. Wade. 2008. Traumatic brain injury during Operation Iraqi Freedom: Findings from the United States Navy-Marine Corps Combat Trauma Registry. *Journal of Neurosurgery* 108(5):950-957.

Galovski, T., and J. Lyons. 2004. Psychological sequelae of combat violence: A review of the impact of PTSD on the veteran family and possible interventions. *Aggression and Violent Behavior* 9(5):477-501.

Gatchel, R. J., and A. Okifuji. 2006. Evidence-based scientific data documenting the treatment and cost-effectiveness of comprehensive pain programs for chronic nonmalignant pain. *Journal of Pain* 7(11):779-793.

Gatchel, R. J., D. D. McGeary, A. Peterson, M. Moore, K. LeRoy, W. C. Isler, A. S. Hryshko-Mullen, and T. Edell. 2009. Preliminary findings of a randomized controlled trial of an interdisciplinary military pain program. *Military Medicine* 174(3):270-277.

Gaylord, K. M., J. B. Holcomb, and M. E. Zolezzi. 2009. A comparison of posttraumatic stress disorder between combat casualties and civilians treated at a military burn center. *Journal of Trauma-Injury Infection & Critical Care* 66(4 Suppl):S191-S195.

Geiss Trusz, S., A. W. Wagner, J. Russo, J. Love, and D. F. Zatzick. 2011. Assessing barriers to care and readiness for cognitive behavioral therapy in early acute care PTSD interventions. *Psychiatry* 74(3):207-223.

Gibbs, D. A., S. L. Martin, L. L. Kupper, and R. E. Johnson. 2007. Child maltreatment in enlisted soldiers' families during combat-related deployments. *Journal of the American Medical Association* 298(5):528-535.

Gilbody, S., P. Bower, J. Fletcher, D. Richards, and A. J. Sutton. 2006. Collaborative care for depression—a cumulative meta-analysis and review of longer-term outcomes. *Archives of Internal Medicine* 166(21):2314-2321.

Guzman, J., R. Esmail, K. Karjalainen, A. Malmivaara, E. Irvin, and C. Bombardier. 2001. Multidisciplinary rehabilitation for chronic low back pain: Systematic review. *British Medical Journal* 322(7301):1511-1516.

Harman, D. R., T. I. Hooper, and G. D. Gackstetter. 2005. Aeromedical evacuations from Operation Iraqi Freedom: A descriptive study. *Military Medicine* 170(6):521-527.

Haskell, S. G., A. Heapy, M. C. Reid, R. K. Papas, and R. D. Kerns. 2006. The prevalence and age-related characteristics of pain in a sample of women veterans receiving primary care. *Journal of Women's Health* 15(7):862-869.

Hearst, N., T. B. Newman, and S. B. Hulley. 1986. Delayed effects of the military draft on mortality. A randomized natural experiment. *New England Journal of Medicine* 314(10):620-624.

Heinrich, R. L., M. J. Cohen, B. D. Naliboff, G. A. Collins, and A. D. Bonebakker. 1985. Comparing physical and behavior therapy for chronic low back pain on physical abilities, psychological distress, and patients' perceptions. *Journal of Behavioral Medicine* 8(1):61-78.

Hesdorffer, D. C., S. L. Rauch, and C. A. Tamminga. 2009. Long-term psychiatric outcomes following traumatic brain injury: A review of the literature. *Journal of Head Trauma Rehabilitation* 24(6):452-459.

Hester, R. K., D. D. Squires, and H. D. Delaney. 2005. The drinker's check-up: 12-month outcomes of a controlled clinical trial of a stand-alone software program for problem drinkers. *Journal of Substance Abuse Treatment* 28(2):159-169.

Hines, D. A., and E. M. Douglas. 2011. Symptoms of posttraumatic stress disorder in men who sustain intimate partner violence: A study of helpseeking and community samples. *Psychology of Men and Masculinity* 12(2):112-127.

Hoffman, B. M., R. K. Papas, D. K. Chatkoff, and R. D. Kerns. 2007. Meta-analysis of psychological interventions for chronic low back pain. *Health Psychology* 26(1):1-9.

Hoge, C. W., C. A. Castro, S. C. Messer, D. McGurk, D. I. Cotting, and R. L. Koffman. 2004. Combat duty in Iraq and Afghanistan, mental health problems, and barriers to care. *New England Journal of Medicine* 351(1):13-22.

Holbrook, T. L., D. B. Hoyt, R. Coimbra, B. Potenza, M. Sise, and J. P. Anderson. 2005. Long-term posttraumatic stress disorder persists after major trauma in adolescents: New data on risk factors and functional outcome. *Journal of Trauma-Injury Infection and Critical Care* 58(4):764-769.

Holroyd, K. A., F. J. O'Donnell, M. Stensland, G. L. Lipchik, G. E. Cordingley, and B. W. Carlson. 2001. Management of chronic tension-type headache with tricyclic antidepressant medication, stress management therapy, and their combination: A randomized controlled trial. *Journal of the American Medical Association* 285(17):2208-2215.

HUD (Department of Housing and Urban Development) and VA (Department of Veterans Affairs). 2010. *Veteran homelessness: A supplemental report to the 2009 annual homeless assessment report to Congress.* http://hudhre.info/documents/2010AHARVeterans Report.pdf (accessed January 30, 2012).

Institute for Clinical Systems Improvement. 2009. *Assessment and management of chronic pain.* Bloomington, MN: Institute for Clinical Systems Improvement.

IOM (Institute of Medicine). 2008. *Gulf War and health: Physiologic, psychologic, and psychosocial effects of deployment-related stress.* Washington, DC: The National Academies Press.

IOM. 2010. *Provision of mental health counseling services under TRICARE.* Washington, DC: The National Academies Press.

IOM. 2011. *Cognitive rehabilitation therapy for traumatic brain injury: Evaluating the evidence.* Washington, DC: The National Academies Press.

Iverson, K. M., J. L. Gradus, P. A. Resick, M. K. Suvak, K. F. Smith, and C. M. Monson. 2011. Cognitive–behavioral therapy for PTSD and depression symptoms reduces risk for future intimate partner violence among interpersonal trauma survivors. *Journal of Consulting and Clinical Psychology* 79(2):193-202.

Jacobsen, L. K., S. M. Southwick, and T. R. Kosten. 2001. Substance use disorders in patients with posttraumatic stress disorder: A review of the literature. *American Journal of Psychiatry* 158(8):1184-1190.

Jacobson, I. G., M. A. K. Ryan, T. I. Hooper, T. C. Smith, P. J. Amoroso, E. J. Boyko, G. D. Gackstetter, T. S. Wells, and N. S. Bell. 2008. Alcohol use and alcohol-related problems before and after military combat deployment. *Journal of the American Medical Association* 300(6):663-675.

Jakupcak, M., D. Conybeare, L. Phelps, S. Hunt, H. A. Holmes, B. Felker, M. Klevens, and M. E. McFall. 2007. Anger, hostility, and aggression among Iraq and Afghanistan war veterans reporting PTSD and subthreshold PTSD. *Journal of Traumatic Stress* 20(6):945-954.

Jakupcak, M., M. T. Tull, M. J. McDermott, D. Kaysen, S. Hunt, and T. Simpson. 2010. PTSD symptom clusters in relationship to alcohol misuse among Iraq and Afghanistan war veterans seeking post-deployment VA health care. *Addictive Behaviors* 35(9):840-843.

Jordan, B. K., C. R. Marmar, J. A. Fairbank, W. E. Schlenger, R. A. Kulka, R. L. Hough, and D. S. Weiss. 1992. Problems in families of male Vietnam veterans with posttraumatic stress disorder. *Journal of Consulting and Clinical Psychology* 60(6):916-926.

Joshi, G. P., and B. O. Ogunnaike. 2005. Consequences of inadequate postoperative pain relief and chronic persistent postoperative pain. *Anesthesiology Clinics of North America* 23(1):21-36.

Kausch, O., L. Rugle, and D. Y. Rowland. 2006. Lifetime histories of trauma among pathological gamblers. *American Journal on Addictions* 15(1):35-43.

Kennedy, P., and J. Duff. 2001. Post traumatic stress disorder and spinal cord injuries. *Spinal Cord* 39(1):1-10.

Kerns, R. D., J. Otis, R. Rosenberg, and M. C. Reid. 2003. Veterans' reports of pain and associations with ratings of health, health-risk behaviors, affective distress, and use of the healthcare system. *Journal of Rehabilitation Research and Development* 40(5):371-379.

Kessler, R. C., I. Hwang, R. LaBrie, M. Petukhova, N. A. Sampson, K. C. Winters, and H. J. Shaffer. 2008. DSM-IV pathological gambling in the National Comorbidity Survey replication. *Psychological Medicine* 38(9):1351-1360.

Killgore, W. D. S., D. I. Cotting, J. L. Thomas, A. L. Cox, D. McGurk, A. H. Vo, C. A. Castro, and C. W. Hoge. 2008. Post-combat invincibility: Violent combat experiences are associated with increased risk-taking propensity following deployment. *Journal of Psychiatric Research* 42(13):1112-1121.

Kriston, L., L. Holzel, A. K. Weiser, M. M. Berner, and M. Harter. 2008. Meta-analysis: Are 3 questions enough to detect unhealthy alcohol use? *Annals of Internal Medicine* 149(12):879-888.

Kroenke, K., M. Bair, T. Damush, S. Hoke, G. Nicholas, C. Kempf, M. Huffman, J. Wu, and J. Sutherland. 2007. Stepped care for affective disorders and musculoskeletal pain (SCAMP) study: Design and practical implications of an intervention for comorbid pain and depression. *General Hospital Psychiatry* 29(6):506-517.

Kroenke, K., J. Shen, T. E. Oxman, J. W. Williams, Jr., and A. J. Dietrich. 2008. Impact of pain on the outcomes of depression treatment: Results from the respect trial. *Pain* 134(1-2):209-215.

Kroenke, K., J. Wu, M. J. Bair, E. E. Krebs, T. M. Damush, and W. Tu. 2011. Reciprocal relationship between pain and depression: A 12-month longitudinal analysis in primary care. *Journal of Pain* 12(9):964-973.

Kubzansky, L. D. and K. C. Koenen. 2009. Is posttraumatic stress disorder related to development of heart disease? An update. *Cleveland Clinic Journal of Medicine* 76(Suppl 2):S60-S65.

Kubzansky, L. D., K. C. Koenen, A. Spiro, 3rd, P. S. Vokonas, and D. Sparrow. 2007. Prospective study of posttraumatic stress disorder symptoms and coronary heart disease in the Normative Aging Study. *Archives of General Psychiatry* 64(1):109-116.

Kubzansky, L. D., K. C. Koenen, C. Jones, and W. W. Eaton. 2009. A prospective study of posttraumatic stress disorder symptoms and coronary heart disease in women. *Health Psychology* 28(1):125-130.

Kuhn, E., K. Drescher, J. Ruzek, and C. Rosen. 2010. Aggressive and unsafe driving in male veterans receiving residential treatment for PTSD. *Journal of Traumatic Stress* 23(3):399-402.

Kulka, R. A. 1990. *Trauma and the Vietnam War generation: Report of findings from the National Vietnam Veterans Readjustment Study*. New York: Brunner/Mazel.

Lange, R. T., G. L. Iverson, B. L. Brooks, and V. L. Rennison. 2010. Influence of poor effort on self-reported symptoms and neurocognitive test performance following mild traumatic brain injury. *Journal of Clinical & Experimental Neuropsychology* 32(9):961-972.

Lauterbach, D., R. Vora, and M. Rakow. 2005. The relationship between posttraumatic stress disorder and self-reported health problems. *Psychosomatic Medicine* 67(6):939-947.

Ledgerwood, D. M., and N. M. Petry. 2006. Posttraumatic stress disorder symptoms in treatment-seeking pathological gamblers. *Journal of Traumatic Stress* 19(3):411-416.

Lester, P., C. Mogil, W. Saltzman, K. Woodward, W. Nash, G. Leskin, B. Bursch, S. Green, R. Pynoos, and W. Beardslee. 2011. Families OverComing Under Stress: Implementing family-centered prevention for military families facing wartime deployments and combat operational stress. *Military Medicine* 176(1):19-25.

Levens, S., A. M. Dyer, C. Zubritsky, K. Knott, and D. W. Oslin. 2005. Gambling among older, primary-care patients: An important public health concern. *American Journal of Geriatric Psychiatry* 13(1):69-76.

Lew, H. L., J. H. Poole, R. D. Vanderploeg, G. L. Goodrich, S. Dekelboum, S. B. Guillory, B. Sigford, and D. X. Cifu. 2007. Program development and defining characteristics of returning military in a VA polytrauma network site. *Journal of Rehabilitation Research and Development* 44(7):1027-1034.

Lew, H. L., J. D. Otis, C. Tun, R. D. Kerns, M. E. Clark, and D. X. Cifu. 2009. Prevalence of chronic pain, posttraumatic stress disorder, and persistent postconcussive symptoms in OIF/OEF veterans: Polytrauma clinical triad. *Journal of Rehabilitation Research and Development* 46(6):697-702.

Lieberman, A. F., P. Van Horn, and C. G. Ippen. 2005. Toward evidence-based treatment: Child-parent psychotherapy with preschoolers exposed to marital violence. *Journal of the American Academy of Child & Adolescent Psychiatry* 44(12):1241-1248.

Lin, E. H., W. Katon, M. Von Korff, L. Tang, J. W. Williams, Jr., K. Kroenke, E. Hunkeler, L. Harpole, M. Hegel, P. Arean, M. Hoffing, R. Della Penna, C. Langston, and J. Unutzer. 2003. Effect of improving depression care on pain and functional outcomes among older adults with arthritis: A randomized controlled trial. *Journal of the American Medical Association* 290(18):2428-2429.

Lin, E. H., L. Tang, W. Katon, M. T. Hegel, M. D. Sullivan, and J. Unutzer. 2006. Arthritis pain and disability: Response to collaborative depression care. *General Hospital Psychiatry* 28(6):482-486.

Linton, S. J., and M. Ryberg. 2001. A cognitive-behavioral group intervention as prevention for persistent neck and back pain in a non-patient population: A randomized controlled trial. *Pain* 90(1-2):83-90.

Litz, B. T., N. Stein, E. Delaney, L. Lebowitz, W. P. Nash, C. Silva, and S. Maguen. 2009. Moral injury and moral repair in war veterans: A preliminary model and intervention strategy. *Clinical Psychology Review* 29(8):695-706.

MacDermid, S., R. Schwarz, A. Faber, J. Adkins, M. Mishkind, and H. Weiss. 2005. Military fathers on the front lines. In *Situated fathering: A focus on physical and social spaces*, edited by W. Marsiglio, K. Roy, and G. L. Fox. Oxford, UK: Rowman and Littlefield. Pp. 209-234.

Maes, M., J. Mylle, L. Delmeire, and C. Altamura. 2000. Psychiatric morbidity and comorbidity following accidental man-made traumatic events: Incidence and risk factors. *European Archives of Psychiatry and Clinical Neuroscience* 250(3):156-162.

Marshall, B. D. L., M. R. Prescott, I. Liberzon, M. B. Tamburrino, J. R. Calabrese, and S. Galea. 2012. Coincident posttraumatic stress disorder and depression predict alcohol abuse during and after deployment among Army National Guard soldiers. *Drug and Alcohol Dependence*, Feb. 16 [Epub ahead of print].

Martin, S. L., D. A. Gibbs, R. E. Johnson, K. Sullivan, M. Clinton-Sherrod, J. L. Walters, and E. D. Rentz. 2010. Substance use by soldiers who abuse their spouses. *Violence Against Women* 16(11):1295-1310.

Masini, B. D., S. M. Waterman, J. C. Wenke, B. D. Owens, J. R. Hsu, and J. R. Ficke. 2009. Resource utilization and disability outcome assessment of combat casualties from Operation Iraqi Freedom and Operation Enduring Freedom. *Journal of Orthopaedic Trauma* 23(4):261-266.

Mayer, T. G., D. McGeary, and R. J. Gatchel. 2003. Chronic pain management through functional restoration for spinal disorders. In *Adult and pediatric spine*, edited by J. Frymoyer and S. Wiesel, 3rd ed. Philadelphia, PA: Lippincott, Williams, and Wilkins. Pp. 323-333.

McAllister, T. W. 2009. Psychopharmacological issues in the treatment of TBI and PTSD. *Clinical Neuropsychologist* 23(8):1338-1367.

McCarren, M., G. R. Janes, J. Goldberg, S. A. Eisen, W. R. True, and W. G. Henderson. 1995. A twin study of the association of post-traumatic stress disorder and combat exposure with long-term socioeconomic status in Vietnam veterans. *Journal of Traumatic Stress* 8(1):111-124.

McCarroll, J. E., Z. Fan, J. H. Newby, and R. J. Ursano. 2008. Trends in US Army child maltreatment reports: 1990-2004. *Child Abuse Review* 17:108-118.

McGeary, D., M. Moore, C. A. Vriend, A. L. Peterson, and R. J. Gatchel. 2011. The evaluation and treatment of comorbid pain and PTSD in a military setting: An overview. *Journal of Clinical Psychology in Medical Settings* 18(2):155-163.

McGuire, J., R. A. Rosenheck, and W. J. Kasprow. 2011. Patient and program predictors of 12-month outcomes for homeless veterans following discharge from time-limited residential treatment. *Administration and Policy in Mental Health* 38(3):142-154.

McKibben, J. B., M. G. Bresnick, S. A. Wiechman Askay, and J. A. Fauerbach. 2008. Acute stress disorder and posttraumatic stress disorder: A prospective study of prevalence, course, and predictors in a sample with major burn injuries. *Journal of Burn Care & Research* 29(1):22-35.

McMillan, T. M., W. H. Williams, and R. Bryant. 2003. Post-traumatic stress disorder and traumatic brain injury: A review of causal mechanisms, assessment, and treatment. *Neuropsychological Rehabilitation* 13(1-2):149-164.

Melcer, T., G. J. Walker, M. Galarneau, B. Belnap, and P. Konoske. 2010. Midterm health and personnel outcomes of recent combat amputees. *Military Medicine* 175(3):147-154.

Merskey, H., and N. Bogduk. 1994. *IASP task force on taxonomy.* Seattle, WA: International Association for the Study of Pain.

MHAT IV (Mental Health Advisory Team IV). 2006. *Mental health advisory team (MHAT) IV Operation Iraqi Freedom 05-07: Final report.* Washington, DC: Office of the Surgeon Multinational Force-Iraq, Office of the Surgeon General, United States Army Medical Command.

MHAT VII. 2011. *Joint mental health advisory team 7 (J-MHAT 7) Operation Enduring Freedom 2010.* Washington, DC: Office of the Surgeon General, United States Army Medical Command, Office of the Command Surgeon HQ, USCENTCOM, Office of the Command Surgeon, US Forces Afghanistan (USFOR-A).

Michaels, A. J., C. E. Michaels, C. H. Moon, J. S. Smith, M. A. Zimmerman, P. A. Taheri, and C. Peterson. 1999. Posttraumatic stress disorder after injury: Impact on general health outcome and early risk assessment. *Journal of Trauma-Injury Infection & Critical Care* 47(3):460-466; discussion 466-467.

Monson, C. M., P. P. Schnurr, P. A. Resick, M. J. Friedman, Y. Young-Xu, and S. P. Stevens. 2006. Cognitive processing therapy for veterans with military-related posttraumatic stress disorder. *Journal of Consulting and Clinical Psychology* 74(5):898-907.

Moser, R. S., P. Schatz, and B. D. Jordan. 2005. Prolonged effects of concussion in high school athletes. *Neurosurgery* 57(2):300-306; discussion 300-306.

Najavits, L. M. 2002. *Seeking safety: A treatment manual for PTSD and substance abuse,* 1st ed. New York: Gilford Press.

Najavits, L. M. 2009. Seeking safety: An implementation guide. In *The clinician's guide to evidence-based practice*, edited by A. Rubin and D. W. Springer. Hoboken, NJ: John Wiley.

Norman, S. B., A. J. Means-Christensen, M. G. Craske, C. D. Sherbourne, P. P. Roy-Byrne, and M. B. Stein. 2006. Associations between psychological trauma and physical illness in primary care. *Journal of Traumatic Stress* 19(4):461-470.

Norman, S. B., K. C. Wilkins, S. F. Tapert, A. J. Lang, and L. M. Najavits. 2010. A pilot study of seeking safety therapy with OEF/OIF veterans. *Journal of Psychoactive Drugs* 42(1):83-87.

O'Donnell, M. L., M. Creamer, and P. Pattison. 2004. Posttraumatic stress disorder and depression following trauma: Understanding comorbidity. *American Journal of Psychiatry* 161(8):1390-1396.

O'Donnell, M. L., M. Creamer, P. Elliott, C. Atkin, and T. Kossmann. 2005. Determinants of quality of life and role-related disability after injury: Impact of acute psychological responses. *Journal of Trauma-Injury Infection and Critical Care* 59(6):1328-1334.

Omalu, B. I., S. T. DeKosky, R. L. Minster, M. I. Kamboh, R. L. Hamilton, and C. H. Wecht. 2005. Chronic traumatic encephalopathy in a national football league player. *Neurosurgery* 57(1):128-134; discussion 128-134.

Otis, J. D., R. McGlinchey, J. J. Vasterling, and R. D. Kerns. 2011. Complicating factors associated with mild traumatic brain injury: Impact on pain and posttraumatic stress disorder treatment. *Journal of Clinical Psychology in Medical Settings* 18(2):145-154.

O'Toole, B. I., and S. V. Catts. 2008. Trauma, PTSD, and physical health: An epidemiological study of Australian Vietnam veterans. *Journal of Psychosomatic Research* 64(1):33-40.

Owens, B. D., J. F. Kragh, Jr., J. C. Wenke, J. Macaitis, C. E. Wade, and J. B. Holcomb. 2008. Combat wounds in Operation Iraqi Freedom and Operation Enduring Freedom. *Journal of Trauma-Injury Infection & Critical Care* 64(2):295-299.

Paris, R., E. R. DeVoe, A. M. Ross, and M. L. Acker. 2010. When a parent goes to war: Effects of parental deployment on very young children and implications for intervention. *American Journal of Orthopsychiatry* 80(4):610-618.

Paris, R., M. L. Acker, A. M. Ross, and E. R. DeVoe. 2011. Building "Strong Families Strong Forces," a home-based intervention for military families with very young children. *Zero to Three Journal* 32(2):36-43.

Pat-Horenczyk, R., O. Peled, T. Miron, D. Brom, Y. Villa, and C. M. Chemtob. 2007. Risk-taking behaviors among Israeli adolescents exposed to recurrent terrorism: Provoking danger under continuous threat? *American Journal of Psychiatry* 164(1):66-72.

PCMH (President's Commission on Mental Health). 1978. *Mental health problems of Vietnam era veterans,* Vol. 3. Washington, DC: U.S. Government Printing Office.

Perlman, S. E., S. Friedman, S. Galea, H. P. Nair, M. Eros-Sarnyai, S. D. Stellman, J. Hon, and C. M. Greene. 2011. Short-term and medium-term health effects of 9/11. *Lancet* 378(9794):925-934.

Poundja, J., D. Fikretoglu, and A. Brunet. 2006. The co-occurrence of posttraumatic stress disorder symptoms and pain: Is depression a mediator? *Journal of Traumatic Stress* 19(5):747-751.

Praxis International. 2010. *St. Paul blueprint for safety*. http://praxisinternational.org/praxis_blue_print_for_safety.aspx (accessed February 29, 2012).

Prigerson, H. G., M. J. Horowitz, S. C. Jacobs, C. M. Parkes, M. Aslan, K. Goodkin, B. Raphael, S. J. Marwit, C. Wortman, R. A. Neimeyer, G. Bonanno, S. D. Block, D. Kissane, P. Boelen, A. Maercker, B. T. Litz, J. G. Johnson, M. B. First, and P. K. Maciejewski. 2009. Prolonged grief disorder: Psychometric validation of criteria proposed for DSM-V and ICD-11. *PLoS Medicine* 6(8):e1000121.

Qureshi, S. U., J. M. Pyne, K. M. Magruder, P. E. Schulz, and M. E. Kunik. 2009. The link between post-traumatic stress disorder and physical comorbidities: A systematic review. *Psychiatric Quarterly* 80(2):87-97.

Radnitz, C. L., L. Hsu, D. D. Tirch, J. Willard, L. B. Lillian, S. Walczak, J. Festa, L. Perez-Strumolo, C. P. Broderick, M. Binks, I. Schlein, N. Bockian, L. Green, and A. Cytryn. 1998a. A comparison of posttraumatic stress disorder in veterans with and without spinal cord injury. *Journal of Abnormal Psychology* 107(4):676-680.

Radnitz, C. L., L. Hsu, J. Willard, L. Perez-Strumolo, J. Festa, L. B. Lillian, S. Walczak, D. D. Tirch, I. S. Schlein, M. Binks, and C. P. Broderick. 1998b. Posttraumatic stress disorder in veterans with spinal cord injury: Trauma-related risk factors. *Journal of Traumatic Stress* 11(3):505-520.

Ramchand, R., G. N. Marshall, T. L. Schell, and L. H. Jaycox. 2008. Posttraumatic distress and physical functioning: A longitudinal study of injured survivors of community violence. *Journal of Consulting and Clinical Psychology* 76(4):668-676.

Rentz, E. D., S. W. Marshall, D. Loomis, C. Casteel, S. L. Martin, and D. A. Gibbs. 2007. Effect of deployment on the occurrence of child maltreatment in military and nonmilitary families. *American Journal of Epidemiology* 165(10):1199-1206.

Ritchie, E. C. 2012. Suicide and the United States Army: Perspectives from the former psychiatry consultant to the Army surgeon general. *Cerebrum* (January/February 2012).

Robertson, I. A., and S. M. Fitzpatrick. 2008. The future of cognitive neurorehabilitation. In *Cognitive neurorehabilitation*, edited by D. T. Stuss, G. Winocur, and I. H. Robertson. Cambridge, UK: Cambridge University Press.

Robichaux, R. J., and J. E. McCarroll. 2011. Family maltreatment and military deployment. In *Combat and operational behavioral health*, edited by E. C. Ritchie. Ft. Detrick, MD: Borden Institute. Pp. 535-542.

Room, R., T. Babor, and J. Rehm. 2005. Alcohol and public health. *Lancet* 365(9458):519-530.

Rosenheck, R., and P. Nathan. 1985. Secondary traumatization in children of Vietnam veterans. *Hospital & Community Psychiatry* 36(5):538-539.

Roth, R. S., M. E. Geisser, and R. Bates. 2008. The relation of post-traumatic stress symptoms to depression and pain in patients with accident-related chronic pain. *Journal of Pain* 9(7):588-596.

Ruff, R. 2005. Two decades of advances in understanding of mild traumatic brain injury. *Journal of Head Trauma Rehabilitation* 20(1):5-18.

Ruff, R. L., S. S. Ruff, and X. F. Wang. 2008. Headaches among Operation Iraqi Freedom/ Operation Enduring Freedom veterans with mild traumatic brain injury associated with exposures to explosions. *Journal of Rehabilitation Research and Development* 45(7):941-952.

Ruscio, A. M., F. W. Weathers, L. A. King, and D. W. King. 2002. Male war-zone veterans' perceived relationships with their children: The importance of emotional numbing. *Journal of Traumatic Stress* 15(5):351-357.

Santiago, P. N., J. E. Wilk, C. S. Milliken, C. A. Castro, C. E. Engel, and C. Hoge. 2010. Screening for alcohol misuse and alcohol-related behaviors among combat veterans. *Psychiatric Services* 61(6):575-581.

Sareen, J., T. Houlahan, B. J. Cox, and G. J. G. Asmundson. 2005. Anxiety disorders associated with suicidal ideation and suicide attempts in the National Comorbidity Survey. *Journal of Nervous and Mental Disease* 193(7):450-454.

Savoca, E., and R. Rosenheck. 2000. The civilian labor market experiences of Vietnam-era veterans: The influence of psychiatric disorders. *Journal of Mental Health Policy and Economics* 3(4):199-207.

Saxon, A. J., T. M. Davis, K. L. Sloan, K. M. McKnight, M. E. McFall, and D. R. Kivlahan. 2001. Trauma, symptoms of posttraumatic stress disorder, and associated problems among incarcerated veterans. *Psychiatric Services* 52(7):959-964.

Sayer, N. A., D. X. Cifu, S. McNamee, C. E. Chiros, B. J. Sigford, S. Scott, and H. L. Lew. 2009. Rehabilitation needs of combat-injured service members admitted to the VA polytrauma rehabilitation centers: The role of PM&R in the care of wounded warriors. *PM&R* 1(1):23-28.

Scherrer, J. F., W. S. Slutske, H. Xian, B. Waterman, K. R. Shah, R. Volberg, and S. A. Eisen. 2007. Factors associated with pathological gambling at 10-year follow-up in a national sample of middle-aged men. *Addiction* 102(6):970-978.

Schneiderman, A. I., E. R. Braver, and H. K. Kang. 2008. Understanding sequelae of injury mechanisms and mild traumatic brain injury incurred during the conflicts in Iraq and Afghanistan: Persistent postconcussive symptoms and posttraumatic stress disorder. *American Journal of Epidemiology* 167(12):1446-1452.

Schnurr, P. P., M. J. Friedman, C. C. Engel, E. B. Foa, M. T. Shea, B. K. Chow, P. A. Resick, V. Thurston, S. M. Orsillo, R. Haug, C. Turner, and N. Bernardy. 2007. Cognitive behavioral therapy for posttraumatic stress disorder in women—a randomized controlled trial. *Journal of the American Medical Association* 297(8):820-830.

Schnyder, U., H. Moergeli, R. Klaghofer, and C. Buddeberg. 2001. Incidence and prediction of posttraumatic stress disorder symptoms in severely injured accident victims. *American Journal of Psychiatry* 158(4):594-599.

Shalev, A. Y., S. Freedman, T. Peri, D. Brandes, T. Sahar, S. P. Orr, and R. K. Pitman. 1998. Prospective study of posttraumatic stress disorder and depression following trauma. *American Journal of Psychiatry* 155(5):630-637.

Shear, K., E. Frank, P. R. Houck, and C. F. Reynolds, 3rd. 2005. Treatment of complicated grief: A randomized controlled trial. *Journal of the American Medical Association* 293(21):2601-2608.

Shear, M. K., A. Zuckoff, and E. Frank. 2001. The syndrome of traumatic grief. *CNS Spectrums* 6(4):339-346.

Shemesh, E., R. Yehuda, O. Milo, I. Dinur, A. Rudnick, Z. Vered, and G. Cotter. 2004. Posttraumatic stress, nonadherence, and adverse outcome in survivors of a mycocardial infarction. *Psychosomatic Medicine* 66:521-526.

Simon-Arndt, C. M., S. L. Hurtado, and L. A. Patriarca-Troyk. 2006. Acceptance of web-based personalized feedback: User ratings of an alcohol misuse prevention program targeting U.S. Marines. *Journal of Health Communication* 20(1):13-22.

Slep, A. M. S., H. M. Foran, R. E. Heyman, and J. D. Snarr. 2011. Risk factors for clinically significant intimate partner violence among active-duty members. *Journal of Marriage and Family* 73: 486-501.

Smith, M. W., P. P. Schnurr, and R. A. Rosenheck. 2005. Employment outcomes and PTSD symptom severity. *Mental Health Services Research* 7(2):89-101.

Spencer, R. J., L. L. Drag, S. J. Walker, and L. A. Bieliauskas. 2010. Self-reported cognitive symptoms following mild traumatic brain injury are poorly associated with neuropsychological performance in OIF/OEF veterans. *Journal of Rehabilitation Research & Development* 47(6):521-530.

Spiro, A., P. Schnurr, and C. M. Aldwin. 1994. Combat-related posttraunatic stress disorder symptoms in older men. *Psychology and Aging* 9(1):17-26.

Starr, A. J., W. R. Smith, W. H. Frawley, D. S. Borer, S. J. Morgan, C. M. Reinert, and M. Mendoza-Welch. 2004. Symptoms of posttraumatic stress disorder after orthopaedic trauma. *Journal of Bone & Joint Surgery—American Volume* 86-A(6):1115-1121.

Stein, M. B., and T. W. McAllister. 2009. Exploring the convergence of posttraumatic stress disorder and mild traumatic brain injury. *American Journal of Psychiatry* 166(7):768-776.

STRONG STAR (South Texas Research Organization Network Guiding Studies on Trauma and Resilience). 2012. *STRONGSTAR research projects: Finding the best ways to prevent and treat combat-related PTSD.* https://delta.uthscsa.edu/strongstar/research.asp (accessed January 30, 2012).

Styka, A. N., D. S. White, R. E. Zumwalt, and S. L. Lathrop. 2010. Trends in adult suicides in New Mexico: Utilizing data from the New Mexico Violent Death Reporting System. *Journal of Forensic Sciences* 55(1):93-99.

Taft, C. T., L. A. King, D. W. King, G. A. Leskin, and D. S. Riggs. 1999. Partners' ratings of combat veterans' PTSD symptomatology. *Journal of Traumatic Stress* 12(2):327-334.

Tanielian, T. L., and L. Jaycox. 2008. *Invisible wounds of war: Psychological and cognitive injuries, their consequences, and services to assist recovery.* Arlington, VA: RAND Corporation.

Terrio, H., L. A. Brenner, B. J. Ivins, J. M. Cho, K. Helmick, K. Schwab, K. Scally, R. Bretthauer, and D. Warden. 2009. Traumatic brain injury screening: Preliminary findings in a US Army brigade combat team. *Journal of Head Trauma Rehabilitation* 24(1):14-23.

Teten, A. L., J. A. Schumacher, C. T. Taft, M. A. Stanley, T. A. Kent, S. D. Bailey, N. J. Dunn, and D. L. White. 2010. Intimate partner aggression perpetrated and sustained by male Afghanistan, Iraq, and Vietnam veterans with and without posttraumatic stress disorder. *Journal of Interpersonal Violence* 25(9):1612-1630.

Thomas, J. L., J. E. Wilk, L. A. Riviere, D. McGurk, C. A. Castro, and C. W. Hoge. 2010. Prevalence of mental health problems and functional impairment among active component and National Guard soldiers 3 and 12 months following combat in Iraq. *Archives of General Psychiatry* 67(6):614-623.

Tinney, G., and K. M. West. 2011. *Safety on the homefront: Adequately addressing violence in families impacted by military service.* Los Angeles, CA: University of Southern California Center for Innovation and Research on Veterans and Military Families.

Turk, D. C., and A. Okifuji. 2002. Psychological factors in chronic pain: Evolution and revolution. *Journal of Consulting and Clinical Psychology* 70(3):678-690.

U.S. Army. 2010a. *Health promotion, risk reduction, and suicide prevention.* Washington, DC: Department of the Army.

U.S. Army. 2010b. *Pain management task force report: Providing a standardized DOD and VHA vision and approach to pain management to optimize the care for warriors and their families.* Falls Chruch, VA: Office of the Army Surgeon General.

VA (Department of Veterans Affairs). 2009. *The assessment and treatment of individuals with history of traumatic brain injury and post-traumatic stress disorder: A systematic review of the evidence.* Washington, DC: VA Health Services Research and Development Service.

VA. 2010a. *Report of (VA) consensus conference: Practice recommendations for treatment of veterans with comorbid TBI, pain, and PTSD.* Washington, DC: VA National Center for PTSD.

VA. 2010b. *Report of VA consensus conference: Practice recommendations for treatment of veterans with comorbid substance abuse and PTSD.* Washington, DC: VA National Center for PTSD.

VA. 2012a. *Healthcare inspection. Prosthetic limb care in VA facilities.* Washington, DC: VA Office of the Inspector General. http://www.va.gov/oig/pubs/VAOIG-11-02138-116.pdf (accessed May 22, 2012).

VA. 2012b. *Strength at home.* http://www.strengthathome.com/ (accessed January 30, 2012).

VA. 2012c. *The National Center on Homelessness Among Veterans.* http://www.va.gov/homeless/NationalCenter.asp (accessed February 29, 2012.)

VA and DoD (Department of Defense). 2009. *VA/DOD clinical practice guideline for management of concussion and mild traumatic brain injury.* Washington, DC: Department of Veterans Affairs and Department of Defense. April.

VA and DoD. 2010. *VA/DOD clinical practice guideline for management of post-traumatic stress.* Washington, DC: Department of Veterans Affairs and Department of Defense.

Vaccarino, V., C. McClure, B. D. Johnson, D. S. Sheps, V. Bittner, T. Rutledge, L. J. Shaw, G. Sopko, M. B. Olson, D. S. Krantz, S. Parashar, O. C. Marroquin, and C. N. Merz. 2008. Depression, the metabolic syndrome and cardiovascular risk. *Psychosomatic Medicine* 70(1):40-48.

van Tulder, M. W., R. Ostelo, J. W. Vlaeyen, S. J. Linton, S. J. Morley, and W. J. Assendelft. 2000. Behavioral treatment for chronic low back pain: A systematic review within the framework of the Cochrane back review group. *Spine* 25(20):2688-2699.

von Känel, R., U. Hepp, B. Kraemer, R. Traber, M. Keel, L. Mica, and U. Schnyder. 2007. Evidence for low-grade systemic proinflammatory activity in patients with posttraumatic stress disorder. *Journal of Psychiatric Research* 41(9):744-752.

von Känel, R., U. Hepp, R. Traber, B. Kraemer, L. Mica, M. Keel, B. T. Mausbach, and U. Schnyder. 2008. Measures of endothelial dysfunction in plasma of patients with posttraumatic stress disorder. *Psychiatry Research* 158(3):363-373.

Wadsworth, S. M., and D. Riggs, eds. 2010. *Risk and resilience in U.S. military families,* 1st ed. New York: Springer.

Wall, S. E. 2006. Neuropsychological dysfunction following repeat concussions in jockeys. *Journal of Neurology, Neurosurgery & Psychiatry* 77(4):518-520.

Washington, D. L., E. M. Yano, J. McGuire, V. Hines, M. Lee, and L. Gelberg. 2010. Risk factors for homelessness among women veterans. *Journal of Health Care for the Poor and Underserved* 21(1):82-91.

Weaver, C. M., J. A. Trafton, R. D. Walser, and R. E. Kimerling. 2007. Pilot test of seeking safety treatment with male veterans. *Psychiatric Services* 58(7):1012-1013.

Weaver, F. M., S. P. Burns, C. T. Evans, L. M. Rapacki, B. Goldstein, and M. C. Hammond. 2009. Provider perspectives on soldiers with new spinal cord injuries returning from Iraq and Afghanistan. *Archives of Physical Medicine and Rehabilitation* 90(3):517-521.

Weis, D. R., and G. H. Manos. 2007. Prevalence and epidemiology of pathological gambling at Naval Medical Center Portsmouth psychiatry clinic. *Military Medicine* 172(7):782-786.

Weisberg, R. B., S. E. Bruce, J. T. Machan, R. C. Kessler, L. Culpepper, and M. B. Keller. 2002. Nonpsychiatric illness among primary care patients with trauma histories and posttraumatic stress disorder. *Psychiatric Services* 53(7):848-854.

Weller, L. A. 2005. Group therapy to treat substance use and traumatic symptoms in female veterans. *Federal Practitioner* 11.

Westermeyer, J., J. Canive, J. Garrard, P. Thuras, and J. Thompson. 2005. Lifetime prevalence of pathological gambling among American Indian and Hispanic American veterans. *American Journal of Public Health* 95(5):860-866.

Wilk, J. E., P. D. Bliese, P. Y. Kim, J. L. Thomas, D. McGurk, and C. W. Hoge. 2010. Relationship of combat experiences to alcohol misuse among U.S. soldiers returning from the Iraq war. *Drug & Alcohol Dependence* 108(1-2):115-121.

Williams, J., M. Herman-Stahl, S. L. Calvin, M. Pemberton, and M. Bradshaw. 2009. Mediating mechanisms of a military web-based alcohol intervention. *Drug & Alcohol Dependence* 100(3):248-257.

Wood, R. L. 2004. Understanding the "miserable minority": A diasthesis-stress paradigm for post-concussional syndrome. *Brain Injury* 18(11):1135-1153.

Yaffe, K., E. Vittinghoff, K. Lindquist, D. Barnes, K. E. Covinsky, T. Neylan, M. Kluse, and C. Marmar. 2010. Postraumatic stress disorder and risk of dementia among US veterans. *Archives of General Psychiatry* 67(6):608-613.

Zatzick, D. F., and S. Galea. 2007. An epidemiologic approach to the development of early trauma focused intervention. *Journal of Traumatic Stress* 20(4):401-412.

Zatzick, D. F., C. R. Marmar, D. S. Weiss, W. S. Browner, T. J. Metzler, J. M. Golding, A. Stewart, W. E. Schlenger, and K. B. Wells. 1997. Posttraumatic stress disorder and functioning and quality of life outcomes in a nationally representative sample of male Vietnam veterans. *American Journal of Psychiatry* 154(12):1690-1695.

Zatzick, D. F., P. Roy-Byrne, J. Russo, F. P. Rivara, R. Droesch, A. Wagner, C. Dunn, G. J. Jurkovich, E. Uehara, and W. Katon. 2004. A randomized effectiveness trial of stepped collaborative care for acutely injured trauma survivors. *Archives of General Psychiatry* 61(May):498-506.

Zatzick, D., G. J. Jurkovich, F. P. Rivara, J. Wang, M. Y. Fan, J. Joesch, and E. Mackenzie. 2008a. A national US study of posttraumatic stress disorder, depression, and work and functional outcomes after hospitalization for traumatic injury. *Annals of Surgery* 248(3):429-435.

Zatzick, D. F., G. J. Jurkovich, M. Y. Fan, D. Grossman, J. Russo, W. Katon, and F. P. Rivara. 2008b. Association between posttraumatic stress and depressive symptoms and functional outcomes in adolescents followed up longitudinally after injury hospitalization. *Archives of Pediatrics & Adolescent Medicine* 162(7):642-648.

Zatzick, D. F., F. P. Rivara, G. J. Jurkovich, C. W. Hoge, J. Wang, M. Y. Fan, J. Russo, S. G. Trusz, A. Nathens, and E. J. Mackenzie. 2010. Multisite investigation of traumatic brain injuries, posttraumatic stress disorder, and self-reported health and cognitive impairments. *Archives of General Psychiatry* 67(12):1291-1300.

Zatzick, D., F. Rivara, G. Jurkovich, J. Russo, S. G. Trusz, J. Wang, A. Wagner, K. Stephens, C. Dunn, E. Uehara, M. Petrie, C. Engel, D. Davydow, and W. Katon. 2011. Enhancing the population impact of collaborative care interventions: Mixed method development and implementation of stepped care targeting posttraumatic stress disorder and related comorbidities after acute trauma. *General Hospital Psychiatry* 33(2):123-134.

Zatzick, D., F. Rivara, G. Jurkovich, J. Russo, A. Wagner, J. Wang, C. Dunn, S. Lord, M. Petrie, S. O'Connor, and W. Katon. 2012. A randomized stepped care intervention trial targeting posttraumatic stress disorder for surgically hospitalized injury survivors. *Annals of Surgery*. Accepted for publication.

9

Access to Care

The purpose of this chapter is to examine the available evidence on barriers to (that is, factors that reduce use of) and facilitators of (that is, factors that increase use of) high-quality care for posttraumatic stress disorder (PTSD) in military and veteran populations. The chapter first provides an overview of the types of barriers to high-quality PTSD care followed by a historical overview of research on barriers to and facilitators of PTSD treatment and related comorbid conditions for veterans in previous wars, beginning with Vietnam. The chapter then reviews the empirical literature on barriers to and facilitators of care, distinguishing between barriers experienced by service members and veterans in three markedly different health care service delivery environments: in the theater of war, in military treatment facilities in the United States, and in the Department of Veteran Affairs (VA) health care system.

Although the existence of barriers to PTSD care (such as stigma) is widely recognized, empirical evidence on some aspects of these barriers remains sparse. In this chapter, the committee chose to review and place an emphasis on peer-reviewed materials. It also chose to augment peer-reviewed literature with information from military reports (for example, the Mental Health Advisory Team [MHAT] reports), presentations to the committee, and site visit meetings.

A 2008 study by the RAND Corporation of psychologic injuries and associated treatment in military and veteran populations found that 14% of Operation Enduring Freedom (OEF) and Operation Iraqi Freedom (OIF) veterans had screened positive for PTSD. The study also found that only slightly more than half the veterans who had psychologic injuries, including

PTSD, received "minimally adequate" treatment for these injuries (Tanielian and Jaycox, 2008). The authors of the report were unable to determine the percentage of veterans with a PTSD diagnosis who received high-quality care for PTSD, but their research strongly suggested that there was a large gap between the number of service members and veterans who had PTSD and the number who received high-quality care for it. That gap represents extensive human suffering and lost productivity. One possible reason for the gap between those who need care and those who are receiving high-quality care is the existence of barriers that prevent access to high-quality care.

BARRIERS TO CARE

Research on posttraumatic care for active-duty service members and veterans has identified a large number of possible barriers to and facilitators of care. Barriers to care exist at the patient, provider, and institutional levels. For example, patient barriers could include concern about the employment effects of seeking treatment for PTSD, a perception that mental health care is ineffective, a lack of information on resources for care, financial concerns, and logistical problems, such as travel distance (Hoge et al., 2004, 2006; Milliken et al., 2007; Warner et al., 2011). For providers, barriers could include lack of training, lack of time, and treatment location issues, such as transportation in the theater of war (MHAT VII, 2011a,b; Sayer et al., 2009b; Warner et al., 2011). At the organizational level, barriers could include rigid organizational requirements for screening and treatment and the competing demands of force readiness in the Department of Defense (DoD). Treatment programs requiring significant time commitments, such as the 3-week Functional and Occupational Rehabilitation Treatment program, are a challenge to receiving treatment because commanders may be hesitant to approve leave for such long periods of time.

Although such external barriers as logistics and financial pressures exist, barriers to care may also be internal and be related to a person's attitudes and beliefs (Curry et al., 2011). Some internal barriers are closely related to the construct of stigma. Stigma has been defined as a negative and erroneous stereotype about a person (Corrigan and Penn, 1999). The stigma process has been further described as consisting of cues, prejudice, and discrimination (Corrigan, 2004) and may be categorized as public stigma or self-stigma. In public stigma, a naive public exhibits prejudice toward a stigmatized group; self-stigma occurs when members of a stigmatized group internalize public stigma (Corrigan and Watson, 2002). The stigma attached to having a mental illness and receiving a psychiatric diagnosis has been the subject of extensive study in military and in civilian contexts (Britt et al., 2007; Corrigan, 2004; Corrigan and Penn, 1999; Corrigan and Watson, 2002; Hoge et al., 2004; Warner et al., 2011).

An additional type of barrier in the DoD and the VA occurs in the translation of research findings into practice. Factors that contribute to this kind of barrier include application to target settings, research-design issues, and a combination of these (Glasgow and Emmons, 2007). From a public-health perspective, such barriers result from an inability to generalize the results of research studies to representative samples of patients, providers, and practice settings (Zatzick and Galea, 2007).

Another barrier to accessing care is that active-duty service members may have difficulty in keeping regularly scheduled appointments for treatment or may not be able to complete a full treatment regimen because of deployment, transfer of duty station, or work schedule. On the basis of such variations, the committee decided to structure its analysis around separate considerations of the barriers and facilitators in the three most common service sectors for PTSD care: in the theater of war, in domestic DoD settings, and in VA facilities, as illustrated in Figure 9-1.

Adding to the complexity of treating some cases of PTSD, are the high rates of co-occurring medical and psychosocial conditions. Some treatments, however, such as prolonged exposure therapy, are effective for both PTSD and for frequently co-occurring conditions such as depression, other anxiety disorders, alcohol and drug use disorders, and mild traumatic brain injury (TBI). In addition, there is ample evidence that community mental health providers who are not expert in cognitive behavior therapy or PTSD can deliver these treatments effectively.

There have been several assessments of barriers to the use of mental health care in military and veteran populations. As part of the National Vietnam Veterans Readjustment Study, conducted during the 1980s, Kulka (1990) asked veterans about their reasons for not seeking treatment for

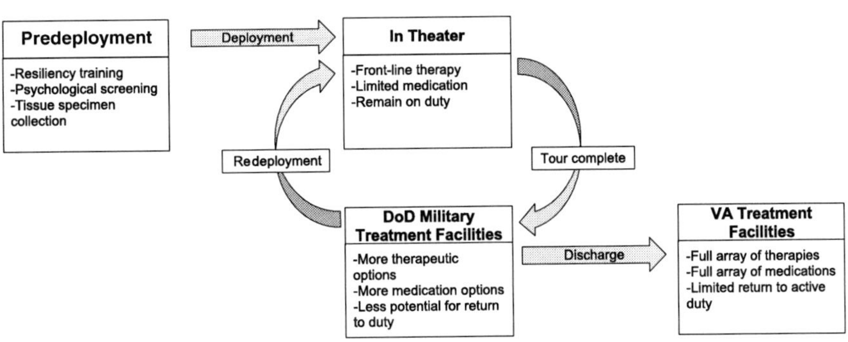

FIGURE 9-1 PTSD services throughout the military life cycle.

their mental health issues. The most frequently cited reasons were the "hope or belief that the individual could solve the problem on his own" and "the hope or belief that the problem would get better on its own." Vietnam veterans who had PTSD sought mental health care at a higher rate than other veterans, but the authors cautioned that this finding did not support claims that the PTSD programs at that time were sufficient in either quality or accessibility (Kulka, 1990). A report from the Institute of Medicine described barriers to delivery of adequate mental health service for 1990–1991 Gulf War veterans who had unexplained physical symptoms (IOM, 2000). They outlined barriers at the provider level, such as competing demands on provider time. They also identified more tacit barriers, such as lack of provider recognition of the symptom complex as a diagnosable entity and reluctance of patients to discuss their illness. Embedding mental health treatment in primary care settings might help to ameliorate specific barriers, particularly the stigma associated with presenting to specialty mental health settings (IOM, 2000).

A 2008 RAND report on treatment for and the burden of psychologic and cognitive injuries in OEF and OIF, *The Invisible Wounds of War,* looked at inadequacies in access to care and in the quality of mental health care for the current Iraq and Afghanistan cohort of veterans (Burnam et al., 2008). Burnam et al. (2008) identified two categories of barriers: the first are structural or financial barriers, and include limited availability of services and financial limitations; the second are personal or social barriers, which include personal values and military culture (Figure 9-2).

Several barriers to and facilitators of mental health care in the DoD and the VA health care systems were identified through focus groups and interviews with health providers and OEF and OIF service members and veterans, including reservists and National Guardsmen. Service members rarely considered seeking mental health care in the military health care system because of privacy concerns related to perceived stigma. Many people stated that if they needed care, they would choose to see an off-base provider or seek counseling from a peer or chaplain. The potential loss of a security clearance, loss of professional opportunities, and the adverse judgment of peers were among the feared outcomes most commonly identified. Another barrier was the tendency to not immediately report mental health problems after deployment so as to avoid delay in reuniting with their families. In the words of one focus group participant, "I lied on my post-deployment forms. Whatever got me back to my family quicker" (Burnam et al., 2008). One facilitator of care was the availability of fellow OEF and OIF veterans with whom to share mental health concerns.

Burnam et al. (2008) used the Institute of Medicine (IOM) definition of high-quality care as safe, effective, patient-centered, timely, efficient, and equitable (IOM, 2001). They concluded that a substantial gap existed

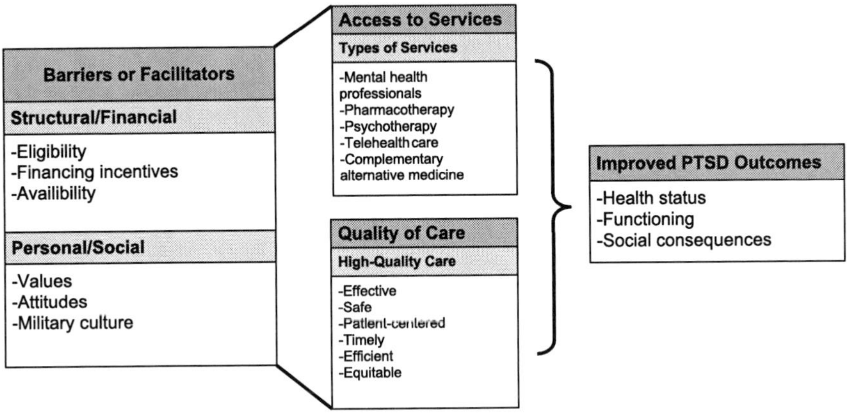

FIGURE 9-2 Barriers to, facilitators of, and access to care for PTSD and related comorbid presentations.
SOURCE: Tanielian and Jaycox, 2008; adapted with permission from RAND Corporation.

between the need for and the use of mental health services for active-duty service members. For veterans who were receiving services in the VA system, the report suggested that improving access would require addressing two major challenges: expanding service capacity and appealing to younger veterans. The authors concluded that both the VA and the DoD should undertake substantial efforts to monitor and enhance the quality of care received by patients who have PTSD.

In the Department of Defense

As discussed in Chapter 4, service members and veterans who have PTSD live, work, and receive mental health care in various settings, ranging from combat zones to specialized PTSD treatment facilities in the VA. Each setting may have specific barriers to and facilitators of care. For example, the use of pharmacotherapy varies markedly depending on the treatment setting (in the theater of war, on U.S. military bases, and in the VA). There are many restrictions on psychiatric medications that a service member may use because of potentially hazardous side effects. Lithium, for example, may not be used in the theater of war, although it is prescribed stateside for service members and is routinely prescribed by the VA. Serotonin reuptake inhibitors, especially selective serotonin and serotonin/norepinephrine—prescribed for depression, anxiety, PTSD, and some other disorders—are prescribed in the VA and in the DoD, but long-term use may adversely affect a service member's career. In the Navy, sailors and marines on selective serotonin reuptake inhibitors cannot carry firearms or deploy unless granted a waiver by their prescribing provider. For other types of psychiatric medications, waivers may be issued case by case by psychiatrists, but the waivers must be consistent with DoD or service-specific guidelines (U.S. Navy, 2009). For some job categories, such as pilot, the use of psychiatric medications while one is on flight status is prohibited (U.S. Air Force, 2009).

In the Theater of War

In the context of service delivery in the theater of war, the best available sources of information on barriers to and facilitators of mental health care are MHAT reports. The series of reports documents improvements in access to mental health treatment in combat settings and the increased need for this treatment for service members who have had multiple deployments. The MHAT reports also show there is persistent stigma and logistical barriers to accessing PTSD care for service members in the theater of war.

In 2003, the first MHAT was assembled and surveyed 756 OIF soldiers, 82% of whom had engaged in combat (MHAT I, 2003). Almost half the soldiers surveyed reported they did not know how to obtain needed mental health services. Only one-third of soldiers who reported they wanted mental health services received the care they needed. That initial MHAT survey recommended immediate improvements in delivery of mental health services, including appointment of in-theater behavioral health consultants and provision of services closer to soldiers' units (MHAT I, 2003).

Later MHAT surveys have continued to document improvements, but they also have identified barriers to receiving high-quality mental health care in the theater of war. For example, the MHAT II survey, conducted in 2005, found that 40% of soldiers who had mental health problems reported receiving some formal mental health services during their deployment, but stigma and organizational barriers, such as time off to receive care and location of facilities, continued to limit access for many soldiers in the theater of war (MHAT II, 2005).

The MHAT VI survey, conducted in 2009 in Iraq and Afghanistan, differed from previous MHAT surveys in a number of ways. The MHAT VI survey was designed to randomly sample preselected platoons, and sampled units were from both support and sustainment units, and maneuver battalions. Current data were compared with data collected in earlier MHAT surveys to investigate service delivery trends. Of enlisted soldiers in Iraq who reported mental health problems, an estimated 7% (support and sustainment sample) and 15% (maneuver sample) did not know that mental health services were available, 16% of support and sustainment soldiers and 29% of maneuver soldiers thought that it was difficult to get an appointment, 36% and 50% thought that it would be difficult to get time off from work for treatment, 9% and 29% had logistic barriers to obtaining treatment, 15% and 24% were discouraged by their leaders from using mental health services, and 13% and 12% did not know where to get help (MHAT VI, 2009). Sampling of support and sustainment units, and maneuver units deployed to Afghanistan yielded similar results (MHAT VI, 2009).

Undertaken in 2010, the joint MHAT VII (surveyed soldiers and marines) extended the findings and assessment methods of previous MHAT surveys. MHAT VII respondents reported the highest level of combat exposures of any MHAT respondents. MHAT VII also reported higher numbers of multiple deployments than MHAT VI. Soldiers on their third and fourth deployments reported increased psychologic problems and use of psychotropic medications than soldiers on their first and second deployments, and overall 4% of respondents reported using psychotropic medications. Although enlisted soldiers who screened positive for any mental health problem reported substantial reductions in barriers to mental health care from what was found in MHAT VI, 29% still reported embarrassment as a factor in not seeking mental health services, 29% reported that it would harm their career, 42% reported that their units would have less confidence in them, 46% reported that their leaders might treat them differently, 34% thought that their leaders might blame them for the problem, and approximately 50% reported that they would be seen as weak. Furthermore, 27% reported that mental health services were not available, 29% reported difficulty in getting appointments, 48% reported that it would be difficult to get time off from work for appointments, and 32% reported that it would be too difficult to get to the mental health specialists' locations. The number of soldiers who reported "I did not know where to get help" (16%) and "my leaders discouraged me from getting services" (14%) were relatively similar to those in the MHAT VI survey. Marines had more mental health concerns in 2010 than in 2006 or 2007 and perceived fewer barriers to mental health care, including reduced stigma associated with receiving mental health care. Mental health providers noted that outreach efforts had been successful in providing behavioral health services outside combat stress control unit locations. Multiple barriers to telehealth delivery were noted by service members and mental health providers (MHAT VII, 2011a,b). Those results show that barriers to seeking care improved but remained.

In Garrison

In one of the earliest studies of soldiers and marines serving in OEF and OIF, Hoge et al. (2004) described mental health service use, stigma, and other barriers to care in four active-duty combat infantry units returning to the United States after deployment. Soldiers and marines who screened positive for mental health problems reported significantly higher rates of perceived barriers than those who screened negative. Of those who screened positive for PTSD, depression, or anxiety disorders, 38% of soldiers deployed to Afghanistan, 43% of soldiers deployed to Iraq, and 45% of marines deployed to Afghanistan expressed interest in receiving help; 23%, 40%, and 29% of persons in these respective groups had seen a health care provider in the preceding year, and those that had seen a mental health provider in the past year ranged from 13% in soldiers deployed to Afghanistan to 27% for soldiers deployed to Iraq. Hoge et al. (2004) concluded that efforts to address barriers to and stigma surrounding mental health treatment in the military should include outreach, education, and changes in service-delivery models, such as integration of mental health services into primary care settings in garrison (that is, on permanent military installations).

In a cross-sectional investigation of mental health problems in active-duty service members returning from Iraq and Afghanistan, Hoge et al. (2006) reported that 19% of OIF and 11% of OEF service members reported a mental health problem and that 31% of OIF veterans had at least one mental health visit in the first year after deployment. Approximately 56% of OIF and 48% of OEF service members who were referred for mental health treatment received it. In a follow-up longitudinal assessment of mental health problems and service use, Milliken et al. (2007) found that 20.3% of active-duty and 42.4% of reserve component soldiers required mental health treatment based on their responses to the post-deployment health assessment (PDHA) and post-deployment health reassessment (PDHRA) after returning from Iraq. Furthermore, soldiers were much more likely to report PTSD symptoms on the PDHRA than on the PDHA, and about half of those who reported PTSD symptoms on the PDHA had improved by the time they took the PDHRA.

Warner et al. (2011) assessed reporting of mental health symptoms and needs for care in 2,500 returning OEF and OIF veterans. Study participants completed both the PDHA and an anonymous survey. Items in both surveys were used to assess the presence of PTSD, depression, and suicidal ideation. Reported symptoms of depression, PTSD, and suicide were 2–4 times higher on the anonymous survey than on the PDHA. More than 20% of soldiers who screened positive for PTSD or depression reported discomfort in answering routine PDHA screening items honestly. Those who screened positive for PTSD or depression also had increased perceptions of stigma and barriers. Those results empirically demonstrate the potential effect of stigma on the reporting of mental health symptoms and care seeking. McGeary et al. (2011) documented that persistent concerns of stigma and fear of potential long-term implications, including separation from the military, also inhibit reporting.

A series of other studies examined barriers and stigma associated with receiving mental health care in active-duty military populations. Wright et al. (2009) found that improved unit leadership ratings and high unit cohesion were associated with lower perceptions of stigma and diminished barriers to care; the association persisted after adjustment for mental health symptom levels. Kim et al. (2010) found that active-duty soldiers who reported a mental health problem perceived greater stigma and had significantly lower rates of service use than did National Guard soldiers. Negative beliefs about mental health care and diminished perceptions of unit social support were associated with decreased visits for mental health counseling and education (Pietrzak et al., 2009). Olmsted et al. (2011) determined that soldiers in treatment perceived greater stigma than soldiers not receiving treatment. Two common barriers to receiving care were not being able to ask for help and not being able to admit to having a problem (Stecker et al., 2007).

Research on barriers to, stigma associated with, and facilitators of PTSD care for active-duty service members seeking care stateside has focused on DoD facilities or has not specified the source of care, but service members can also receive care through the TRICARE purchased-care program. Multiple reports have raised concerns about access to and adequacy of mental health services available from TRICARE contract network providers, including the availability of providers who are willing to see TRICARE beneficiaries, the familiarity of TRICARE mental health providers with military culture, and the training and expertise of TRICARE mental health providers (APA, 2007; DoD, 2007; IOM, 2010). The 2010 IOM report on TRICARE and licensed professional counseling found an absence of guidelines or designated scope of practice for a wide array of behavioral health providers who treat TRICARE patients; this led to a recommendation that TRICARE evaluate its goals for level of preparedness and training of all its health care providers. A GAO report (2011a) reviewed access to TRICARE Standard and Extra providers, including an analysis of concerns about access to mental health providers. The report acknowledged the DoD's efforts in response to earlier reports to address access problems but concluded that serious barriers to access mental health providers, particularly psychiatrists, nevertheless continue. Data for accurately assessing the shortfall in providers or the success of recent DoD initiatives to improve access are still inadequate. Data for determining the degree to which providers have the appropriate training and expertise to treat combat-related PTSD are also lacking.

In its reports to Congress, the DoD has noted the increased use of TRICARE contract mental health providers (GAO, 2011a), which is consistent with what the committee found on its site visit to Fort Hood in September 2011. During the site visit, mental health staff acknowledged to the committee that a substantial and increasing number of active-duty personnel have been referred to TRICARE contract providers because of inadequate staffing in the military mental health clinics to meet the needs of service members seeking PTSD care.

In the Department of Veterans Affairs

Sayer et al. (2009a,b) used qualitative interviews with patients and providers to document barriers to and facilitators of care for veterans who have PTSD and are seen in the VA. They conducted in-depth interviews with veterans who were filing claims related to service-connected disability. The investigation identified multiple barriers to treatment, including beliefs that discouraged seeking mental health treatment, concerns about the ability of the health care system to meet a patient's needs, lack of knowledge about PTSD, treatment access, and trauma-related avoidance. Facilitators of VA services included recognition and acceptance of PTSD, availability of help, beliefs that encouraged seeking treatment, system facilitation (such as promotion of help-seeking by primary care providers), and encouragement of treatment seeking by members of a patient's social network.

In a study of barriers experienced by providers, Sayer et al. (2009b) interviewed 40 providers in VA clinical teams that provide specialized services for TBI or PTSD. Providers were asked questions about referral processes, assessment and treatment challenges, terminology, comorbidities, and collaborations. They found screening and referral challenges that included false negative TBI screening results; assessment challenges derived from retrospective evaluations of TBI, PTSD, and functional impairments; secondary gain issues; high no-show rates; uncertainty about evidence-based PTSD treatments for mild TBI; lack of coordination of care with other VA services; and questionable availability of services, including psychiatric staffing. Although these two studies are small, they could serve as a model for assessing barriers to PTSD care in the VA.

In 2011, the GAO identified four key barriers that might prevent veterans from seeking mental health care at VA facilities: stigma and beliefs about mental health care, lack of understanding or awareness of mental health care, logistical challenges to accessing mental health care, and concerns about VA health care in general (GAO, 2011b). On the basis of a literature review and interviews with officials of the VA and veteran service organizations, particular concerns included perception by veterans that seeking help would negatively affect their careers, that treatment may be painful and bring up bad memories, and that they would be able to solve their problems without treatment. The VA and veteran service organization officials also noted that barriers affected different demographic groups differently, for example, younger veterans might think that only older veterans go to the VA for health care, women may perceive the VA health care system as primarily male-oriented, National Guard and reservists may have more concerns about privacy and stigma, and veterans who live in rural locations may have greater distances to travel to receive care.

A 2011 survey of VA mental health care providers in five Veteran Integrated Service Networks (VISNs) found many perceived system barriers to veterans' seeking mental health care (VA, 2011). Of the 272 providers surveyed (a mixture of social workers, psychologists, psychiatrists, and nurses), 63% could schedule an appointment for a new patient within 14 days in their clinic, but 18% could not see a new veteran for at least 30 days, and 7% thought the waiting time would be longer than 60 days. Some also noted long waiting times for established patients: 25% could see an established patient at the earliest preferred date, 36% within 14 days of the preferred date, 22% within a month, 11% in more than a month, and 7% in more than 60 days. Providers also noted there were waiting times for referrals to specialty mental health care, such as for PTSD or substance abuse. Most (71%) of the providers thought that current staffing levels were inadequate. When they were asked about other system barriers to provision of mental health care, 46% cited a need for more off-hours appointments (evenings and weekends), 27% said that participating in compensation and pension examinations took time they could otherwise spend with patients, and 25% cited shortages of other staff (clerical and scheduling) (VA, 2011).

In a nonrandomized study of rural veterans of all eras who had never enrolled for VA health benefits or had not used VA health services in the preceding 2 years, the primary veteran-reported barrier to accessing health care of any kind was perceived cost (Davis et al., 2011). Of veterans whose last deployment was in Iraq, Afghanistan, or Kuwait, 22% reported a delay in obtaining or an inability to obtain mental health care compared with 5.6% of veterans who had been deployed elsewhere. The study authors suggested that lack of mental health screening and evaluation may also be a barrier to obtaining mental health care.

BARRIERS TO DELIVERY OF EVIDENCE-BASED CARE

As noted in Chapter 7, the VA/DoD clinical practice guideline and other practice guidelines have identified psychosocial treatments—specifically prolonged exposure (PE) and cognitive processing therapy (CPT)—and pharmacologic treatments as having the strongest evidence base for treatment for PTSD. The VA has trained over 4,000 clinicians who provide care in many settings (such as specialized programs, mental health clinics, and Vet Centers) in PE and CPT. The VA has reported adequate capacity to provide CPT or PE for all OEF and OIF veterans who have PTSD and are enrolled in the Veterans Health Administration, and it plans to train an additional 400 staff in these therapies in 2012 to have the capacity to treat veterans of all eras who have PTSD (Schiffner, 2011). Recently, the VA announced that it plans to hire 1,600 nurses, psychiatrists, psychologists, social workers, and other mental health staff and about 300 administrative support staff (VA, 2012b). Challenges and barriers to delivering CPT and PE identified through surveys of trained providers and program evaluations include the need to modify training to be intensive and experiential with interaction between trainers and trainees, the need to allow continuing consultation and mentorship with experts for at least 6 months after initial training, the need to monitor and quantify treatment provided, the need for adequate time to deliver treatment according to protocol, and the need to be supported by local management (Karlin et al., 2010; Schiffner, 2011).

To address some of those barriers, the VA has trained master trainers to deliver the initial training in each VISN and to serve as local mentors and consultants. By augmenting the VA computerized clinical record to document the number of veterans who have PTSD and are given at least 8 hours of psychotherapy within a 14-week period, the VA will be able to assess performance measures, such as availability and adequacy of CPT and PE treatment at local facilities and in the overall VA system (Schiffner, 2011). Some of the same challenges to implementing VA training initiatives for psychotherapies are relevant to evidence-based pharmacologic treatment for PTSD. Pharmacologic treatment for PTSD can be prescribed by clinicians in multiple venues—including specialized programs, mental health clinics, and primary care practices—and pharmacologic training must be broadly implemented for these providers.

Similar challenges to and solutions for training VA providers in evidence-based treatments for PTSD may be applicable to DoD mental health care. These challenges include the barriers experienced in specific populations (such as deployed troops), comorbid PTSD presentations, substance abuse and dependence, and the need for stabilization and engagement through stepped-care treatment protocols (see Chapter 8).

Some specific active-duty and veteran subpopulations experience different barriers to PTSD care from the veteran population as a whole. For example, Westermeyer et al. (2002) reported that American Indian veterans were less likely to use VA mental health services than other mental health services because of barriers to accessing care, such as lack of VA outreach to them, distrust of the VA, and lack of resources to access the VA. Similarly, women, racial- and ethnic-minority populations, victims of sexual assault sustained during military service, severely wounded veterans, residents of rural areas, and National Guard and reserve populations may all encounter additional barriers to care (Stecker et al., 2007). Data on the prevalence and causes of these population-specific barriers are lacking, but treatment programs and other interventions need to take them into account for optimal effectiveness. The committee recognizes the importance of barriers to high-quality care experienced by various populations and anticipates further examination of this subject in phase 2 of its study.

As documented in other chapters, evidence-based treatment for PTSD should be provided as soon as feasible, before the disorder becomes chronic or symptoms worsen. The DoD and the VA have made progress in early screening of service members and veterans, respectively, who have or are at risk for PTSD. That progress should be followed by timely access to evidence-based care that integrates evidence-based treatments into a stepped-care, multimodal treatment plan, for example, combining cognitive behavioral therapy with couples therapy. During early engagements with service members or veterans, mental health providers need to be able to treat those who are in crisis while assessing the need for long-term, evidence-based treatment.

FACILITATORS OF CARE FOR PTSD

This chapter has focused primarily on barriers to accessing care for PTSD. In this section, the committee discusses new approaches that are being used or studied to improve the delivery of mental health services to military and veteran populations. The DoD and the VA are in the forefront of exploring innovative methods for reaching service members, veterans, and their families who are in need of PTSD treatment but for whom the traditional office visit to a mental health provider is not possible. Among the approaches is the use of computers to deliver high-quality person-to-person therapy.

Computing and information technology can address logistical barriers and stigma issues that are present in all service-delivery settings. It has been implemented to different degrees by both the DoD and the VA, which have given users opportunities to access and interact with computing applications (and care providers) for the delivery of clinical services, to participate in anonymous mental health screening, and to access tools that are designed to foster self-awareness and promote a sense of urgency in seeking care. Those opportunities are available to users regardless of their physical location or the time of day. The challenge is to create technologic tools that can provide benefits to users in ways that are ethically sound.

Treatment Delivery Technologies

The rapid and broad adoption of computing and mobile technologies may be opportune in view of the demands that the OEF and OIF conflicts have placed on the DoD and the VA health care systems. Since 2004, numerous recommendations (APA, 2007; DoD, 2007; Dole and Shalala, 2007;

IOM, 2007; Tanielian and Jaycox, 2008) have cited two major needs for improvement: support for randomized controlled trials (RCTs) that assess the efficacy, effectiveness, and implementation of treatment methods and lead to wider dissemination of evidenced-based approaches; and identification and implementation of ways to enhance health care dissemination and delivery for military personnel and their families in ways that provide better awareness of and access to care while reducing stigma.

Telemental Health-Based Interventions

Telemental health (TMH or telemedicine) approaches take advantage of recent advances in computer and information technology that support user interaction with clinicians or clinical applications via low-cost, high-bandwidth connectivity with the Internet. TMH methods constitute more of a delivery medium for providing services to users in remote locations and are not specific to any one model of assessment or treatment. The core methods of TMH delivery are videoteleconferencing (real-time synchronous interaction with a live provider over the Internet), interaction with Internet-based sites that can provide screening assessments and general clinical information (for example, DCoE, 2012, or VA, 2012a), and in some cases programmed guides that allow users to embark on self-managed mental health programming, sometimes supported by additional synchronous or asynchronous interaction with a clinical provider.

In recent years, there has been growing recognition of the value of TMH technologies—such as videoconferencing, Internet use, or telephone use—to conduct therapy for patients who have PTSD (Frueh et al., 2007a). These approaches decrease the burdens of travel time, costs, and time away from work or family and could improve access to services for traditionally underserved populations (for example, patients in rural settings and people who have transportation difficulties or physical disabilities) and people in regions that may be difficult for therapists to reach (such as combat zones). Continuing advances in low-cost, faster, and more sophisticated Internet technologies have led to a substantial investment in TMH infrastructure by government agencies (Godleski et al., 2008), and a growing literature details the structure and mechanics of a variety of TMH applications, as well as research into their effectiveness and efficiency (Frueh et al., 2000; Monnier et al., 2003; Norman, 2006; Richardson et al., 2009).

Videoconferencing

Early research has shown that videoconferencing can be implemented cost-effectively (Bose et al., 2001; Elford et al., 2000; Fortney et al., 2005). Much attention has focused on this medium for providing evidence-based treatments to veterans, and the VA is promoting telemedicine as an important means of providing care to veterans who live in remote areas (IOM, 2005). Several uncontrolled studies have indicated that telemedicine has resulted in a reduction in PTSD symptoms in veterans (Deitsch et al., 2000; Germain et al., 2009; Morland et al., 2004). For example, Tuerk et al. (2011) administered PE to veterans via videoconferencing and compared responses with those in a sample of veterans who were treated with PE in a standard clinical setting. There were few differences between the two formats, apart from the weekly express posting of the audiorecording of the PE session to the patient. Although the trial was not an RCT, it demonstrated that this delivery mode was safe and resulted in effect sizes comparable with those observed in patients treated the traditional way.

In an initial group-based RCT that compared videoconferencing with standard PE treatment, Frueh et al. (2007b) reported videoconferencing and face-to-face therapy resulted in comparable reductions in symptoms; however, patients who had videoconferencing reported less comfort with therapy and poorer adherence to homework exercises than their counterparts who received treatment in person. A larger nonrandomized study of 89 patients found that whereas telemedicine delivered PE resulted in significant symptom reduction, it was not as effective as face-to-face treatment (Gros et al., 2011b). Encouraging findings also came from a strongly designed RCT that found comparable results in treating anger in veterans who had PTSD via telemedicine and with in-person therapy (Morland et al., 2010). Such results have supported a growing recognition of the potential usefulness of delivering PE via a telemedicine approach. Large well-controlled trials with OIF and OEF veterans that will permit more definitive conclusions about the effectiveness of this medium are under way (Gros et al., 2011a).

Internet-Based Interventions

Several RCTs of Internet-based treatments for PTSD have been conducted. Litz et al. (2007) assessed DE-STRESS, an 8-week Internet-delivered CBT program, in a military population. Participants were randomly assigned to the DE-STRESS group or an Internet-based supportive counseling program. DE-STRESS entailed therapist-guided exploration of self-monitoring triggers, development of a hierarchy of trauma triggers, stress management, in vivo exposure, trauma writing sessions, and relapse prevention. The treatment group had significantly greater decreases in symptoms of PTSD, depression, and anxiety 6 months after treatment; however, the overall dropout rate was 30%, which is high and reduces the benefit of the intervention (Cukor et al., 2009).

Another Internet-based treatment, Interapy (Lange et al., 2000, 2001, 2003), is a CBT approach that uses exposure and cognitive restructuring techniques. Interapy involves 2 sessions a week for 5 weeks, during which participants have 10 writing sessions lasting 45 minutes each to describe their trauma in detail, work on cognitive reappraisal, and address their perception of the effect of the trauma on their lives. The largest assessment of Interapy was conducted in a community sample of 69 subjects and 32 wait list controls (Lange et al., 2003). The treatment group improved significantly more than the controls, and there were large effect sizes for PTSD symptoms and general psychopathologic conditions. However, many of the traumas reported in this population may not have met criterion A for PTSD (such as losing a loved one, divorce, or a personal attack). Interapy and DE-STRESS share several intervention components, including repeated writing about the traumatic experience and provision of various levels of therapist assistance (Cukor et al., 2009).

Hirai and Clum (2005) used an Internet-based, 8-week self-help program for traumatic event-related consequences (SHTC) to compare people who had experienced a traumatic event, but had only subclinical PTSD symptoms, with a wait list control group. No therapist aid was provided. SHTC consisted of CBT modules, such as psychoeducation; relaxation training, including breathing retraining, muscle relaxation, and imagery-induced relaxation; cognitive restructuring; and exposure. Participants had to master the material in each module independently before proceeding to the next module. Treatment decreased avoidance behavior, frequency of intrusive symptoms, state anxiety, and depressive symptoms and increased coping skills and coping self-efficacy significantly more than the wait list condition. However, given the low symptom severity in the sample, it is not possible to determine whether a person who has more severe PTSD would benefit from the program without some provider contact.

A recent meta-analysis of outcomes of Internet-based programs for anxiety disorders found that among four wait-list–controlled studies of PTSD yielded preliminary support for the use of Internet-based approaches for PTSD (Reger and Gahm, 2009). In a literature review, Richardson et al. (2009) also found strong evidence of patient satisfaction and successful clinical assessment with Internet-based programs. However, both groups of authors concluded that more evidence is needed on the effectiveness of these approaches for specific mental health diagnoses, such as depression and anxiety disorders. Future research on such Internet-based therapies as DE-STRESS, Interapy, and SHTC should focus on the effectiveness of CBT techniques delivered online to more severely traumatized populations, factoring in ethical and legal considerations regarding the amount of provider contact (Tate and Zabinski, 2004). It should be noted that evidence from research on other mental health problems indicates that rates of attrition after Internet-based interventions are higher in the absence of provider contact to facilitate completion (Gros et al., 2011b).

The pressure of increased demands on the DoD and the VA health care systems and the need to break down barriers to care and to reduce costs will probably support continued interest and research in TMH. From an economics perspective, research has demonstrated cost reductions in providing care with telemedicine and Internet-based applications (Harley, 2006; Jong, 2004; Persaud et al., 2005; Shore et al., 2007a), and this trend will probably continue with advances in low-cost, high-fidelity computer and information technology. However, large-scale studies using robust design and sampling methodology is needed to identify the clinical interventions that can be delivered in this format effectively and ethically. Richardson et al. (2009) report that several telemedicine services for mental health care have been operating for more than 12 years, such as Virginia's Appal-Link network, South Australia's Rural and Remote Mental Health Service, and services at the University of Arizona; the University of California, Davis; the University of Michigan; and the University of Nebraska. More robust quantitative indicators of the success or failure of large-scale programs like those may soon be available.

Telemedicine programs will necessarily demand attention to ethical and practice issues. Practice guidelines are gradually emerging (Rizzo et al., 2004; Shore and Manson, 2004; Shore et al., 2007b) to address such issues as protection of privacy and security, standard-of-care assurances, cross-state licensure, practice behavior and treatment approaches, and clinical risk management. Those issues will inform decision making with respect to when care can be delivered via computer and information technology or in person safely and effectively (Hyler and Gangure, 2004; McGinty et al., 2006; Miller et al., 2005; Schopp et al., 2006; Shore et al., 2007b).

Novel technologies being developed to enhance TMH systems will require both clinical and ethical scrutiny. For example, advanced online systems have recently been developed that leverage artificially intelligent "virtual humans" to serve as health care guides and personal screening agents (Rizzo et al., 2011). These systems are undergoing evaluations with service members, veterans, and their families to determine whether such interactive virtual human representations that can be anonymously accessed and interacted with will promote awareness of service options. Such awareness may help people who otherwise might not seek care to jump-start the search for help with a live provider.

Other Facilitators

A recent development has the potential to expand treatment opportunities for service members who have PTSD at bases without large hospitals or mental health care. The National Defense Authorization Act for 2012 lifted a restriction against mental health consultations across state lines and exempts the requirement that health care providers be licensed in the state in which their patients are treated. Although the state licensure requirements for military health care providers providing care in federal facilities are exempt, the new exemption includes care provided at any location.

A further facilitator to care is the incorporation of PTSD screening, diagnosis, and treatment into primary care settings at military treatment facilities. For example, the U.S. Army RESPECT-Mil model (see Chapters 4 and 6) provides service members with an annual opportunity to discuss any PTSD symptoms with a primary care clinician without the stigma of going to a mental health clinic. Integrated primary care and mental health teams are also being used by the other services such as the Air Force Behavioral Health Optimization Program. Similar collaborative care models are also being implemented in the VA. The development of such models has the potential to greatly expand access to and the acceptability of mental health care for service members and veterans.

SUMMARY

Many service members and veterans have PTSD, so there is a growing demand for PTSD treatment services in the DoD and the VA. However, many of the service members and veterans do not seek or successfully access those services. Although there are some published studies of the use of PTSD services and programs in the DoD and the VA, the committee found there is a need for more empirical data on barriers to accessing high-quality PTSD care for military and veteran populations. Information and data related to barriers experienced by service members transitioning from the DoD into the VA health care system and the nature and impact of stigma that is perceived by service members and veterans are lacking.

An overarching goal of the committee's analysis of barriers and facilitators is to identify ways of improving access to high-quality care. In phase 2, the committee will continue to assess barriers to PTSD care, including barriers that are sex specific, race specific, or ethnicity specific. The committee believes that a sound conceptual framework that comprehensively elucidates barriers to and facilitators of access to high-quality PTSD services can result in effective change.

REFERENCES

APA (American Psychological Association). 2007. *The psychological needs of U.S. military service members and their families: A preliminary report.* Presidential Task Force on Military Deployment Services for Youth, Families and Service Members. Washington, DC: American Psychological Association.

Bose, U., P. McLaren, A. Riley, and A. Mohammedali. 2001. The use of telepsychiatry in the brief counseling of non-psychotic patients from an inner-London general practice. *Journal of Telemedicine and Telecare* 7:S8-S10.

Britt, T. W., T. M. Greene-Shortridge, and C. A. Castro. 2007. The stigma of mental health problems in the military. *Military Medicine* 172(2):157-161.

Burnam, M. A., L. S. Meredith, T. C. Helmus, R. M. Burns, R. A. Cox, E. D'Amico, L. T. Martin, M. E. Vaiana, K. M. Williams, and M. R. Yochelson. 2008. Systems of care: Challenges and opportunities to improve access to high-quality care. In *Invisible wounds of war: Psychological and cognitive injuries, their consequences, and services to assist recovery*, edited by T. L. Tanielian and L. Jaycox. Arlington, VA: RAND Corporation.

Corrigan, J. D. 2004. How stigma interferes with mental health care. *American Psychologist* 59(7):614-625.

Corrigan, P. W., and D. L. Penn. 1999. Lessons from social psychology on discrediting psychiatric stigma. *American Psychologist* 54(9):765-776.

Corrigan, P. W., and A. C. Watson. 2002. The paradox of self-stigma and mental illness. *Clinical Psychology—Science and Practice* 9(1):35-53.

Cukor, J., J. Spitalnick, J. Difede, A. Rizzo, B. O. Rothbaum. 2009. Emerging treatments for PTSD. *Clinical Psychology Review* 29(8):715-726.

Curry, M. A., P. Renker, S. Robinson-Whelen, R. B. Hughes, P. Swank, M. Oschwald, and L. E. Powers. 2011. Facilitators and barriers to disclosing abuse among women with disabilities. *Violence & Victims* 26(4):430-444.

Davis, L. L., S. Kertesz, A. Mahaney-Price, M. Martin, K. Tabb, K. Pettey, S. McNeal, U. Granstaff, K. Hamner, M. Powell, M. Hilgeman, A. Snow, M. Stanton, P. Parmelee, M. Litaker, and M. Hawn. 2011. Alabama veterans rural health initiative: A preliminary evaluation of unmet health care needs. *Journal of Rural Social Sciences* 26(3):74-100.

DCoE (Defense Centers of Excellence). 2012. *Afterdeployment.org*. http://www.afterdeployment.org/ (accessed January 24, 2012).

Deitsch, S. E., B. C. Frueh, and A. B. Santos. 2000. Telepsychiatry for post-traumatic stress disorder. *Journal of Telemedicine and Telecare* 6(3):184-186.

DoD (Department of Defense). 2007. *An achievable vision: Report of the Department of Defense Task Force on Mental Health*. Falls Church, VA: Defense Health Board.

Dole, B., and D. Shalala. 2007. *Report of the President's Commission on Care for America's Returning Wounded Warriors*. Washington, DC: White House.

Elford, R., H. White, R. Bowering, A. Ghandi, B. Maddiggan, K. St John, M. House, J. Harnett, R. West, and A. Battcock. 2000. A randomized, controlled trial of child psychiatric assessments conducted using videoconferencing. *Journal of Telemedicine and Telecare* 6(2):73-82.

Fortney, J. C., D. E. Steffick, J. F. Burgess, M. L. Maciejewski, and L. A. Petersen. 2005. Are primary care services a substitute or complement for specialty and inpatient services? *Health Services Research* 40(5):1422-1442.

Frueh, B. C., S. E. Deitsch, A. B. Santos, P. B. Gold, M. R. Johnson, N. Meisler, K. M. Magruder, and J. C. Ballenger. 2000. Procedural and methodological issues in telepsychiatry research and program development. *Psychiatric Services* 51(12):1522-1527.

Frueh, B. C., A. L. Grubaugh, J. D. Elhai, and T. C. Buckley. 2007a. US Department of Veterans Affairs disability policies for posttraumatic stress disorder: Administrative trends and implications for treatment, rehabilitation, and research. *American Journal of Public Health* 97(12):2143-2145.

Frueh, B. C., J. Monnier, E. Yim, A. L. Grubaugh, M. B. Hamner, and R. G. Knapp. 2007b. A randomized trial of telepsychiatry for post-traumatic stress disorder. *Journal of Telemedicine and Telecare* 13(3):142-147.

GAO (U.S. Government Accountability Office). 2011a. *Defense health care: Access to civilian providers under TRICARE standard and extra.* Washington, DC: GAO.

GAO. 2011b. *VA mental health: Number of veterans receiving care, barriers faced, and efforts to increase access.* Washington, DC: GAO.

Germain, V., A. Marchand, S. Bouchard, M.-S. Drouin, and S. Guay. 2009. Effectiveness of cognitive behavioural therapy administered by videoconference for posttraumatic stress disorder. *Cognitive Behaviour Therapy* 38(1):42-53.

Glasgow, R. E., and K. M. Emmons. 2007. How can we increase translation of research into practice? Types of evidence needed. *Annual Review of Public Health* 28:413-433.

Godleski, L., J. E. Nieves, A. Darkins, and L. Lehmann. 2008. VA telemental health: Suicide assessment. *Behavioral Sciences & the Law* 26(3):271-286.

Gros, D. F., M. Strachan, K. J. Ruggiero, R. G. Knapp, B. C. Frueh, L. E. Egede, C. W. Lejuez, P. W. Tuerk, and R. Acierno. 2011a. Innovative service delivery for secondary prevention of PTSD in at-risk OIF-OEF service men and women. *Contemporary Clinical Trials* 32(1):122-128.

Gros, D. F., M. Yoder, P. W. Tuerk, B. E. Lozano, and R. Acierno. 2011b. Exposure therapy for PTSD delivered to veterans via telehealth: Predictors of treatment completion and outcome and comparison to treatment delivered in person. *Behavior Therapy* 42(2):276-283.

Harley, J. 2006. Economic evaluation of a tertiary telepsychiatry service to an island. *Journal of Telemedicine & Telecare* 12(7):354-357.

Hirai, M., and G. A. Clum. 2005. An Internet-based self-change program for traumatic event related fear, distress, and maladaptive coping. *Journal of Traumatic Stress* 18(6):631-636.

Hoge, C. W., C. A. Castro, S. C. Messer, D. McGurk, D. I. Cotting, and R. L. Koffman. 2004. Combat duty in Iraq and Afghanistan, mental health problems, and barriers to care. *New England Journal of Medicine* 351(1):13-22.

Hoge, C. W., J. L. Auchterlonie, and C. S. Milliken. 2006. Mental health problems, use of mental health services, and attrition from military service after returning from deployment to Iraq or Afghanistan. *Journal of the American Medical Association* 295(9):1023-1032.

Hyler, S. E., and D. P. Gangure. 2004. Legal and ethical challenges in telepsychiatry. *Journal of Psychiatric Practice* 10(4):272-276.

IOM (Institute of Medicine). 2000. *Protecting those who serve: Strategies to protect the health of deployed U.S. forcess.* Washington, DC: National Academy Press.

IOM. 2001. *Crossing the quality chasm: A new health system for the 21st century.* Washington, DC: National Academy Press.

IOM. 2005. *Quality through collaboration: The future of rural health.* Washington, DC: The National Academies Press.

IOM. 2007. *PTSD compensation and military service.* Washington, DC: The National Academies Press.

IOM. 2010. *Provision of mental health counseling services under TRICARE.* Washington, DC: The National Academies Press.

Jong, M. 2004. Managing suicides via videoconferencing in a remote northern community in Canada. *International Journal of Circumpolar Health* 63(4):422-428.

Karlin, B. E., J. I. Ruzek, K. M. Chard, A. Eftekhari, C. M. Monson, E. A. Hembree, P. A. Resick, and E. B. Foa. 2010. Dissemination of evidence-based psychological treatments for posttraumatic stress disorder in the Veterans Health Administration. *Journal of Traumatic Stress* 23(6):663-673.

Kim, P. Y., J. L. Thomas, J. E. Wilk, C. A. Castro, and C. W. Hoge. 2010. Stigma, barriers to care, and use of mental health services among active duty and national guard soldiers after combat. *Psychiatric Services* 61(6):582-588.

Kulka, R. A. 1990. *Trauma and the Vietnam War generation: Report of findings from the National Vietnam Veterans Readjustment Study.* New York: Brunner/Mazel.

Lange, A., B. Schrieken, J.-P. van de Ven, B. Bredeweg, P. M. G. Emmelkamp, J. van der Kolk, L. Lydsdottir, M. Massaro, and A. Reuvers. 2000. "Interapy": The effects of a short protocolled treatment of posttraumatic stress and pathological grief through the Internet. *Behavioural and Cognitive Psychotherapy* 28(02):175-192.

Lange, A., J. P. van de Ven, B. Schrieken, and P. M. G. Emmelkamp. 2001. Interapy. Treatment of posttraumatic stress through the Internet: A controlled trial. *Journal of Behavior Therapy and Experimental Psychiatry* 32(2):73-90.

Lange, A., D. Rietdijk, M. Hudcovicova, J. P. van de Ven, B. Schrieken, and P. M. G. Emmelkamp. 2003. Interapy: A controlled randomized trial of the standardized treatment of posttraumatic stress through the Internet. *Journal of Consulting and Clinical Psychology* 71(5):901-909.

Litz, B. T., C. C. Engel, R. A. Bryant, and A. Papa. 2007. A randomized, controlled proof-of-concept trial of an Internet-based, therapist-assisted self-management treatment for posttraumatic stress disorder. *American Journal of Psychiatry* 164(11):1676-1683.

McGeary, D., M. Moore, C. A. Vriend, A. L. Peterson, and R. J. Gatchel. 2011. The evaluation and treatment of comorbid pain and PTSD in a military setting: An overview. *Journal of Clinical Psychology in Medical Settings* 18(2):155-163.

McGinty, K. L., S. A. Saeed, S. C. Simmons, and Y. Yildirim. 2006. Telepsychiatry and e-mental health services: Potential for improving access to mental health care. *Psychiatric Quarterly* 77(4):335-342.

MHAT I (Mental Health Advisory Team). 2003. *Operation Iraqi Freedom (OIF) mental health advisory team (MHAT)*. Washington, DC: Office of the Surgeon General, United States Army Medical Command.

MHAT II. 2005. *Operation Iraqi Freedom (OIF-II) mental health advisory team (MHAT-II)*. Washington, DC: Office of the Surgeon General, United States Army Medical Command.

MHAT VI. 2009. *Mental health advisory team (MHAT) VI Operation Iraqi Freedom 07-09*. Washington, DC: Office of the Surgeon, Multinational Force-Iraq and Office of the Surgeon General, United States Army Medical Command.

MHAT VII. 2011a. *Joint mental health advisory team 7 (J-MHAT 7) Operation Iraqi Freedom 2010*. Washington, DC: Office of the Surgeon General, United States Army Medical Command, Office of the Command Surgeon HQ, USCENTCOM, Office of the Command Surgeon, US Forces Afghanistan (USFOR-A).

MHAT VII. 2011b. *Joint mental health advisory team 7 (J-MHAT 7) Operation Enduring Freedom 2010*. Washington, DC: Office of the Surgeon General, United States Army Medical Command, Office of the Command Surgeon HQ, USCENTCOM, Office of the Command Surgeon, US Forces Afghanistan (USFOR-A).

Miller, T. W., D. C. Burton, K. Hill, G. Luftman, L. J. Veltkemp, and M. Swope. 2005. Telepsychiatry: Critical dimensions for forensic services. *Journal of the American Academy of Psychiatry and the Law* 33(4):539-546.

Milliken, C. S., J. L. Auchterlonie, and C. W. Hoge. 2007. Longitudinal assessment of mental health problems among active and reserve component soldiers returning from the Iraq war. *Journal of the American Medical Association* 298(18):2141-2148.

Monnier, J., R. G. Knapp, and B. C. Frueh. 2003. Recent advances in telepsychiatry: An updated review. *Psychiatric Services* 54(12):1604-1609.

Morland, L. A., K. Pierce, and M. Y. Wong. 2004. Telemedicine and coping skills groups for Pacific Island veterans with post-traumatic stress disorder: A pilot study. *Journal of Telemedicine and Telecare* 10(5):286-289.

Morland, L. A., C. J. Greene, C. S. Rosen, D. Foy, P. Reilly, J. Shore, Q. He, and B. C. Frueh. 2010. Telemedicine for anger management therapy in a rural population of combat veterans with posttraumatic stress disorder: A randomized noninferiority trial. *Journal of Clinical Psychiatry* 71(7):855-863.

Norman, S. 2006. The use of telemedicine in psychiatry. *Journal of Psychiatric and Mental Health Nursing* 13(6):771-777.

Olmsted, K. L. R., J. M. Brown, J. R. Vandermaas-Peeler, S. J. Tueller, R. E. Johnson, and D. A. Gibbs. 2011. Mental health and substance abuse treatment stigma among soldiers. *Military Psychology* 23(1):52-64.

Persaud, D. D., S. Jreige, C. Skedgel, J. Finley, J. Sargeant, and N. Hanlon. 2005. An incremental cost analysis of telehealth in Nova Scotia from a societal perspective. *Journal of Telemedicine & Telecare* 11(2):77-84.

Pietrzak, R. H., D. C. Johnson, M. B. Goldstein, J. C. Malley, and S. M. Southwick. 2009. Perceived stigma and barriers to mental health care utilization among OEF-OIF veterans. *Psychiatric Services* 60(8):1118-1122.

Reger, M. A., and G. A. Gahm. 2009. A meta-analysis of the effects of Internet- and computer-based cognitive-behavioral treatments for anxiety. *Journal of Clinical Psychology* 65(1): 53-75.

Richardson, L. K., B. C. Frueh, A. L. Grubaugh, L. Egede, and J. D. Elhai. 2009. Current directions in videoconferencing tele-mental health research. *Clinical Psychology-Science and Practice* 16(3):323-338.

Rizzo, A. A., D. Strickland, and S. Bouchard. 2004. The challenge of using virtual reality in telerehabilitation. *Telemedicine Journal & E-Health* 10(2):184-195.

Rizzo, A., T. D. Parsons, B. Lange, P. Kenny, J. G. Buckwalter, B. Rothbaum, J. Difede, J. Frazier, B. Newman, J. Williams, and G. Reger. 2011. Virtual reality goes to war: A brief review of the future of military behavioral healthcare. *Journal of Clinical Psychology in Medical Settings* 18(2):176-187.

Sayer, N. A., G. Friedemann-Sanchez, M. Spoont, M. Murdoch, L. E. Parker, C. Chiros, and R. Rosenheck. 2009a. A qualitative study of determinants of PTSD treatment initiation in veterans. *Psychiatry* 72(3):238-255.

Sayer, N. A., N. A. Rettmann, K. F. Carlson, N. Bernardy, B. J. Sigford, J. L. Hamblen, and M. J. Friedman. 2009b. Veterans with history of mild traumatic brain injury and post-traumatic stress disorder: Challenges from provider perspective. *Journal of Rehabilitation Research & Development* 46(6):703-716.

Schiffner, S. 2011. *Data request on mental health providers in the VA, provider training, and the use of complementary and alternative medicine and treatments.* Response to data request by the Committee on the Assessment of Ongoing Efforts in the Treatment of PTSD. October 18, 2011. Washington, DC.

Schopp, L. H., G. Demiris, and R. L. Glueckauf. 2006. Rural backwaters or front-runners? Rural telehealth in the vanguard of psychology practice. *Professional Psychology: Research and Practice* 37(2):165-173.

Shore, J. H., and S. M. Manson. 2004. Telepsychiatric care of American Indian veterans with post-traumatic stress disorder: Bridging gaps in geography, organizations, and culture. *Telemedicine Journal (now Telemedicine and E-Health)* 10:64-69.

Shore, J. H., E. Brooks, D. M. Savin, S. M. Manson, and A. M. Libby. 2007a. An economic evaluation of telehealth data collection with rural populations. *Psychiatric Services* 58(6):830-835.

Shore, J. H., D. M. Hilty, and P. Yellowlees. 2007b. Emergency management guidelines for telepsychiatry. *General Hospital Psychiatry* 29(3):199-206.

Stecker, T., J. C. Fortney, F. Hamilton, and I. Ajzen. 2007. An assessment of beliefs about mental health care among veterans who served in Iraq. *Psychiatric Services* 58(10):1358-1361.

Tanielian, T. L., and L. Jaycox. 2008. *Invisible wounds of war: Psychological and cognitive injuries, their consequences, and services to assist recovery.* Arlington, VA: RAND Corporation.

Tate, D. F., and M. F. Zabinski. 2004. Computer and Internet applications for psychological treatment: Update for clinicians. *Journal of Clinical Psychology* 60(2):209-220.

Tuerk, P. W., M. Yoder, A. Grubaugh, H. Myrick, M. Hamner, and R. Acierno. 2011. Prolonged exposure therapy for combat-related posttraumatic stress disorder: An examination of treatment effectiveness for veterans of the wars in Afghanistan and Iraq. *Journal of Anxiety Disorders* 25(3):397-403.

U.S. Air Force. 2009. *Medical examinations and standards.* Air Force Instruction 48-123. Washington, DC: U.S. Air Force.

U.S. Navy. 2009. *Subject: Small arms training and qualification.* OPNAVINST 3591.1F. Washington, DC: U.S. Navy.

VA (Department of Veterans Affairs). 2011. *A query of VA mental health professionals.* http://graphics8.nytimes.com/packages/pdf/opinion/editorial/VAMentalHealth.pdf (accessed January 8, 2012).

VA. 2012a. *Mission and overview.* National Center for PTSD. http://www.ptsd.va.gov/about/mission/mission-and-overview.asp (accessed March 3, 2012).

VA. 2012b. *VA to increase mental health staff by 1,900.* http://www.va.gov/opa/pressrel/pressrelease.cfm?id=2302 (accessed April 12, 2012).

Warner, C. H., G. N. Appenzeller, T. A. Grieger, S. Belenkly, J. Breitback, J. Parker, C. M. Warner, and C. W. Hoge. 2011. Importance of anonymity to encourage honest reporting in mental health screening after combat deployment. *Archives of General Psychiatry* 68:1065-1071.

Westermeyer, J., J. Canive, P. Thuras, D. Chesness, and J. Thompson. 2002. Perceived barriers to VA mental health care among upper midwest American Indian veterans—description and associations. *Medical Care* 40(1):62-71.

Wright, K. M., O. Cabrera, P. D. Bliese, A. B. Adler, C. W. Hoge, and C. A. Castro. 2009. Stigma and barriers to care in soldiers postcombat. *Psychological Services* 6(2):108-116.

Zatzick, D. F., and S. Galea. 2007. An epidemiologic approach to the development of early trauma focused intervention. *Journal of Traumatic Stress* 20(4):401-412.

10

Findings and Recommendations

The committee was asked by Congress to consider the efforts of the Department of Defense (DoD) and the Department of Veterans Affairs (VA) to prevent posttraumatic stress disorder (PTSD) and to screen, diagnose, treat, and rehabilitate service members and veterans who have PTSD. The number of service members and veterans of all eras who have symptoms of PTSD is immense; of the 2.6 million service members who have been deployed to Iraq and Afghanistan alone since October 2001, about 13% to 20% are expected to develop PTSD.

In this phase 1 report, the committee provides an overview of the management of PTSD in the DoD and the VA, citing selected examples of programs and services that are available to service members, veterans, and their families; describes some of the innovations that are being explored for the prevention and diagnosis of and treatment for PTSD; and highlights substantial data gaps in and barriers to the evaluation, implementation, and use of the services. The committee's findings led to recommendations that could, in the short and long term, improve the management of PTSD for service members, veterans, and their families. To emphasize recommendations that were, in many cases, applicable to both the DoD and the VA and that addressed programs, services, and facilities in both health care systems, the committee grouped its recommendations into five action items:

- **Analyze: Collect data on the implementation, delivery, and effectiveness of all prevention, screening, diagnosis, treatment, and rehabilitative services that are currently in use.**

- **Implement: Encourage and support the use of evidence-based methods for PTSD screening, treatment, and rehabilitation.**
- **Innovate: Instigate research to provide evidentiary support for the effectiveness of emerging prevention methods, treatments, and rehabilitative services.**
- **Overcome: Remove barriers to the delivery of screening, diagnosis, treatments, and rehabilitative services.**
- **Integrate: Screen for, assess, and treat PTSD comorbidities.**

The committee summarizes below some of its findings in this report that support those broad recommendations and presents more specific recommendations for implementing them.

ANALYZE

A. The DoD and the VA should collect data on the implementation, delivery, and effectiveness of all prevention, screening, diagnosis, treatment, and rehabilitative services that are currently in use.

The committee requested information from the DoD and the VA about PTSD programs and services offered by the departments, including the number of service members and veterans in each department who have received a diagnosis of PTSD. Although the need for PTSD services in the next few years in both the DoD and the VA is uncertain, tracking the prevalence of PTSD for this population of service members and veterans should not be difficult. The DoD and the VA, with their comprehensive electronic medical records, have the ability to track, collate, and analyze data on PTSD programs and services for those receiving care in their facilities. For the DoD, this information should be collected both in garrison as well as in deployed locations. Data may also be collected for subpopulations of service members and veterans, such as those with co-occurring conditions, women, or older veterans, to help tailor treatments for those groups.

The RESPECT-Mil program, initiated by the U.S. Army (see Chapters 4 and 6), is an example of a screening program that is being implemented servicewide (DoD, 2011). Although all soldiers are screened in the primary care setting under this program, data on long-term effectiveness are lacking. Follow-up will be necessary to ensure that service members who may not present initially with symptoms of PTSD, and therefore may not be referred for treatment, are not overlooked if they become symptomatic later or become more open to receive treatment.

Treatments for PTSD are being practiced and evaluated in a variety of venues, including DoD specialty clinics, VA medical centers, and civilian settings. Many researchers are engaged in collecting data on both established and experimental treatments for PTSD, but many gaps remain to be addressed. Among them are gaps in data on the effectiveness of such complementary and alternative treatments for PTSD as yoga, the timing of evidence-based treatment, long-term follow-up to assess relapse and treatment effects, and the integration of psychosocial and pharmacologic therapies. Randomized controlled trials (RCTs) would be the best approach to assess the efficacy of PTSD treatments. The committee recognizes, however, that there are considerable costs involved in conducting RCTs, in terms of not only money but also time and people. Therefore, small open trials or pilot studies might be a cost-effective approach to identify initially those treatments most likely to provide positive outcomes or populations most likely to benefit from them.

The committee commends the DoD and the VA for the development of the joint *VA/DoD Clinical Practice Guideline for Management of Post-Traumatic Stress* (VA and DoD, 2010) that presents the evidence base for numerous PTSD treatments, but notes that there is little information on adherence to its use by DoD or VA mental health providers (Kirchner, 2011). Adherence to this guideline by mental health providers in the DoD and VA will help ensure that patients who have PTSD are first treated with therapies shown to be effective in a variety of populations. Other treatments may be used as adjuncts or as second-line treatments should the well-established treatments prove to be ineffective for some patients.

Rehabilitation of service members and veterans who have PTSD has not received the attention that has been given to other elements of treatment. Many service members returning from the conflicts in Iraq and Afghanistan present with comorbid conditions ranging from apparent physical injuries, such as amputations, to subtle but more common problems, such as mild traumatic brain injury (TBI) and depression. Tracking the efficacy of diagnosis of and treatment for PTSD in light of the additional medical problems can be daunting, but such information will help refine future treatments for both PTSD and comorbid conditions. Furthermore, as described in Chapter 8, PTSD affects all aspects of a service member's life, including employment and family relationships. Dealing with those myriad problems requires a coordinated effort to identify service members and families that are at risk, to provide access to services, and to ensure programs and services are appropriate and effective. Data-gathering efforts may be difficult, particularly in the case of veterans who are in the National Guard and reserves, who live in the community and may not have ready access to VA facilities and their electronic medical records, or who may see private practitioners. To address the issues of collecting data to improve military readiness, identifying at-risk individuals and populations, and implementing effective programs for treating and rehabilitating service members and veterans, the committee offers the following recommendation:

A1. To study the efficacy of treatment and to move toward measurement-based PTSD care in the DoD and the VA, assessment data should be collected before, during, and after treatment and should be entered into patients' medical records. This information should be made accessible to researchers with appropriate safeguards to ensure patient confidentiality.

Because of the immense scope of the PTSD problem, and the need to implement solutions immediately given that the conflict in Afghanistan is ongoing and the effects are immediate, a broad range of prevention, screening, diagnosis, treatment, and rehabilitation programs have been implemented by the DoD and the VA. The U.S. Army is instituting a servicewide stress prevention program, Comprehensive Soldier Fitness, with the goal of preventing or reducing the prevalence of PTSD in service members (U.S. Army, 2012a). The Air Force (Morgan and Garmon Bibb, 2011), and Navy and Marine Corps (Meredith et al., 2011; Nash, 2011) have similar programs to improve resilience and to better prepare service members for the rigors of deployment. However, the programs are still in the implementation phase, and their efficacy is not yet known. The collection of such data will be critical for improving military readiness for conflicts.

Although the DoD has also been a leader in promoting the prevention of sexual assault and harassment (see Chapter 5) and in initiating programs to help military families deal with the stress of having a family member deployed to a combat zone, little research has been published on the efficacy of its efforts. Follow-up may be difficult in the case of service members who have prolonged medical problems, including PTSD, who typically leave the service and enter the VA health care system, where the psychosocial sequelae—such as intimate partner violence, criminal activity, and unemployment or underemployment—may be more obvious and pressing but long-term outcomes are difficult to assess. Some VA treatment programs and services enlist families in the treatment and rehabilitation of veterans who have PTSD, including Vet Centers that provide such family services as marital and employment counseling.

The committee applauds the collaborative efforts of the DoD and the VA in the development of the *VA/DoD Clinical Practice Guideline for Management of Post-Traumatic Stress* (2010), discussed in Chapter 7, and the joint guidelines for other medical conditions that are frequently comorbid with PTSD such as those for postdeployment health, concussion and mild TBI, substance use disorder, major depressive disorder, and several types of pain (for example, VA and DoD, 2009). These guidelines are recommended for use by health care providers in both the DoD (U.S. Army, 2012b) and the VA (Kirchner, 2011). Other collaborative efforts include a number of conferences on military health issues. The committee is aware of at least one program, the Federal Recovery Coordination Program, that was jointly developed by the DoD and the VA "to assist some of the most severely wounded, ill, and injured service members, veterans, and their families." However, two GAO reports (2011a,b) cited challenges in program enrollment, staffing needs, caseloads, and placement locations. The reports indicated there were substantial coordination problems with other DoD and VA programs that could result in duplication of effort, inefficiency, and confusion of enrollees. A third GAO report (2011c) on integrating DoD and VA care coordination programs was also critical of the lack of collaboration between the two departments in terms of case management and care coordination. The committee notes that although the Federal Recovery Coordination Program only serves about 2,000 service members and veterans, such efforts need to be carefully scrutinized as to their effectiveness before they are implemented more broadly; however, lack of such effective programs also leaves many service members and veterans underserved.

The DoD and the VA have developed and implemented many programs and policies and have each dedicated portions of their research budgets to fund novel studies in an attempt to address prevention, screening, diagnosis, treatment, and rehabilitation for PTSD. Many of the PTSD prevention and treatment programs in the DoD and the VA are or will be undergoing evaluation. Knowledge of the results will be critical for informing programs in other facilities so that ineffective programs may be discontinued and effective programs implemented. But not all such evaluations receive wide dissemination, particularly in the peer-reviewed literature. Those observations and others noted in the report led the committee to the following recommendation:

> **A2. The DoD and the VA should institute programs of research to evaluate the efficacy, effectiveness, and implementation of all their PTSD screening, treatment, and rehabilitation services, including research in different populations of active-duty personnel and veterans; the effectiveness of DoD prevention services should also be assessed. The DoD and the VA should coordinate, evaluate, and review these efforts continually and routinely and should disseminate the findings widely.**

IMPLEMENT

B. Encourage and support the use of evidence-based methods for PTSD screening, treatment, and rehabilitation.

As described in Chapters 6, 7, and 8, there are many evidence-based approaches that may be used to screen, treat, and rehabilitate service members and veterans who have PTSD. In Chapter 6, the committee discussed the many screening and diagnostic tools that have been used to identify service members, veterans, and civilians who have symptoms of PTSD. Because many of those symptoms are also present in other mental health disorders, particularly anxiety and depression, it is important to differentiate PTSD so the best treatments can be used. Thus, there is a need for validated tools for screening, assessing, and diagnosing PTSD and comorbid mental health disorders accurately.

The committee recognized in Chapters 4 and 6 that all service members who deploy complete a predeployment and two postdeployment health assessments; the postdeployment assessments, conducted immediately and 3–6 months after return from deployment, include a screen for PTSD symptoms. Service members who screen positive for PTSD are not required to receive treatment, but they do meet with a provider who reviews the postdeployment health risk assessment with them and gives them referrals to mental health services, if need be, before signoff can occur. Whether the service member then seeks care for his or her mental health problem is unknown. Therefore, the committee considered such a screening by a primary care physician (whom a service member must see once a year as part of his or her periodic health assessment) to be a critical part of the PTSD care continuum. Many National Guard and reservists also may not see military mental health providers but rather see their own civilian primary care physicians or use TRICARE primary care physicians. Unlike the primary care physicians in military treatment facilities, civilian physicians are not required to screen for PTSD and may not even know their patients are veterans. The prompt in the electronic medical record for a VA provider to ask a veteran about PTSD symptoms once a year presents a good opportunity for a veteran to discuss any late-developing mental health issues without having to initiate the conversation.

B1. PTSD screening should be conducted at least once a year when primary care providers see service members at DoD military treatment facilities or at any TRICARE provider locations, as is currently done when veterans are seen in the VA.

Although both the DoD and the VA have training programs for mental health providers in evidence-based treatments, the committee heard from mental health practitioners during its site visit to Fort Hood, Texas, and through the professional experience of several committee members that in the VA and the DoD that not all clinicians who treat service members and veterans have been trained in all these treatments, nor do they necessarily use them. Nevertheless, the committee found that DoD and VA mental health providers may not always be familiar with military culture, posing a barrier to their understanding of the service member's treatment needs. Many service members informed the committee they were unable to attend treatment sessions because of their duties.

The VA has established a comprehensive training program for evidence-based psychosocial treatment for PTSD for its mental health providers (see Chapter 4). It had enlisted national experts to train about 3,300 VA clinicians in cognitive processing therapy (CPT), 1,500 in prolonged exposure (PE), and 800 in both by the end of 2011, and there are plans to train an additional 400 (Schiffner, 2011). Recently, the VA announced that it plans to hire an additional 1,900 nurses, psychiatrists, psychologists, social workers, and other mental health staff, which also has implications for training (VA, 2012). Training in the VA includes intensive workshops followed by consultation with senior staff to increase the likelihood that trained therapists will actually use the treatment with their patients. The VA reports it has adequate staffing capacity to provide CPT or PE for PTSD to all veterans of the Iraq and Afghanistan conflicts and is close to having full capacity to provide these therapies to all VA users. Vet Center staff members are also receiving training in PE and CBT. The increased use of mental health services notably by Operation Enduring Freedom (OEF) and Operation Iraqi Freedom (OIF) veterans has also meant that some clinicians do not have the time available to use resource-intensive treatments, such as CPT and PE, even if they are trained to do so (see Chapter 4). However, there are other evidence-based treatments, most notably pharmacotherapy, that are highly recommended by the VA/DoD guideline, but no comparable national training program for their use has been implemented. The VA also acknowledged there are other barriers to implementing evidence-based care after the practitioner is trained (Schiffner, 2011).

The committee learned from the VA that it plans to add a template to its medical records to track psychotherapy progress notes (Desai, 2011). The committee does not know if the DoD has similar plans. Lack of a system to identify which treatments, other than pharmaceuticals, were provided to which patients makes it difficult to determine the extent to which CPT or PE therapy is being used at the local level and the outcomes of the treatments.

New guidance from the DoD assistant secretary of defense for health affairs requires that training of DoD mental health providers be tracked (DoD, 2010), but there are no specifics on how such tracking is to be conducted or to whom the data are reported (see Chapter 4). Training in the DoD includes how to adjust treatments to meet a service member's needs and the use of alternative treatments. The required training also includes an online course in military culture and terminology. Continuing education is encouraged but not required. Because the DoD guidance was issued so recently (in 2010), no information is available on how the training has been implemented or on its results—that is, how many providers have been trained or mentored.

INNOVATE

C. Instigate research providing evidentiary support for the use of emerging prevention methods, treatments, and rehabilitative services.

The use of emerging programs and services for the prevention of PTSD in service members and veterans and treatment and rehabilitation of those who have it was discussed in Chapters 5, 7, and 8, respectively. The committee was struck by the number of complementary and alternative medicine (CAM) treatments that are being proposed for managing PTSD, but was also surprised by the lack of rigorous evidence of their effectiveness. The committee heard from several service members that their experiences with CAM treatment such as yoga were beneficial for their PTSD.

With regard to preventing PTSD, the DoD uses several programs to improve resilience and hardiness in service members before, during, and after deployment to a combat zone. In particular, the U.S. Army's Comprehensive Soldier Fitness program (U.S. Army, 2012) and the Marine Corps' Operational Stress Control and Readiness program (Nash, 2011) are being instituted throughout those services to help soldiers deal with the stresses of deployment. The Air Force (Morgan and Garmon Bibb, 2011) and Navy (Meredith et al., 2011) are initiating similar programs to help service members adjust to the rigors of combat and enhance their coping and leadership skills. As noted in Chapter 5, although those programs build on widely used resilience programs, such as Battlemind (Adler et al., 2009), no pilot studies have been conducted to determine whether this type of program reduces the incidence of PTSD.

Both the DoD and the VA are receptive to the use of emerging treatments for PTSD in their populations. The DoD has been in the forefront in developing early treatment interventions for service members exposed to traumatic events in combat zones. It has developed programs to include mental health providers in the theater of war and as close to the front lines as possible to counsel service members and prevent the exacerbation of stress reactions. A number of CAM treatments are being proposed and are being used for managing PTSD, but as with early treatment interventions, there is a lack of empirical evidence for their effectiveness.

The differing missions of the DoD and the VA result in different approaches to rehabilitation for service members, veterans, and their families. For example, the Comprehensive Soldier Fitness program has a component to help families cope with the added stresses resulting from their service members' deployment. The VA is able to provide a variety of services to veterans who have PTSD, including employment counseling and assistance with housing and education. Both the DoD and the VA are addressing the issue of comorbid conditions with respect to treatment and rehabilitation.

The DoD and the VA have specialized mental health programs for service members and veterans who have PTSD, respectively, that may be provided in inpatient or outpatient settings. The treatment programs, such as the RESET program described to the committee at Fort Hood, have been developed specifically for military personnel who have PTSD. Data on efficacy and effectiveness of many of these specialized programs are being collected, but they have not been evaluated or disseminated, so many new programs may be "reinventing the wheel" at different locations, and this might lead to redundancy and inefficiency. Evaluation methods and metrics have not been standardized, making comparisons among programs within and between the DoD and the VA difficult.

Although most service members live and work close to or on military bases, and thus are near a military treatment facility of some level, gaps in the delivery of treatment are of particular concern. Delivery of PTSD treatment is also a challenge for service members deployed in theaters of combat.

The VA serves a more dispersed population than does the DoD, inasmuch as veterans may live in cities, small towns, or rural areas that have differing access to mental health care. The VA is responsible for long-term care of those who have permanent disabilities when they leave the military, including both psychologic and physical disabilities. Complicating the delivery of mental health care to those and other veterans is that many of them are members of the National Guard and reserves who may seek care from civilian, non-VA, and non-DoD providers.

As discussed in Chapter 9, both the DoD and the VA are exploring and in some cases implementing telemedicine, that is, the use of computers and technology for screening and providing interactive therapy for service members or veterans who may be reluctant to engage in or cannot access face-to-face therapy. Telemedicine may also offer promise for service members and veterans who fear the stigma of being in mental health clinics or for those in the theater of war, where opportunities for counseling may be sporadic. Computer-delivered virtual reality programs for PE therapy are also being evaluated (for example, Reger et al., 2011).

C1. Specialized intensive PTSD programs and other approaches for the delivery of PTSD care, including combining different treatment approaches and such emerging treatments as complementary and alternative medicine and couple and family therapy, need to be rigorously evaluated throughout DoD facilities (including TRICARE

providers) and VA facilities for efficacy, effectiveness, and cost. More rigorous assessment of symptom improvements (for example, such outcome metrics as follow-up rates) and of functional improvements (for example, improvements in physical comorbidities, memory, and return to duty) is needed. The evaluations of these programs should be made publicly available.

Chapter 3 provides an overview of the neurobiology of PTSD. Many advances have been made in understanding the stress response, particularly the roles of cortisol and the hypothalamic-pituitary-adrenal axis, but much remains to be discovered. Research into the neurobiologic mechanisms of PTSD is providing important knowledge to guide the development and use of pharmaceuticals for PTSD treatment, including selective serotonin reuptake inhibitors, catecholamines, and glucocorticoids (for example, Mueller et al., 2009; Norrholm and Jovanovic, 2010; Putman and Roelofs, 2011). Although there are no validated biomarkers of PTSD, this field of research has the potential to identify people who are at risk for PTSD, to diagnose it, and to provide the most effective treatments for it, whether psychosocial, pharmacologic, or otherwise. Biomarkers may also be of use in identifying people who are at risk for relapse or symptom exacerbation. The role of genetics in the development and treatment of PTSD is another promising field; for example, the use of gene expression patterns could be used to distinguish between those who have and those who do not have PTSD. Such knowledge could ultimately help to prevent PTSD, target effective PTSD treatments, improve quality of life, and reduce treatment costs.

C2. The DoD and the VA should support neurobiology research that might help translate current knowledge of the neurobiology of PTSD to screening, diagnosis, and treatment approaches and might increase understanding of the biologic basis of evidence-based therapies.

OVERCOME

D. Remove barriers to the delivery of screening, diagnosis, treatments, and rehabilitative services.

During its review of the literature and in discussions with service members, veterans, family members, and mental health providers in the DoD and the VA, the committee learned of numerous obstacles and barriers experienced by those who have PTSD when they seek diagnosis, treatment, and rehabilitative services (discussed in detail in Chapter 9). Barriers exist at many levels, from the individual to the organizational, and although many are applicable to any health care system, such as recording treatments in medical records and allocating providers' time, some of the barriers are peculiar to the DoD or the VA. For example, active-duty service members must request permission from their commanders to take time off from their duties to see health care providers, and this can prove difficult if it conflicts with duty requirements.

Not all veterans receive care in VA medical facilities even if they are eligible for care. Of those who do, however, some live and work many miles from the nearest VA health care provider, particularly mental health providers, and this burdens them with the challenge of accessing care. Although both departments are making efforts to reduce barriers to care for service members and veterans, many obstacles to maximizing the use of mental health care in the DoD and the VA remain. As described in Chapter 9, there are innovative approaches for the delivery of PTSD treatments that use telemedicine, but even these innovations have barriers, such as the need for an aging veteran population to have access to and facility with computers, limited Internet access in rural areas, and cost considerations.

The committee recognizes that translating mental health research into practical screening, diagnosis, treatment, and rehabilitation programs for service members and veterans is an obstacle. Applying information on best practices or adapting research findings from a civilian population to an active-duty or veteran population can be challenging, but these are necessary if the unique requirements of treating service members in the theater of war, on a base, and in the community are to be met. For example, the use of some medications commonly prescribed for PTSD in civilian populations or nondeployed service members may be prohibited for some service members in a combat zone or performing some duties. In spite of considerable efforts to reduce stigma for active-duty service members by finding less obvious methods to deliver mental health care, the perception persists that those who seek such care are flawed or that receiving care can be a detriment to a military career.

In Chapter 4, the committee identified many of the PTSD resources, programs, and services that are being used or developed in the DoD and the VA. The committee also talked with mental health providers, service members, veterans, and their families at Fort Hood, in the community, and at its open information-gathering sessions. Recently, the RAND Corporation released a comprehensive compilation of programs in the DoD for psychologic health, including PTSD and TBI (Weinick et al., 2011). The committee found that many programs were base-specific and were being implemented because of a champion's or promoter's interest in them. The committee recognizes that both the DoD and the VA have made considerable efforts to develop "one-stop shops" for mental health services. The DoD has developed www.militaryonesource.com, which provides a variety of counseling services and referrals for service members and their families, and the VA has established www.myhealth.va.gov, a website that links to a variety of services and referrals and provides advice on health.

Chapters 6, 7, and 9 discuss new technologies for the delivery of PTSD screening and treatment. The committee noted that more work needs to be done to evaluate access to and efficacy of these technologies although studies are being conducted. The use of telemedicine for the delivery of PTSD psychosocial therapies is promising and may be of particular benefit for service members in the theater of war and veterans in rural areas.

D1. The DoD and the VA should support research that investigates emerging technologic approaches (mobile, telemedicine, Internet-based, and virtual reality) that may help to overcome barriers to awareness, accessibility, availability, acceptability, and adherence to evidence-based treatments and disseminate the outcomes to a wide audience.

INTEGRATE

E. Screen for, assess, and treat for PTSD comorbidities.

The committee found three types of integration that are necessary to provide the best treatment options for service members and veterans. First, the screening, diagnosis, and treatment of PTSD need to be integrated into a variety of clinical settings, particularly primary care, so those who have symptoms can be identified and treated as soon as appropriate. Second, treatment of PTSD needs to be integrated with treatment of the physical, psychological, and psychosocial co-occurring conditions that often accompany it. Third, there is the need to integrate various treatment options, such as psychotherapy with pharmacotherapy or other treatments, including CAM therapies, to address all aspects of PTSD morbidity.

Although some service members and veterans have a diagnosis of PTSD alone, PTSD often occurs with other mental health conditions or physical disorders that complicate diagnosis and treatment. There is considerable evidence that PTSD is more common among veterans and active-duty service members who are diagnosed with other psychiatric problems such as depression and substance abuse or misuse, medical conditions such as TBI and pain, or who display other problematic psychosocial behaviors such as aggressive driving or intimate partner violence. In Chapter 8, the committee considered screening for, diagnosis of, and treatment and rehabilitation for PTSD in patients who have other health problems as well. In particular, as a result of the conflicts in Iraq and Afghanistan, TBI is frequently comorbid in service members who have PTSD. Other psychiatric and physical conditions that often co-occur with PTSD include substance use disorders (for example, people may self-medicate with pain killers, sleep aids, or alcohol to alleviate their PTSD symptoms), chronic pain from injuries, and depression and anxiety disorders. PTSD may also affect other aspects of a service member's or veteran's life, particularly social and familial relationships. Some common symptoms of PTSD—such as hyperarousal, numbing, and avoidance—may result in an afflicted person's lashing out at or avoiding family members, employers, colleagues, and friends. They may also lead to intimate partner violence, child neglect or abuse, divorce, unemployment, incarceration, and homelessness.

Integrating treatment of PTSD into treatment for comorbid conditions can prove challenging. There are no guidelines to help health and mental health providers to treat people for PTSD and other conditions simultaneously or sequentially. The current *VA/DoD Clinical Practice Guideline for Management of Post-Traumatic Stress* requires that patients be assessed for co-occurring conditions. Patients who have severe or unstable comorbid conditions should be considered for referral to a specialty clinic. If patients have comorbid psychiatric conditions, management of these disorders is also necessary. The VA and the DoD have developed clinical practice guidelines for several of the common PTSD comorbidities—including substance use disorders, major depressive disorder, concussion and mild TBI—and postdeployment health, all of which are referred to in the *VA/DoD Clinical Practice Guideline for Management of Post-Traumatic Stress*. The guideline also recommends a collaborative care strategy be developed in the primary care setting for patients who have comorbidities, with an emphasis on first treating the most severe symptoms and disorders and only calling in specialists as needed. The presence of comorbidities may also influence the choice of PTSD treatment options. The *VA/DoD Clinical Practice Guideline for Management of Concussion/Mild Traumatic Brain Injury* (VA and DoD, 2009), for example, calls for health care providers to screen patients who have mild TBI for PTSD and other psychiatric disorders and to treat them for PTSD as appropriate. The committee recognizes that the guidelines are a valuable reference for health care providers in the DoD and the VA, but had no data on which to assess provider training and implementation of the guidelines.

E1. Research to create an evidence base to guide the integration of treatment for comorbidities with treatment for PTSD should be sponsored by the DoD and the VA. PTSD treatment trials should incorporate assessment of comorbid conditions and of the value of concurrent and sequential care. Effective treatments should be included in updates of the *VA/DoD Clinical Practice Guideline for Management of Post-Traumatic Stress.*

PHASE 2

During phase 1 of this study, the committee reviewed literature and heard from service members and mental health care providers about programs and services in the DoD and the VA on PTSD prevention, screening, diagnosis, assessment, treatment, and rehabilitation. The committee also heard from families of service members about the impact of PTSD on them. During its data-gathering efforts and deliberations, including a visit to Fort Hood, Texas, the committee identified many subjects on which further information was necessary before conclusions could be drawn. Although the committee was not required to make any visits to military installations in phase 1, it believed that in order to refine its data requests for the services, it would be informative to visit a military base before asking for additional data. Subsequently, information was requested from the surgeons general of the Army, Navy, and Air Force; however, such information was largely unavailable to the committee for this phase 1 report. Cost considerations, new neurobiologic findings, and the use of complementary and alternative treatments for PTSD will be reconsidered in more depth in phase 2.

The committee's statement of task for phase 2 requires it to visit three Army bases: Fort Hood and Fort Bliss in Texas and Fort Campbell in Tennessee. The committee anticipates visiting the remaining two Army bases in the fall of 2012. Although most service members who served in Iraq and are serving in Afghanistan are Army soldiers, the Marine Corps also has a substantial presence and has sustained numerous casualties. The Navy and Air Force also have been engaged in these conflicts, but their personnel are far fewer (see Chapter 1). Because of the large number of marines who have fought in Iraq and Afghanistan, the committee hopes to visit a Marine Corps base in phase 2. The enabling legislation for this committee directed it to consider not only active-duty service members but also veterans, and the committee expects to visit at least one VA medical center in phase 2. The committee also expects that those visits will provide it with more information on specialized services and programs, as well as the availability of and need for programs targeted specifically to racial, gender, and ethnic populations.

The committee is not tasked with surveying all military and veteran health facilities for PTSD programs and services. Rather, it hopes through its visits to gain an appreciation of some of the particular issues surrounding the diagnosis of and treatment for PTSD in current and past military personnel. The visits also allow the committee to hear directly from service members, veterans, and their families about programs and services that work well for them and about ones that do not and about possible ways to improve care.

As noted in Chapter 1, the committee has requested information from the DoD and the VA on numbers and demographics of personnel who have PTSD, on treatments they are receiving, on programs being evaluated (or not), and on costs. Some quantitative information has been received, particularly from the VA, but many of the data requests are still outstanding. When the data are received, they will be evaluated and discussed in phase 2. The committee will conduct further literature reviews to identify where results from DoD or VA or civilian PTSD programs have been published. Until the committee receives more substantial information from the DoD on program outcomes, it will be difficult, perhaps impossible, to determine availability of, access to, and efficacy of each DoD PTSD program. The committee will also refine its data requests to the VA to try to clarify the use of and results from its PTSD programs.

REFERENCES

Adler, A. B., P. D. Bliese, D. McGurk, C. W. Hoge, and C. A. Castro. 2009. Battlemind debriefing and battlemind training as early interventions with soldiers returning from Iraq: Randomization by platoon. *Journal of Consulting & Clinical Psychology* 77(5):928-940.

Desai, R. 2011. NEPEC and PTSD program evaluation. Presentation to the Committee on the Assessment of Ongoing Efforts in the Treatment of PTSD. February 28, 2011. Washington, DC.

DoD (Department of Defense). 2010. *Guidance for mental health provider training for the treatment of post-traumatic stress disorder and acute stress disorder.* Memorandum. Washington, DC: Department of Defense, Office of the Assistant Secretary of Defense. December 13.

DoD. 2011. Welcome to the RESPECT-MIL program. *RESPECT Mil Newsletter* Fall. http://www.pdhealth.mil/respect-mil/index1.asp (accessed January 30, 2012).

GAO (U.S. Government Accountability Office). 2011a. *DOD and VA health care—Action needed to strengthen integration across care coordination and case management programs.* GAO-12-129T. Washington, DC: GAO.

GAO. 2011b. *Federal Recovery Coordination Program: Enrollment, staffing, and care coordination pose significant challenges.* GAO-11-572T. Washington, DC: GAO.

GAO. 2011c. *DOD and VA health care: Federal recovery coordination program continues to expand but faces significant challenges.* GAO-11-250. Washington, DC: GAO.

Kirchner, J. E. 2011. *Mental Health QUERI Center Strategic Plan.* North Little Rock, AR: VA, Quality Enhancement Research Initiative (QUERI). December.

Meredith, L. S., C. D. Sherbourne, S. Gaillot, L. Hansell, H. V. Ritschard, A. Parker, and G. Wrenn. 2011. *Promoting psychological resilience in the U.S. military.* Santa Monica, CA: RAND Corporation.

Morgan, B. J., and S. C. Garmon Bibb. 2011. Assessment of military population-based pyschological resilience programs. *Military Medicine* 176(9):976-885.

Mueller, D., L. A. Olivera-Figueroa, D. S. Pine, and G. J. Quirk. 2009. The effects of yohimbine and amphetamine on fear expression and extinction in rats. *Psychopharmacology* 204(4):599-606.

Nash, W. P. 2011. US Marine Corps and Navy combat and operational stress continuum model: A tool for leaders. Chapter 7. In *Textboooks of military medicine: Combat and operational behavioral health*, edited by E. C. Ritchie. Fort Detrick, MD: Office of the Surgeon General, Borden Institute.

Norrholm, S. D., and T. Jovanovic. 2010. Tailoring therapeutic strategies for treating post-traumatic stress disorder symptom clusters. *Neuropsychiatric Disease and Treatment* 6:517-532.

Putman, P.m and K. Roelofs. 2011. Effects of single cortisol administrations on human affect reviewed: Coping with stress through adaptive regulatoin of automatic cognitive processing. *Psychoneuroendocrinology* 36(4):439-448.

Reger, G. M., K. M. Holloway, C. Candy, B. O. Rothbaum, J. Difede, A. A. Rizzo, and G. A. Gahm. 2011. Effectiveness of virtual reality exposure therapy for active duty soldiers in a military mental health clinic. *Journal of Traumatic Stress* 24(1):93-96.

Schiffner, S. 2011. *Data request on mental health providers in the VA, provider training, and the use of complementary and alternative medicine and treatments.* Response to data request by the Committee on the Assessment of Ongoing Efforts in the Treatment of PTSD. October 18, 2011. Washington, DC.

U.S. Army. 2012a. *Comprehensive solder fitness.* http://csf.army.mil/ (accessed January 30, 2012).

U.S. Army. 2012b. *Policy guidance on the assessment and treatment of post-traumatic stress disorder (PTSD). Memorandum for commanders, MEDCOM regional/medical commands.* OTSG/MEDCOM Policy Memo 12-035. Fort Sam Houston, TX: U.S. Army Medical Command. April 10.

VA (Department of Veterans Affairs). 2012. *VA to increase mental health staff by 1,900.* http://www.va.gov/opa/pressrel/pressrelease.cfm?id=2302 (accessed April 12, 2012).

VA and DoD. 2009. *VA/DOD clinical practice guideline for management of concussion and mild traumatic brain injury.* Washington, DC: Department of Veterans Affairs and Department of Defense. April.

VA and DoD. 2010. *VA/DOD clinical practice guideline for management of post-traumatic stress.* Washington, DC: Department of Veterans Affairs and Department of Defense. October.

Weinick, R. M., E. B. Beckjord, C. M. Farmer, K. T. Martin, E. M. Gillen, J. D. Acosta, M. P. Fisher, J. Garnett, G. C. Gonzalez, T. C. Helmus, K. H. Jaycox, K. A. Reynolds, N. Salcedo, and D. M. Scharf. 2011. Programs addressing psychological health and traumatic brain injury among U.S. military servicemembers and their families. Arlington, VA: RAND Corporation.

Appendix A

Committee Member Biographies

Sandro Galea (*Chair*) is a professor and chair of the Department of Epidemiology of the Mailman School of Public Health of Columbia University. He is a physician and epidemiologist and has conducted large studies in several countries focused on the causes of mental disorders, in particular the role of traumatic events in shaping population health. He is especially interested in the determinants of health in urban populations with regard to the multiple levels of influence of social policies, social environment, and molecular and genetic factors. In addition to being an associate editor of two scientific journals, Dr. Galea is the author of more than 300 journal articles, 50 chapters and commentaries, and five books. Dr. Galea has received several honors, including the William Farr Award in Epidemiology, the Robert Wood Johnson Foundation Health Policy Investigator Award, and the John C. Cassel Memorial Lecture. He also serves as a member of the Committee on the Initial Assessment of Readjustment Needs of Military Personnel, Veterans, and Their Families. Dr. Galea received his DrPH from Columbia University, his MPH from Harvard University, and his MD from the University of Toronto.

Kathryn K. Basham is a Smith College School for Social Work professor, codirector of its PhD program, and editor of its *Smith College Studies in Social Work*. Her research focuses on couple and family therapy for survivors of childhood trauma and for service members, veterans, and their families. Dr. Basham is interested in addressing the different sources and effects of trauma in male and female combat veterans who have posttraumatic stress disorder (PTSD) and the effects on the family unit during all phases of the deployment cycle. She has served on two Institute of Medicine (IOM) committees: the Committee on Gulf War and Health: Physiological, Psychologic, and Psychosocial Effects of Deployment-Related Stress and the Committee on Qualifications of Professionals Providing Mental Health Counseling Services Under TRICARE. Dr. Basham recently served on the Steering Committee cosponsored by the Council of Social Work Education to set standards for accredited curricula related to treatment and prevention practices for service members and families affected by military service. In addition to her extensive record of publications and professional presentations, she has received the Distinguished Clinical Practitioner award from the National Academies of Practice. Dr. Basham received her PhD from Smith College.

Larry Culpepper is a professor and chairman of family medicine at the Boston University School of Medicine and chief of family medicine at Boston Medical Center. He has conducted federally funded studies of depression and anxiety and is a Primary Care Fellow of the U.S. Health Resources and Services Administration. He received the Society of Teachers of Family Medicine Excellence in Education Award in 1991, the NAPCRG-STFM Career Research Award in 1997, and the North American Primary Care Research Group Maurice Wood Lifetime Research Award in 2010. Dr. Culpepper is an IOM member. He received his MD from Baylor College of Medicine and his MPH from Boston University.

Jonathan R. Davidson is an emeritus professor of psychiatry and for 20 years served as director of the Anxiety and Traumatic Stress Program of Duke University Medical Center. He has researched and used psychotherapy, pharmacotherapy, and holistic approaches to treat people for mental illnesses. His contributions to the understanding of and treatment for anxiety and traumatic stress have been recognized with the American Psychiatric Association Adolf Meyer Research Award, and he is a Fellow of the American Psychiatric Association, the Royal College of Psychiatrists, the American Psychopathological Association, and the American College of Neuropsychopharmacology. Dr. Davidson has been a member of several advisory boards, committees, National Institute of Mental Health study sections, the National Institutes of Health National Center for Complementary and Alternative Medicine advisory council, and other task forces related to psychiatry, anxiety disorders, and traumatic stress. He has also served as co-chair of the American Psychiatric Association *DSM-IV* Work Group for Posttraumatic Stress Disorder. He has received numerous federal grants to support his research and has been the principal investigator or coinvestigator in more than 70 clinical studies, including a landmark trial of hypericum (St. John's wort) in depression. Dr. Davidson is a member of the IOM Board on the Health of Select Populations. He received his MD from University College Hospital Medical School, London.

Edna B. Foa is a professor of clinical psychology in psychiatry and director of the Center for the Treatment and Study of Anxiety of the University of Pennsylvania. Her academic career has focused on the psychopathology and treatment of anxiety disorders, with an emphasis on obsessive compulsive disorder and PTSD. She has recently been involved in the dissemination of evidence-based treatments for PTSD to community clinics in the United States and abroad. Dr. Foa is recognized as one of the world leaders in the area of anxiety disorders. She developed a theoretical framework called Emotional Processing Theory that delineates the psychological mechanisms of the anxiety disorders and their treatments. She also developed prolonged exposure therapy for PTSD, widely acknowledged for its efficacy and effectiveness in a variety of trauma populations. Dr. Foa was the chair of the *DSM-IV* subcommittee for obsessive compulsive disorder and co-chair the *DSM-IV* subcommittee for PTSD. She has also been the chair for the Treatment Guidelines Task Force of the International Society for Traumatic Stress Disorders. Dr. Foa has published 18 books and more than 300 research articles and book chapters and has lectured extensively around the world. Her work has been recognized with numerous awards and honors. She was named one of *Time* magazine's 100 most influential people for 2010. Dr. Foa received her PhD in clinical psychology and personality from the University of Missouri, Columbia.

Kenneth W. Kizer is the director of the Institute for Population Health Improvement at the University of California, Davis, and Target of Excellence professor of the School of Medicine and Betty Irene Moore School of Nursing. His current research interests include health care quality improvement and patient safety, health care transformation, and veterans and military health issues. He formerly served as the undersecretary for health of the U.S. Department of Veterans Affairs, where he was the chief architect of the transformation of the Veterans Health System in the latter 1990s. His other positions have included being the founding president and CEO of the National Quality Forum and director of the California Department of Health Services. Dr. Kizer is an IOM member and has served as a member of numerous committees during the last 25 years, including most recently the IOM Committee on the Readjustment Needs of Military Personnel, Veterans, and Their Families and the Committee on Smoking Cessation in Military and Veteran Populations. Dr. Kizer is an honors graduate of Stanford University and the University of California, Los Angeles, where he received his MD and MPH.

Karestan C. Koenen is a tenured associate professor in the Department of Epidemiology of Columbia University's Mailman School of Public Health. Her research uses a developmental epidemiologic approach to examine the joint roles of genetic and environmental risk factors, especially those sustained during childhood, in the development and etiology of PTSD. Dr. Koenen is a coinvestigator in the Army Study to Assess Risk and Resilience in Servicemembers, the largest study of mental health risk and resilience ever conducted among military personnel. The study is being conducted by the National Institute of Mental Health, which has contracted with the Harvard School of Public Health. In addition to her teaching and research, Dr. Koenen is an experienced clinician who specializes in empirically validated short-term treatments for PTSD and was a Research Fellow in psychiatric epidemiology. She has received numerous awards for her work, including the Chaim Danieli Young Professional Award for Excellence in Service/Research in Traumatic Stress from the International Society for Traumatic Stress Studies, the Department of Veterans Affairs Special Contribution Award, and an American Sociological Association Citation Award for work on psychologic risks for U.S. veterans of Vietnam. Dr. Koenen earned her PhD in clinical and developmental psychology from Boston University.

Douglas L. Leslie is a health economist and professor of public health sciences and psychiatry at the Pennsylvania State University. In addition to his experience in health services, economics, and pharmacoeconomics, he has worked extensively with the Department of Veterans Affairs, in particular with data from its administrative claims database. The primary focus of his research is the effects of managed care and other fiscal pressures on patterns of service use and costs for the mentally ill. Dr. Leslie's other research interests and expertise include quality of mental health care, adherence to treatment guidelines, and the cost-effectiveness of antipsychotic medications. He has published numerous scientific journal articles and has received several awards for his research, including an Excellence in Mental Health Policy and Economics Research Award from the International Center of Mental Health Policy and Economics. Dr. Leslie received his PhD in economics from Yale University.

Richard A. McCormick is a senior scholar at the Center for Health Care Research and Policy at Case Western Reserve University MetroHealth Medical Center. He served as director of mental health services at Department of Veterans Affairs facilities throughout Ohio and adjoining areas of other states, as a commissioner for the Department of Veterans Affairs Capital Assets Realignment for Enhanced Services Commission, and as co-chair of the Active-Duty Sub-Committee of the Department of Defense Task Force on Mental Health. He is a consultant and scientific board member for two studies of returning National Guard and reserve members and has served as a national consultant for Disabled American Veterans. His research interests include war trauma and related stress reactions and adherence to treatment among the seriously mentally ill who have co-occurring medical problems, alcohol misuse and abuse, and other disorders of impulse control, such as pathologic gambling. Dr. McCormick received his PhD in clinical psychology from Case Western Reserve University.

Mohammed Milad is an associate professor in the Department of Psychiatry at Harvard Medical School and an associate in research psychiatry at Massachusetts General Hospital, where he is also the director of the Behavioral Neuroscience Laboratory. He is investigating the neural mechanisms of fear inhibition in the human brain through the use of functional magnetic resonance imaging studies. His research focuses on the neural circuits of fear extinction and includes the role of meditation in fear modulation, the potential use of transcranial magnetic stimulation, and the role of sleep in the consolidation of fear extinction. Dr. Milad also conducts translational research in rodents and humans to examine the influence of estrogen and other gonadal hormones on the neural circuits of fear extinction. He has been awarded the Positive Neuroscience Award by the Templeton Foundation and named a Kavli Fellow by the National Academy of Sciences. Dr. Milad received his PhD in behavioral neuroscience from the Ponce School of Medicine and Health Sciences in Puerto Rico.

Elspeth C. Ritchie is the chief clinical officer of the Washington, DC, Department of Mental Health. Before joining the department, Colonel Ritchie (retired) served for 5 years as the director of the Proponency of Behavioral Health in the Office of the U.S. Army Surgeon General, and she continues to serve as a psychiatry consultant. She has gained international recognition as an expert in disaster and combat mental health issues and has more than 150 publications, including works on military combat and operational psychiatry, disaster response, and interventions. Col. Ritchie is the senior editor of the *Military Medicine Textbook on Combat and Operational Behavioral Health* and the *Textbook of Forensic Military Mental Health*, and the author of *Interventions Following Mass Violence and Disasters: Strategies for Mental Health Practice*. She has been the recipient of the Bruno Lima Award for Contributions to Psychiatric Care in Times of Disaster and the William C. Porter award from the Association of Military Surgeons of the United States. Col. Ritchie received her MD from George Washington University School of Medicine and Health Sciences and her MPH from the Uniformed Services University of the Health Sciences (USUHS). She is a professor of psychiatry at the USUHS and on the faculty of Saint Elizabeth's Hospital.

Albert Rizzo started the Laboratory for Virtual Reality, Psychology, Rehabilitation, and Social Neuroscience at the University of Southern California (USC) in 1995 after practicing clinically for 9 years. He is currently an associate director at the USC Institute for Creative Technologies and has appointments as a research professor in the USC Department of Psychiatry and at the USC School of Gerontology. Dr. Rizzo's research focus is on the design, development, and evaluation of virtual reality systems targeting clinical assessment, treatment, and rehabilitation. His projects have involved the creation of a virtual reality exposure-therapy system (Virtual Iraq/Afghanistan) for combat-related PTSD in Operation Enduring Freedom and Operation Iraqi Freedom active-duty service members and veterans. He is also working with a team that is creating artificially intelligent virtual patients for training novice clinicians in the skills required for challenging clinical interviews and diagnostic assessments (of sexual assault, patient resistance, suicide lethality, etc.). Dr. Rizzo is an editor of a number of cognition and computer-science journals—including *Presence*, the *Journal of Media Psychology*, and *The International Journal of Virtual Reality*—and has published extensively on the topic of clinical virtual reality. He received his PhD in clinical psychology from the State University of New York at Binghamton.

Barbara O. Rothbaum is a professor of psychiatry and the director of the Trauma and Anxiety Recovery Program and associate vice chair of Clinical Research at Emory University School of Medicine. Her research focuses on innovative cognitive behavioral treatments, including virtual reality, pharmacotherapy, and psychotherapy for PTSD and other anxiety disorders. Dr. Rothbaum has more than 200 publications and two patents and serves as an editorial board member and manuscript reviewer for more than 15 journals. Dr. Rothbaum serves on the Board of Directors of the Anxiety Disorders Association of America and is a past president of the International Society for Traumatic Stress Studies. She received her PhD in clinical psychology from the University of Georgia.

Douglas F. Zatzick is a professor in the Department of Psychiatry and Behavioral Science, associate vice chair for health services research, and medical director of the Inpatient Consultation-Liaison Service at the University of Washington's Harborview Medical Center Burn and Trauma Center. Dr. Zatzick was formerly the chief resident in psychiatry at the San Francisco VA Medical Center and completed a Department of Veterans Affairs–sponsored Robert Wood Johnson Clinical Scholars Fellowship at the University of California, San Francisco. His research focuses on PTSD and co-occurring conditions and on the development of early interventions after traumatic events. Specifically, his work, published in numerous scientific journals, includes clinical epidemiologic studies of ethnoculturally diverse trauma survivors and intervention studies of collaborative-care models to reduce PTSD symptoms and functional disability in physically injured trauma survivors who are treated in trauma-care systems. Dr. Zatzick received his MD from the University of California, San Diego.

Appendix B

Congressional Legislation

National Defense Authorization Act for Fiscal Year 2010
Law #: Public Law 111-84
111th Congress (1st Session)

HR2647 Skelton (D-Mo.) 10/22/09
Enrolled (finally passed both houses)
To authorize appropriations for fiscal year 2010 for military activities of the Department of Defense, for military construction, and for defense activities of the Department of Energy, to prescribe military personnel strengths for such fiscal year, and for other purposes.

SEC. 726. INDEPENDENT STUDY ON POST-TRAUMATIC STRESS DISORDER EFFORTS.

(a) Study Required.—The Secretary of Defense, in consultation with the Secretary of Veterans Affairs, shall provide for a study on the treatment of post-traumatic stress disorder to be conducted by the Institute of Medicine of the National Academy of Sciences or such other independent entity as the Secretary shall select for purposes of the study.

(b) Elements.—The study required by subsection (a) shall include the following:

(1) A list of each operative program and method available for the prevention, screening, diagnosis, treatment, or rehabilitation of post-traumatic stress disorder, including—

(A) the rates of success for each such program or method (including an operational definition of the term "success" and a discussion of the process used to quantify such rates);

(B) based on the incidence of actual diagnoses, an estimate of the number of members of the Armed Forces and veterans diagnosed by the Department of Defense or the Department of Veterans Affairs as having post-traumatic stress disorder and the number of such veterans who have been successfully treated; and

(C) any collaborative efforts between the Department of Defense and the Department of Veterans Affairs to prevent, screen, diagnose, treat, or rehabilitate post-traumatic stress disorder.

(2) The status of studies and clinical trials involving innovative treatments of post-traumatic stress disorder that are conducted by the Department of Defense, the Department of Veterans Affairs, or the private sector, including—

(A) efforts to identify physiological markers of post-traumatic stress disorder;

(B) with respect to efforts to determine causation of post-traumatic stress disorder, brain imaging studies and the correlation between brain region physiology and post-traumatic stress disorder diagnoses and the results (including any interim results) of such efforts;

(C) the effectiveness of alternative therapies in the treatment of post-traumatic stress disorder, including the therapeutic use of animals;

(D) the effectiveness of administering pharmaceutical agents before, during, or after a traumatic event in the prevention and treatment of post-traumatic stress disorder; and

(E) identification of areas in which the Department of Defense and the Department of Veterans Affairs may be duplicating studies, programs, or research with respect to post-traumatic stress disorder.

(3) A description of each treatment program for post-traumatic stress disorder, including a comparison of the methods of treatment by each program, at the following locations:

(A) Fort Hood, Texas.

(B) Fort Bliss, Texas.

(C) Fort Campbell, Tennessee.

(D) Other locations the entity conducting the study considers appropriate.

(4) The respective current and projected future annual expenditures by the Department of Defense and the Department of Veterans Affairs for the treatment and rehabilitation of post-traumatic stress disorder.

(5) A description of gender-specific and racial and ethnic group-specific mental health treatment and services available for members of the Armed Forces, including—

(A) the availability of such treatment and services;

(B) the access to such treatment and services;

(C) the need for such treatment and services; and

(D) the efficacy and adequacy of such treatment and services.

(6) A description of areas for expanded future research with respect to post-traumatic stress disorder.

(7) Any other matters the Secretary of Defense and Secretary of Veterans Affairs consider relevant with respect to the purposes of obtaining a comprehensive scientific assessment of—

(A) the incidence of post-traumatic stress disorder among members of the Armed Forces and veterans;

(B) the availability and effectiveness of various treatment programs and methods available for post-traumatic stress disorder;

(C) the current and future projected costs of such treatment programs and methods; or

(D) additional areas of needed research.

(8) Any other matters the entity conducting the study considers relevant.
(c) Reports.—

(1) INITIAL REPORT.—Not later than July 1, 2012, the entity conducting the study required by subsection (a) shall submit to the Secretary of Defense, the Secretary of Veterans Affairs, and the appropriate committees a report on the study.

(2) RESPONSE.—Not later than January 1, 2013, the Secretary of Defense and the Secretary of Veterans Affairs shall each submit to the appropriate committees a response to the report submitted under paragraph (1), including any recommendations on the treatment of post-traumatic stress disorder based on such report.

(d) Updated Reports Required.—

(1) UPDATED REPORT.—Not later than July 1, 2014, the entity conducting the study required by subsection (a) shall submit to the Secretary of Defense, the Secretary of Veterans Affairs, and the appropriate committees an update of the report required by subsection (c).

(2) UPDATED RESPONSE.—Not later than January 1, 2015, the Secretary of Defense and the Secretary of Veterans Affairs shall each submit to the appropriate committees a response to the updated report submitted under paragraph (1), including any recommendations on the treatment of post-traumatic stress disorder based on such updated report.

(e) Appropriate Committees Defined.—In this section, the term "appropriate committees" means—

(1) the Committee on Armed Services, the Committee on Appropriations, the Committee on Veterans' Affairs, and the Committee on Energy and Commerce of the House of Representatives; and

(2) the Committee on Armed Services, the Committee on Appropriations, the Committee on Veterans' Affairs, and the Committee on Health, Education, Labor, and Pensions of the Senate.

Appendix C

Posttraumatic Stress Disorder Programs in the Department of Defense

TABLE C-1 PTSD Programs in the Department of Defense by Branch of Service

Program Name	DoD wide	Army	Army Reserve	Army National Guard	Air Force	Air Force Reserve	Air National Guard	Navy	Navy Reserve	Marine Corps	Marine Corps Reserve
Adaptive Disclosure Training								X		X	
After Deployment	X										
Air Force Special Operations Command Resiliency Program					X						
Air Force Suicide Prevention Program					X	X	X				
Air Force Wounded Warrior Program					X	X	X				
Air National Guard Psychological Health Program							X				
Army Wounded Warrior Program		X	X	X							
Automated Behavioral Health Clinic Program		X	X	X							
Automated Tools and Outcome Measures	X										
Battlemind		X	X	X							
Brigade Resiliency Teams		X									
Buddy-to-Buddy Program				X			X				
Care Provider Support Programs		X	X	X							
Caregiver Optimization Systems (CAREOPS)		X		X						X	
Center for Deployment Psychology	X										
Center for Spiritual Leadership		X	X	X							
Cognitive-Behavioral Couple Therapy for Combat Street Reactions and Intimate Relationship Problems		X			X						
Cognitive Processing Therapy for PTSD		X									
Combat and Operational Stress Reaction/Staff Resiliency Program								X	X		
Combat Stress Control Team		X	X	X							
Community Behavioral Health Services		X									

Comprehensive Combat and Complex Casualty Care Program	X							X			
Defender's Edge					X						
Deployment Health Clinical Center Specialized Care Program	X										
DESTRESS-PC (Delivery of Self Training and Education for Stressful Situations–Primary Care)	X										
Domestic Violence Among Returning Servicemembers with PTSD	X										
DSTRESS										X	X
Effects of Integration Restoration (iRest) on Sleep and Perceived Stress		X									
Elmendorf Air Force Base TBI Clinic		X			X					X	
Evolution		X			X						
Family Advocacy Program (Army)		X	X	X							
Family Optimization Systems (FAMOPS)		X		X							
Family Strong Hawaii		X	X	X							
Federal Recovery Coordination Program	X										
Fort Bliss Restoration and Resilience Center		X	X	X							
Fort Hood Resilience and Restoration Center's Warrior Combat Stress Reset Program		X	X	X							
HeartMath					X			X		X	
Installation Suicide Response Team		X									
Integrative Pain Center	X										
Integrative Restoration (iRest)	X										
Marine Corps Combat and Operational Stress Control										X	X
Marine Corps Operational Stress Training Program										X	
Marine Corps Wounded Warrior Regiment Psychological Health and TBI Clinical Services Staff								X		X	
Medical Soldier Readiness Processing		X			X						

continued

TABLE C-1 Continued

Program Name	DoD wide	Army	Army Reserve	Army National Guard	Air Force	Air Force Reserve	Air National Guard	Navy	Navy Reserve	Marine Corps	Marine Corps Reserve
Military Pathways	X										
Mind-Body Skills Groups for the Treatment of War Zone Stress in Military and Veteran Populations	X										
Mind-Body Trauma First Aide		X	X	X							
Mobile Telehealth Program	X										
National Center for Telehealth and Technology Mobile Applications	X										
National Guard Psychological Health Program				X			X				
National Guard Transition Assistance Advisors				X			X				
The National Intrepid Center of Excellence	X										
Navy Operational Stress Control								X	X		
Operation BRAVE (Building Resilience and Valuing Empowered) Families		X									
Operational Stress Control and Readiness (OSCAR)										X	X
Outcomes of Prolonged Exposure and Cognitive Processing Therapy Used in the Treatment of Combat Operational Stress in Deployed Locations	X										
Physical Medicine and Integrative Care Services	X										
Post Deployment Open House Program					X	X	X				
Postdeploymenthealth.com	X										
Post-Traumatic Stress Residential Rehabilitation Program		X									
Psychiatric Service Dog Society Research	X										

Psychological Health Pathways Program	X										
PTSD Training Program		X	X	X							
PTSD Treatment in Primary Care Settings	X										
Randomized Exploratory Study to Evaluate Two Acupuncture Methods for the Treatment of Headaches Associated with TBI	X										
Recovery Coordination Program	X										
Re-engineering Healthcare Integration Programs	X	X			X			X			
Reset		X									
RESPECT-MIL		X									
Return to Duty Performance Validation Program (TBI Program)		X	X	X	X						
Returning Warrior Workshops									X		X
Scripps Military Brain Injury Rehabilitation Program	X										
Seeking Safety	X										
Sesame Workshop Military Families Initiative	X										
SimCoach	X										
Soldier 360°		X									
Soldier Evaluation for Life Fitness		X									
STEPS UP (Stepped Enhancement of PTSD Services Using Primary Care)		X									
Stress Gym	X										
Strong Families, Strong Forces	X										
STRONG STAR (South Texas Research Organizational Network Guiding Studies on Trauma and Resilience) Research Consortium	X										
Suicide Awareness Voices of Education					X		X			X	
Theater of War	X										
Third Location Decompression								X			
Traumatic Stress Response Team					X	X	X				
TRICARE Assistance Program	X										

continued

TABLE C-1 Continued

Program Name	DoD wide	Army	Army Reserve	Army National Guard	Air Force	Air Force Reserve	Air National Guard	Navy	Navy Reserve	Marine Corps	Marine Corps Reserve
Virtual Behavioral Telehealth Pilot at Fort Richardson		X									
Virtual Behavioral Telehealth Pilot at Tripler Army Medical Center		X									
Virtual Reality and Innovative Technology Applications	X										
Virtual Reality Graded Exposure Therapy with Physiological Monitoring								X		X	
Virtual Reality Iraq/Afghanistan	X										
Warrior and Family Assistance Center			X								
Warrior Mind Training		X						X		X	
Warrior Resilience & Thriving		X	X	X							
Warrior Restoration Center		X									
Warrior Strengthening Program	X										
Warrior Transition Units		X	X	X							
Warrior's Huddle		X									
Wellness and Resiliency Assessment–Post-Deployment		X	X	X							
Wounded Warrior Regiment										X	
Yellow Ribbon Reintegration Program (Air Force)						X	X				
Yellow Ribbon Reintegration Program (Army)			X	X							

SOURCE: Weinick, R. M., E. B. Beckjord, C. M. Farmer, K. T. Martin, E. M. Gillen, J. D. Acosta, M. P. Fisher, J. Garnett, G. C. Gonzalez, T. C. Helmus, K. H. Jaycox, K. A. Reynolds, N. Salcedo, and D. M. Scharf. 2011. Programs addressing psychological health and traumatic brain injury among U.S. military servicemembers and their families. Arlington, VA: RAND Corporation; adapted with permission from RAND Corporation.